Decision Making in
CARDIOLOGY
An Algorithmic Approach

Decision Making in
CARDIOLOGY
An Algorithmic Approach

Achyut Sarkar MD DM (Cardiology) FACC
Professor of Cardiology
Ex-Institute of Postgraduate Medical Education and Research (IPGME&R)
Consulting Interventional Cardiologist
Woodland Hospital and BM Birla Heart Research Center
Kolkata, West Bengal, India

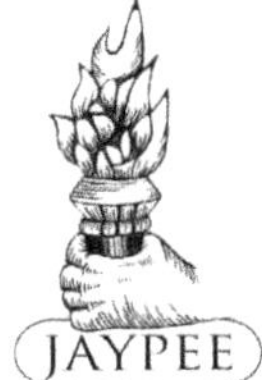

JAYPEE
JAYPEE BROTHERS MEDICAL PUBLISHERS
The Health Sciences Publisher
New Delhi | London

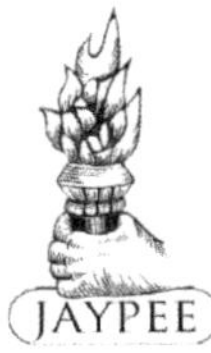 **Jaypee Brothers Medical Publishers (P) Ltd**

Headquarters
EMCA House
23/23-B, Ansari Road, Daryaganj
New Delhi 110 002, India
Landline: +91-11-23272143, +91-11-23272703
+91-11-23282021, +91-11-23245672
E-mail: jaypee@jaypeebrothers.com

Corporate Office
Jaypee Brothers Medical Publishers (P) Ltd.
4838/24, Ansari Road, Daryaganj
New Delhi 110 002, India
Phone: +91-11-43574357
Fax: +91-11-43574314
E-mail: jaypee@jaypeebrothers.com

Overseas Office
JP Medical Ltd.
83, Victoria Street, London
SW1H 0HW (UK)
Phone: +44-20 3170 8910
Fax: +44(0)20 3008 6180
E-mail: info@jpmedpub.com

Website: www.jaypeebrothers.com
Website: www.jaypeedigital.com

Inquiries for bulk sales may be solicited at: jaypee@jaypeebrothers.com

Decision Making in Cardiology: An Algorithmic Approach / Achyut Sarkar
First Edition: **2023**

Preface

Algorithm is a "set of rules that precisely defines a sequence of operation," typically used to perform a computation. Algorithm is an essential language used in artificial intelligence, which is gradually creeping in cardiology, like every field of science and technology. I have tried to express decision-making in cardiology in a language of future, i.e., algorithm. All the common day-to-day problems in cardiology have been discussed. In addition, the emerging issues such as primary electrical abnormalities, sudden cardiac death, cardio-oncology, geriatric cardiology, and sports cardiology have been included. And certainly, the treatise begins with a section on artificial intelligence in cardiology.

Robots are not going to replace us, the cardiologists. Difficult, demeaning, demanding, dangerous, dull—these are the jobs robots will be taking. We will go on practicing clinical cardiology, using their language—algorithm.

Achyut Sarkar

Acknowledgments

I wish to thank M/S Jaypee Brothers Medical Publishers (P) Ltd, New Delhi, India for whom the creation of this book has become possible. I thank my late parents. Their memories are still great inspiration. I thank my daughter Parnisha and son Arjab. Their academic aptitude has always been encouraging to me and Dr Asima Sarkar, my wife who is a great blessing in my life. She has sacrified her invaluable professional time and supported my academic activities. I thank her with immense gratitude.

Contents

SECTION 5: HEART FAILURE

SECTION 6: PULMONARY HYPERTENSION

SECTION 7: MYOCARDITIS AND CARDIOMYOPATHY

SECTION 12: SUDDEN CARDIAC DEATH

SECTION 13: CARDIO-ONCOLOGY

SECTION 14: GERIATRIC CARDIOLOGY

SECTION 15: SPORT CARDIOLOGY

SECTION 16: ACUTE VASCULAR SYNDROME

Artificial Intelligence

CHAPTER 1

Artificial Intelligence: General Approach

INTRODUCTION

In 1950, a renowned mathematician, AM Turing, mentioned this question in a paper[1] which came out in the journal of Mind—"Can machine think?" Artificial intelligence (AI) provides an affirmative answer to the question. That is the simplest way to define AI, which essentially is a branch of computer science dealing with building up smart machines capable of doing tasks which need human intelligence. In a textbook, "Artificial Intelligence: A Modern Approach," author Stuart Russell and Peter Norvig defined AI as "the study of agents that receive percepts from the environment and perform actions." AI can be defined in another way as "algorithms enabled by constraints, exposed by representations that support models targeted at loops that tie thinking, perception, and action together." Machine learning is one of them and deep learning is one of those machine-learning techniques. AI is not without its risk. Stephen Hawking described the impact of unsupervised AI as cataclysmic. "Unless we learn how to prepare for, and avoid potential risks, AI could be the worst event in the history of civilization."

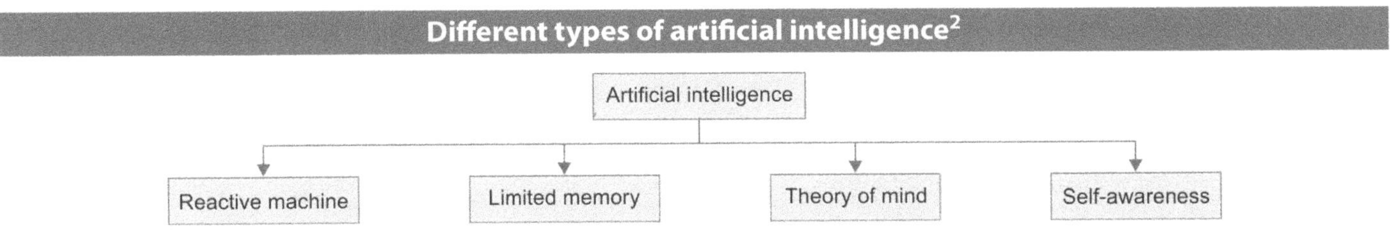

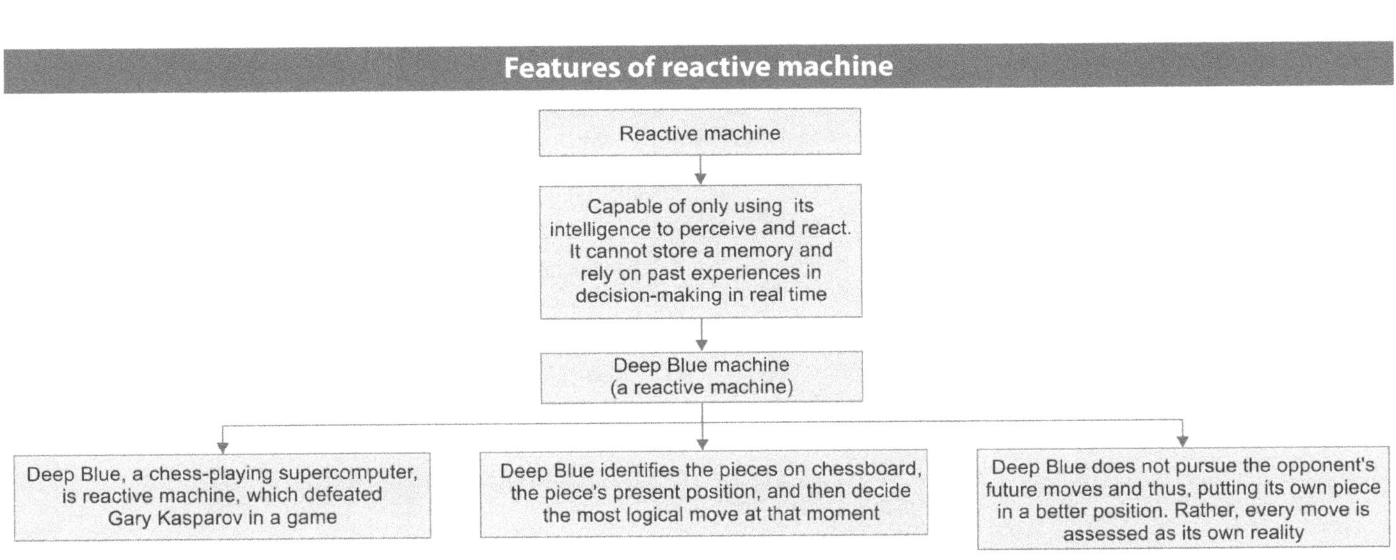

Features of limited memory

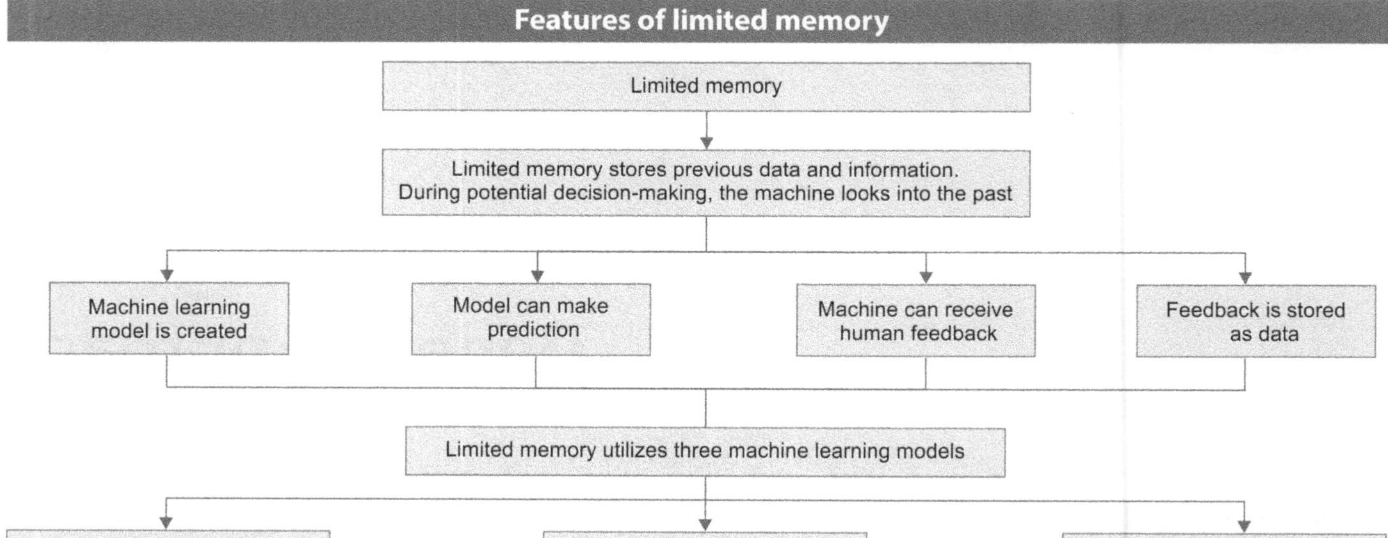

Different category of artificial intelligence[3]

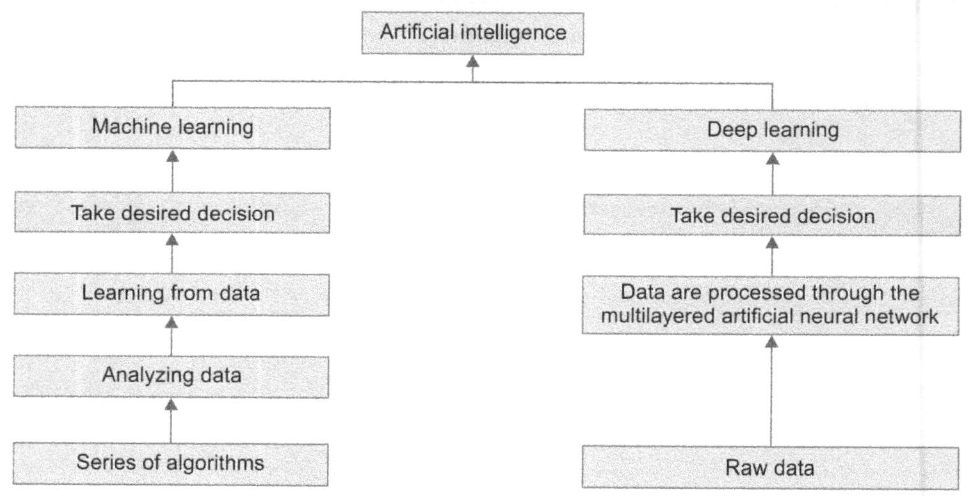

Different types of artificial intelligence according to grade of intelligence

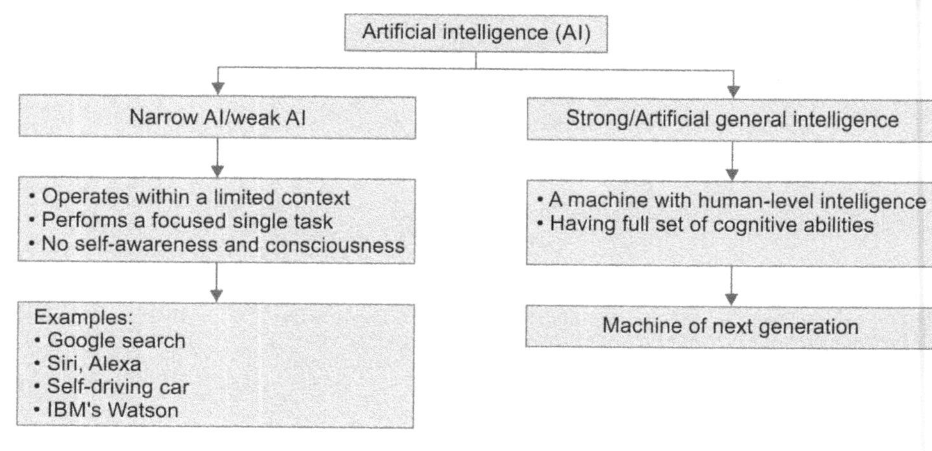

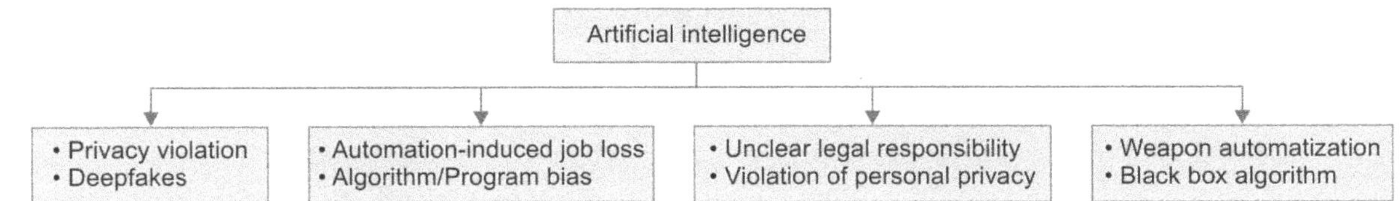

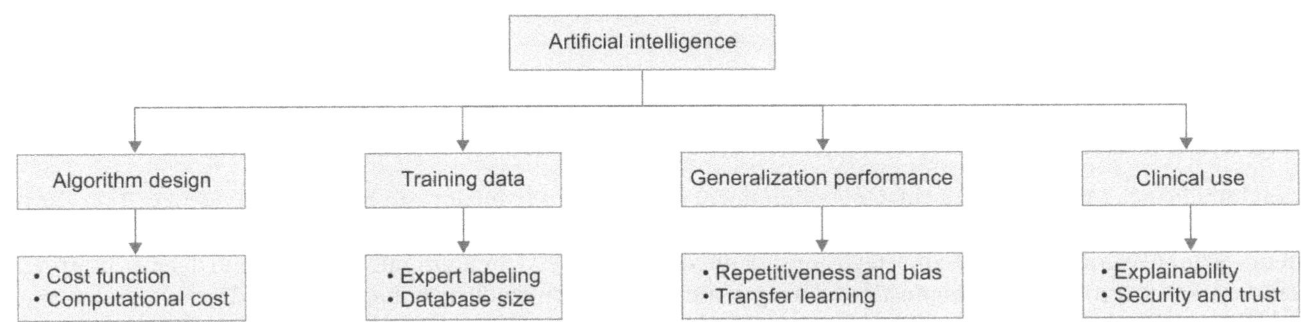

REFERENCES

1. Turing AM. Computing machinery and intelligence. Mind. 1950;49:433-60.
2. Russell S, Norvig P. Artificial intelligence: a modern approach, 3rd edition. London: Pearson Education Limited; 2016.
3. Juarez-Orozco LE, Martinez-Manzanera O, Storti AE, Knuuti J. Machine learning in the evaluation of myocardial ischemia through nuclear cardiology. Curr Cardiovasc Imaging Rep. 2019;12(5).
4. Weese J, Lorenz C. Four challenges in medical image analysis from an industrial perspective. Med Image Anal. 2016;33:44-9.

CHAPTER 2

Artificial Intelligence: Application in Cardiology

INTRODUCTION

Artificial intelligence (AI) is gradually playing a significant participation in health and biomedical research. There are huge data in cardiology, generating from electrocardiogram, different imaging like echocardiogram, computed tomography (CT), magnetic resonance imaging (MRI), and electronic health record (EHR). AI, by automated analysis and deeper interpretation of these data, can improve safety, diagnostic and prognostic prediction in medical management, and intervention in patients with cardiovascular diseases.

The *traditional AI system* is based on fact sheet and research work. The system produces predetermined output. In contrast, *machine learning (ML)* utilizes an algorithm based on a large database and complex statistical input. The heuristic system learns and makes judgement with minimum human intervention. *Deep learning (DL)* is a specific form of ML system, in which the system uses multiple deep neural layers for learning. In the DL system, each layer uses to add the knowledge of the previous layer.[1] The system does not need the support for manual definition of classification rule.

Artificial intelligence, ML, and DL can be performed on desktop supported by graphics processing units (GPUs) designed for gaming. DL can even be performed using cloud service such as Google cloud or Amazon AWS. AI software packages are mostly in open source, like Keras or TensorFlow.

Relationship between artificial intelligence, machine learning, and deep learning

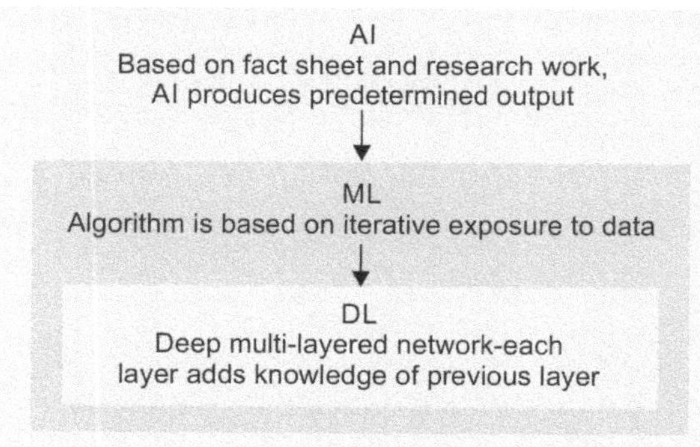

(AI: artificial intelligence; ML: machine learning; DL: deep learning)

How to build up a model for deep learning application in cardiology[2]

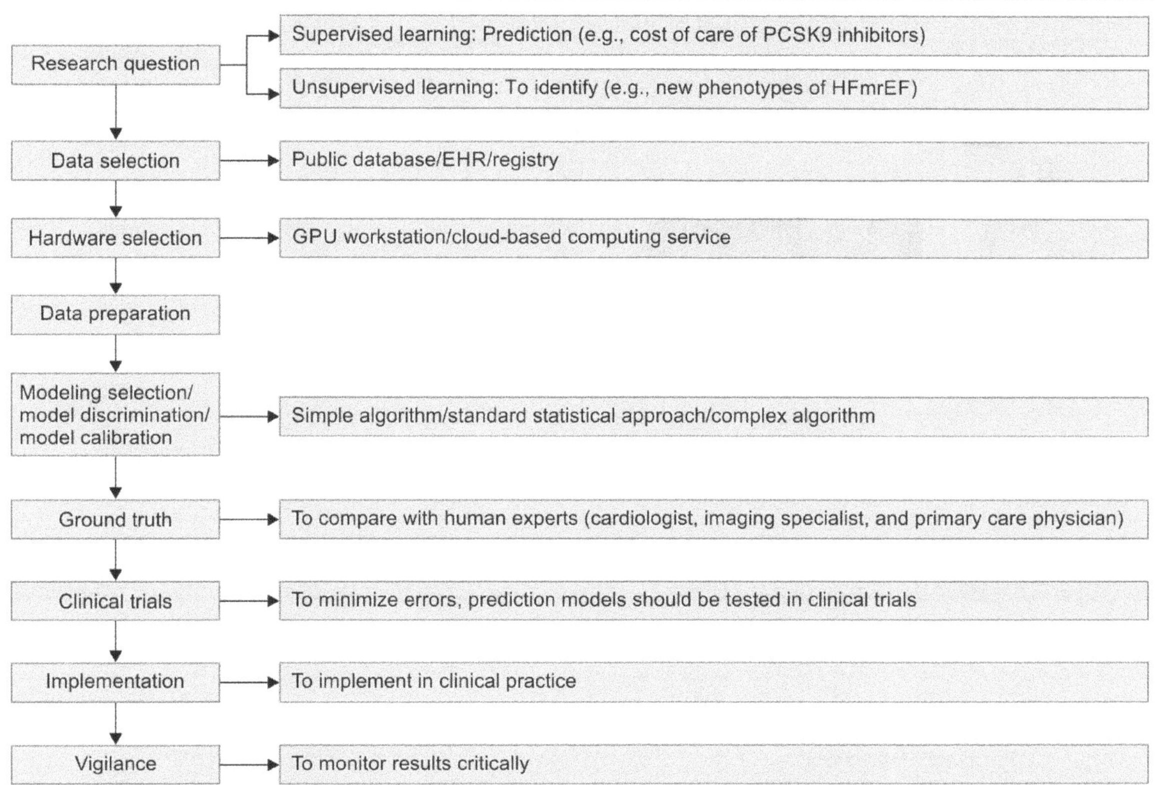

(EHR: electronic health record; HFmrEF: heart failure with mildly reduced EF; PCSK9i: proprotein convertase subtilisin/kexin type 9)

Deep learning model: Rhythm recognition[3]

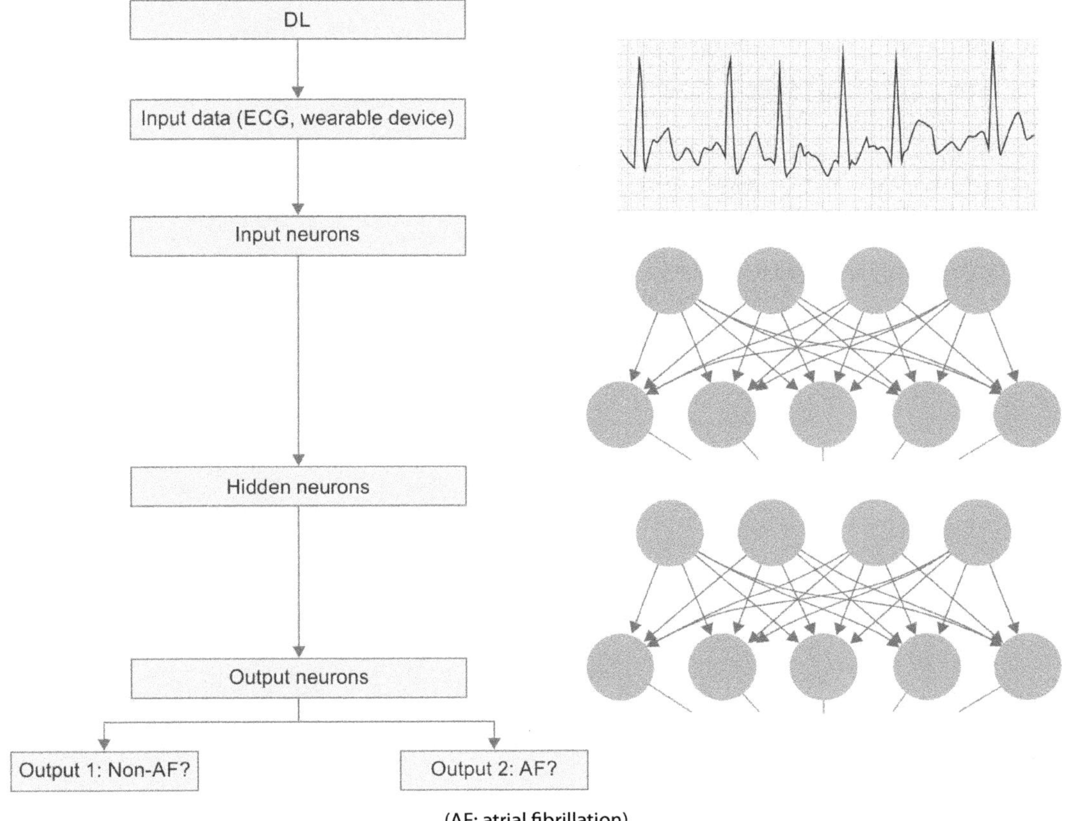

(AF: atrial fibrillation)

Deep learning model for cardiovascular imaging: CCTA and CT-FFR[4]

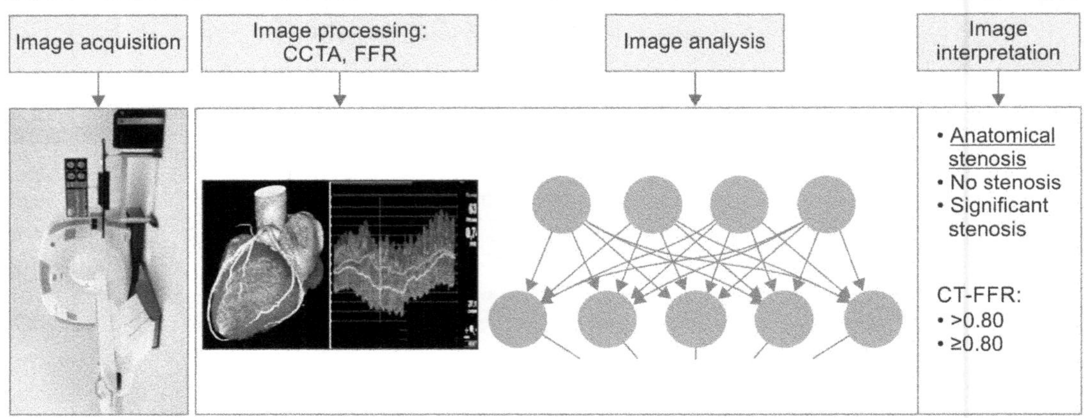

(CCTA: coronary computed tomography angiogram; CT-FFR: computed tomography-functional flow reserve)

Clinical application of deep learning: CCTA and CT-FFR[5]

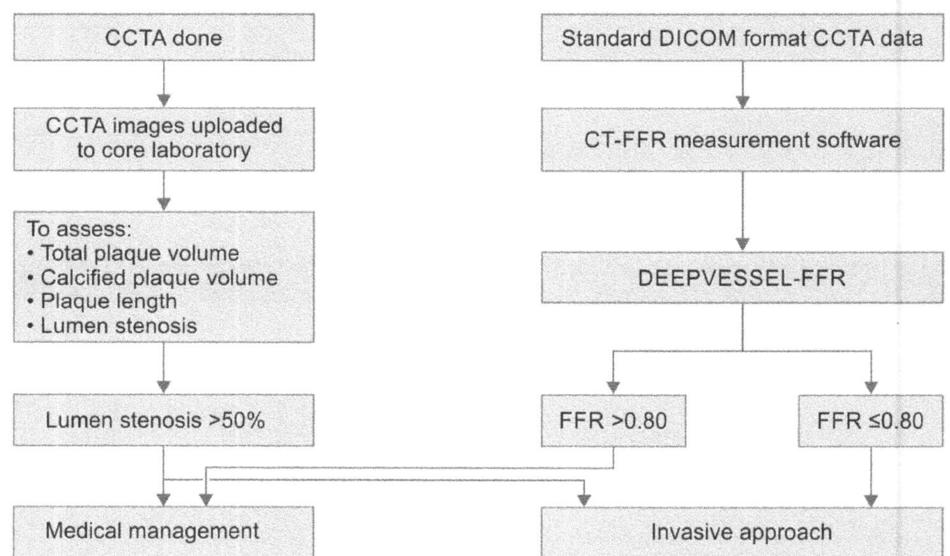

(CCTA: coronary computed tomography angiogram; CT-FFR: computed tomography-functional flow reserve; DICOM: digital imaging and communications in medicine)

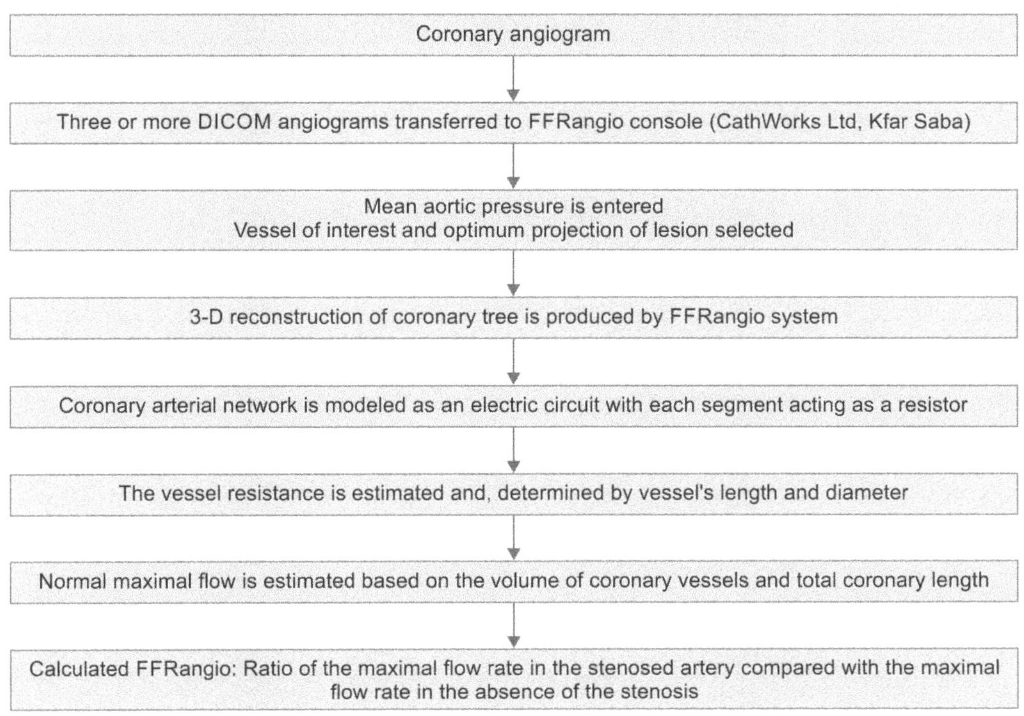

(DICOM: digital imaging and communications in medicine)

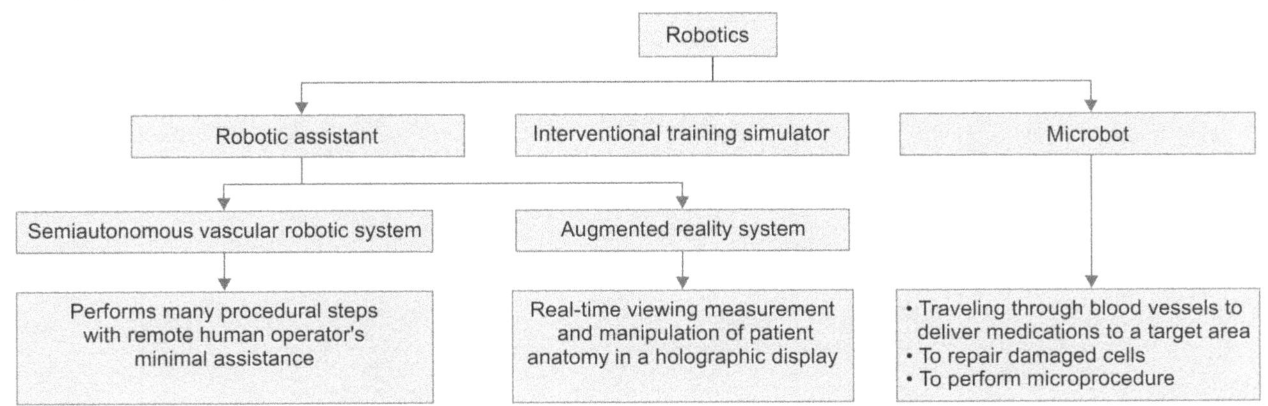

REFERENCES

1. Goodfellow I, Bengio Y, Courville A, Bengio Y. Deep Learning. Cambridge: MIT Press; 2016.
2. Silver D, Huang A, Maddison CJ, Guez A, Sifre L, van den Driessche G, et al. Mastering the game of go with deep neural networks and tree search. Nature. 2016;529:484-9.
3. Xia Y, Wulan N, Wang K, Zhang H. Detecting atrial fibrillation by deep convolutional neural networks. Comput Biol Med. 2018;93:84-92.
4. Wang ZQ, Zhou YJ, Zhao YX, Shi DM, Liu YY, Liu W, et al. Diagnostic accuracy of a deep learning approach to calculate FFR from coronary CT angiography. J Geriatr Cardiol. 2019;16(1):42-8.
5. Li Y, Qiu H, Hou Z, Zheng J, Li J, Yin Y, et al. Additional value of deep learning computed tomographic angiography-based fractional flow reserve in detecting coronary stenosis and predicting outcomes. Acta Radiol. 2022;63(1):133-40.
6. Fearon WF, Achenbach S, Engstrøm T, Assali A, Shlomitz R, Jeremias A, et al. Accuracy of fractional flow reserve derived from coronary angiography. Circulation. 2019;139:477-84.

Hypertension

CHAPTER 3

Essential Hypertension: General Approach

INTRODUCTION

Hypertension has been defined as a numerical level, described differently by different hypertension guidelines. In a simplest way, hypertension can be defined as a level, at which the benefit of treatment outweighs the risk of treatment.

Definition of hypertension: Office blood pressure

Office BP

AHA 2017[1]	ESC 2018[2]	NICE 2019[3]	ISH 2020[4]	WHF 2021[5]	WHO 2021
≥130/80 mm Hg	≥140/90 mm Hg	≥140/90 mm Hg	≥140/90 mm Hg	≥140/90 mm Hg	≥140/90 mm Hg

(AHA: American Heart Association; ESC: European Society of Cardiology; ISH: International Society of Hypertension; NICE: National Institute for Health and Care Excellence; WHF: World Heart Federation; WHO: World Health Organization)

Definition of hypertension: Out-of-office blood pressure

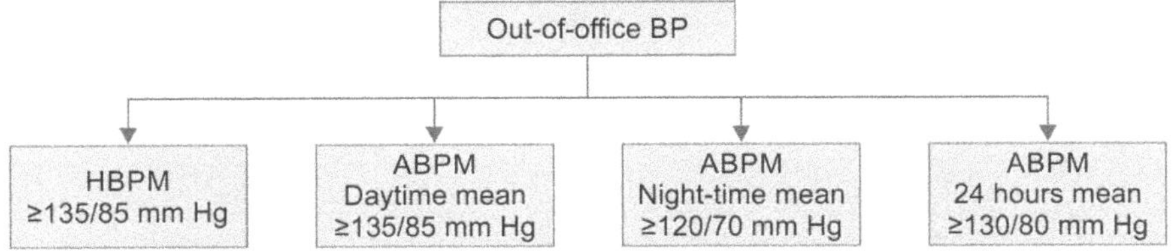

(ABPM: ambulatory blood pressure monitoring; HBPM: home blood pressure monitoring)

Hypertension-related terminology

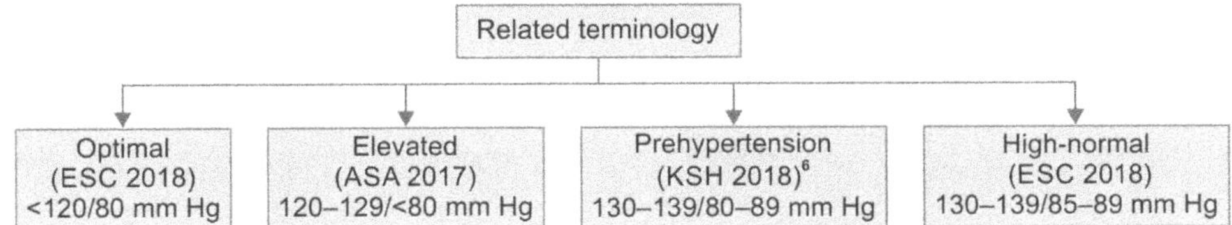

(ASA: American Stroke Association; ESC: European Society of Cardiology; KSH: The Korean Society of Hypertension)

Different set-up for blood pressure recording[7]

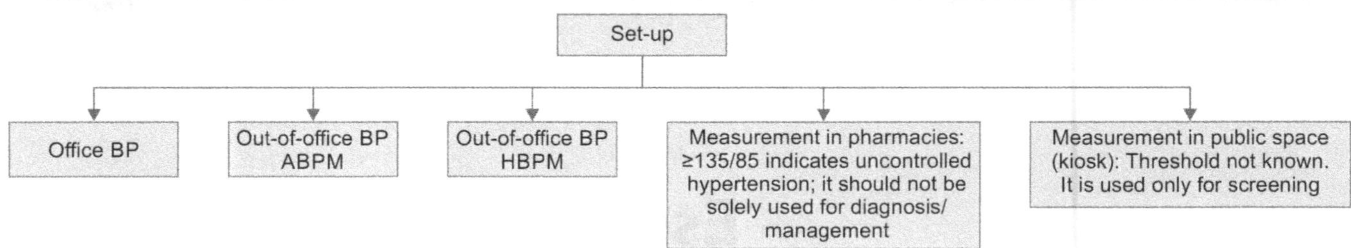

(ABPM: ambulatory blood pressure monitoring; HBPM: home blood pressure monitoring)

Different devices to measure blood pressure

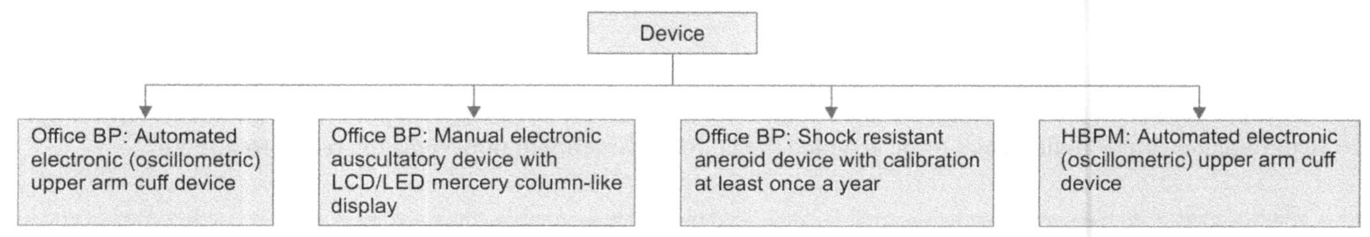

(HBPM: home blood pressure monitoring)

Basic issues to follow during blood pressure measurement

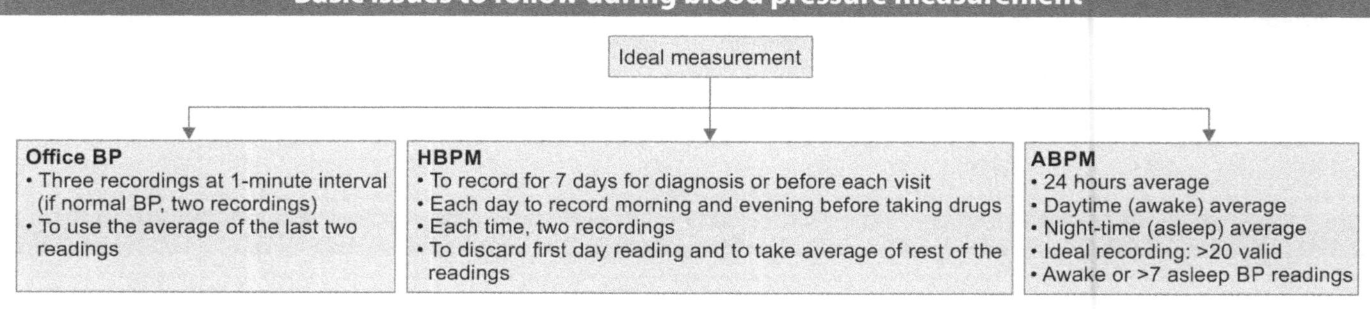

(ABPM: ambulatory blood pressure monitoring; HBPM: home blood pressure monitoring)

How to confirm hypertension

(ABPM: ambulatory blood pressure monitoring; HBPM: home blood pressure monitoring)

How to stage/grade hypertension

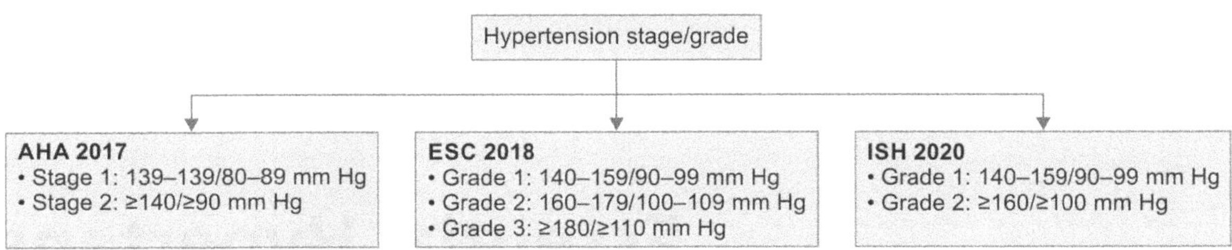

(AHA: American Heart Association; ESC: European Society of Cardiology; ISH: International Society of Hypertension)

Routine laboratory tests in hypertension

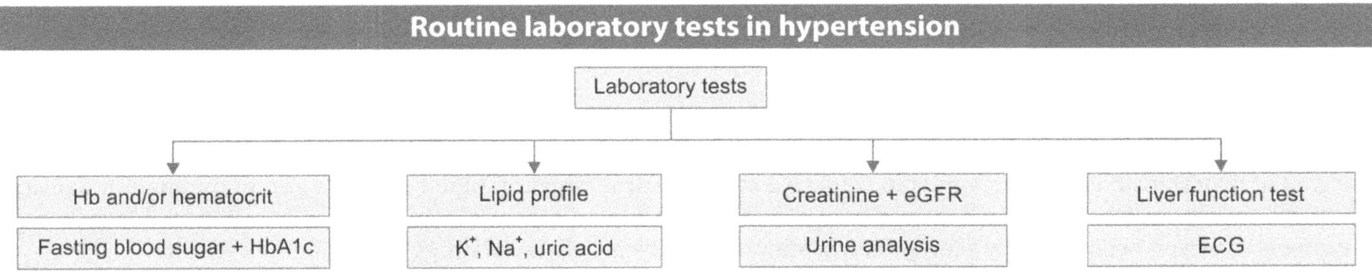

(Hb: hemoglobin; HbA1c: glycated hemoglobin; ECG: electrocardiogram; eGFR: estimated glomerular filtration rate)

Laboratory test to assess hypertension-mediated organ damage

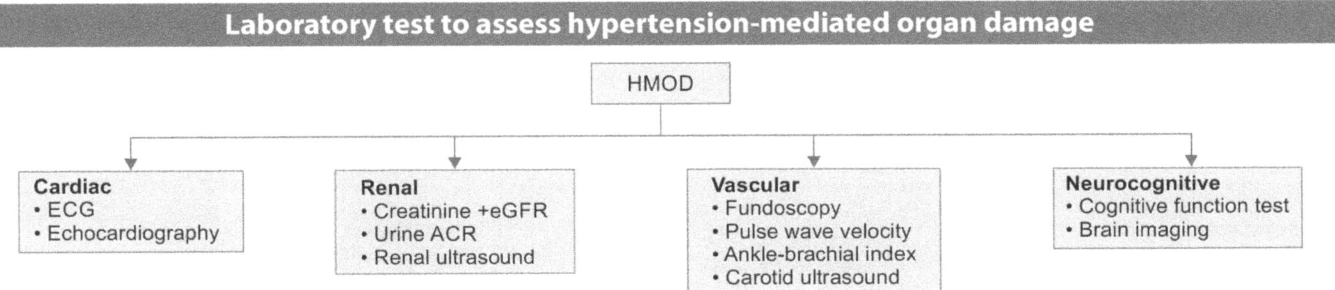

(eGFR: estimated glomerular filtration rate; ACR: albumin-to-creatinine ratio; HMOD: hypertension-mediated organ damage)

REFERENCES

1. Whelton PK, Carey RM, Aronow WS, Casey DE Jr, Collins KJ, Dennison Himmelfarb C, et al. 2017 ACC/AHA/AAPA/ABC/ ACPM/AGS/ APhA/ASH/ASPC/NMA/PCNA guideline for the prevention, detection, evaluation, and management of high blood pressure in adults: executive summary: a report of the American college of cardiology/American heart association task force on clinical practice guidelines. J Am Coll Cardiol. 2018;71(19):2199-269.
2. Williams B, Mancia G, Spiering W, Agabiti Rosei E, Azizi M, Burnier M, et al. 2018 ESC/ESH Guidelines for the management of arterial hypertension. Eur Heart J. 2018;39:3021-104.
3. NICE (2019). Hypertension in adults: diagnosis and management. NICE guideline [NG136]. [online] Available from https://www.nice.org.uk/guidance/ng136 [Last accessed July, 2022].
4. Unger T, Borghi C, Charchar F, Khan NA, Poulter NR, Prabhakaran D, et al. 2020 International society of hypertension global hypertension practice guidelines. Hypertension. 2020;75(6):1334-57.
5. Jeemon P, Séverin T, Amodeo C, Balabanova D, Campbell NR, Gaita D, et al. World heart federation roadmap for hypertension – A 2021 update. Global Heart. 2021;16(1):63.
6. Lee HY, Shin J, Kim GH, Park S, Ihm SH, Kim HC, et al. 2018 Korean Society of hypertension guidelines for the management of hypertension. part II-diagnosis and treatment of hypertension. Clin Hypertens. 2019;25:20.
7. Stergiou GS, Palatini P, Parati G, et al. 2021 European society of hypertension practice guidelines for office and out-of-office blood pressure measurement. J Hypertens. 2021;39:1293-302.

Essential Hypertension: Management

INTRODUCTION

The goal of hypertension management is to achieve a set numerical target of blood pressure and to maintain it. Lifestyle modification is essential part, and when used early, can decrease other disease risk and may avoid the need for drug therapy. The later is however, occurred only a few patients. Majority will eventually need drugs and other intervention.

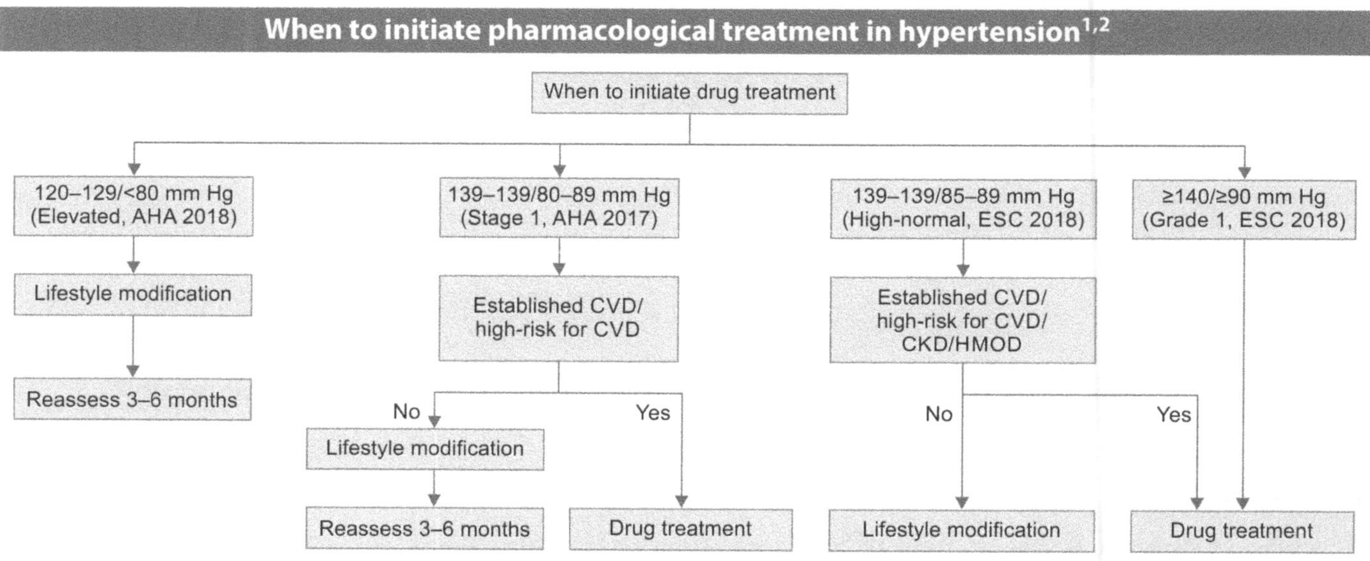

(AHA: American Heart Association; CVD: cardiovascular disease; CKD: chronic kidney disease; ESC: European Society of Cardiology; HMOD: hypertension-mediated organ damage)

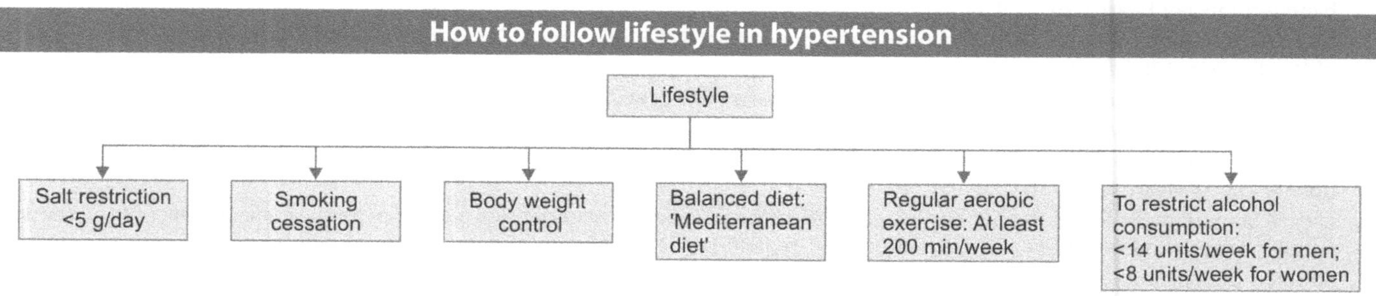

Pharmacological management for hypertension[1-7]

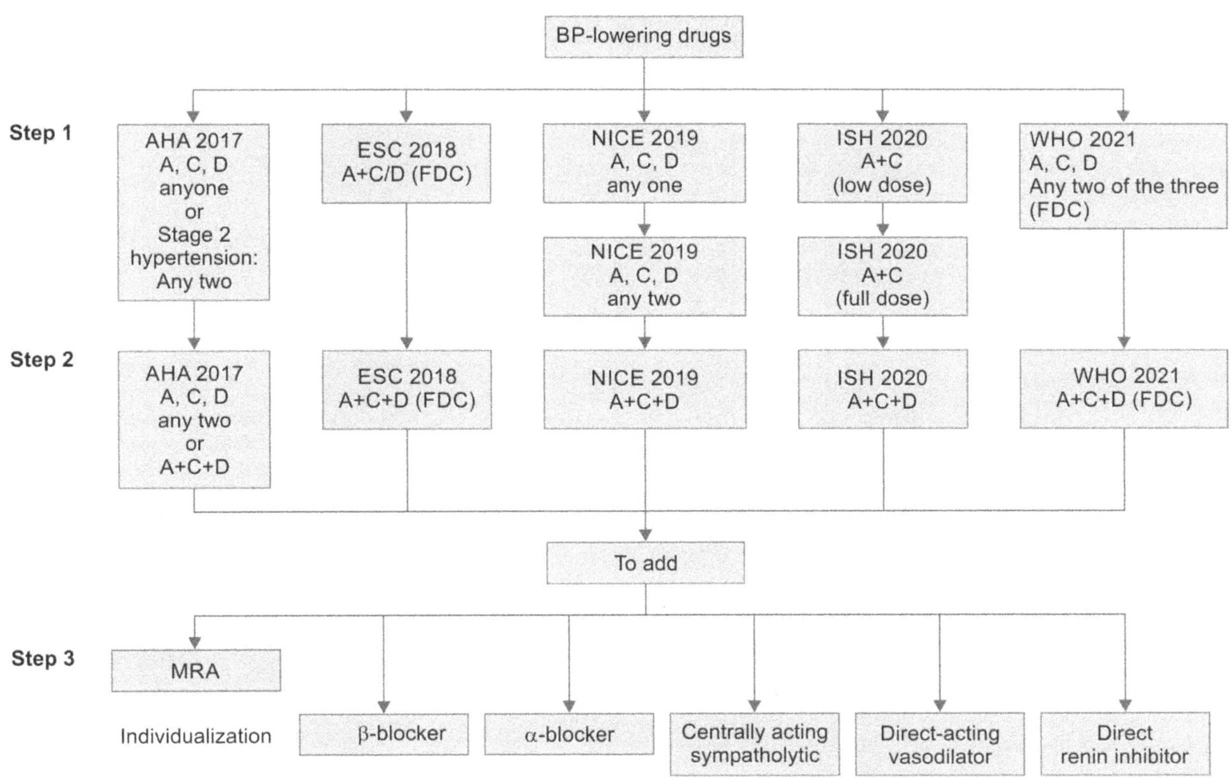

[AHA: American Heart Association; ESC: European Society of Cardiology; ISH: International Society of Hypertension; NICE: National Institute for Health and Care Excellence; A: angiotensin-converting enzyme (ACE) inhibitors/angiotensin receptor blocker (ARB); C: calcium channel blocker; D: thiazide or thiazide-like diuretic; FDC: fixed dose combination; MRA: mineralocorticoid receptor antagonist; WHO: World Health Organization]

Pharmacological management for hypertension: Monotherapy (ESC 2018)

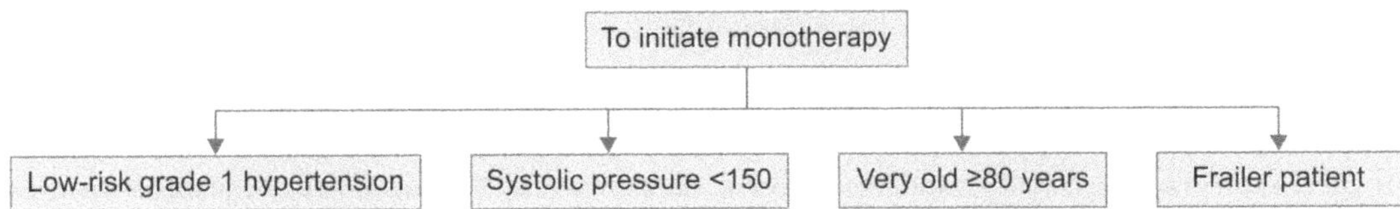

Pharmacological management for hypertension: β-blocker (ESC 2018)

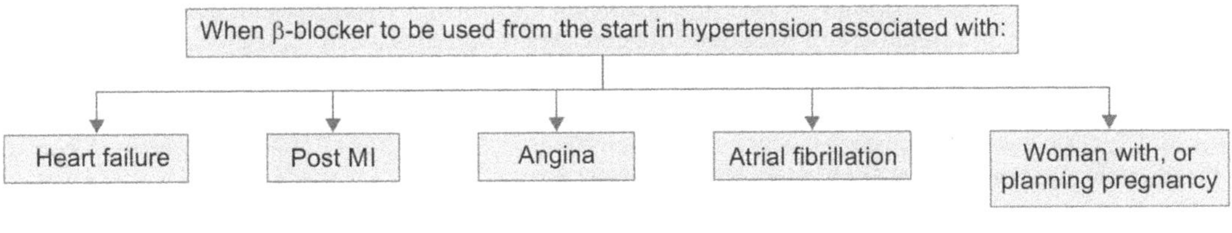

(MI: myocardial infarction)

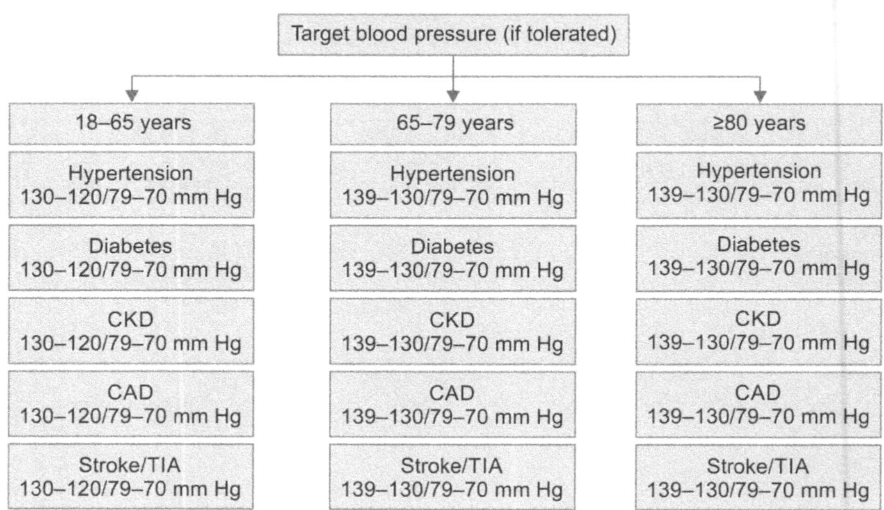

(CAD: coronary artery disease; CVD: cardiovascular disease; CKD: chronic kidney disease; TIA: transient ischemic attack)

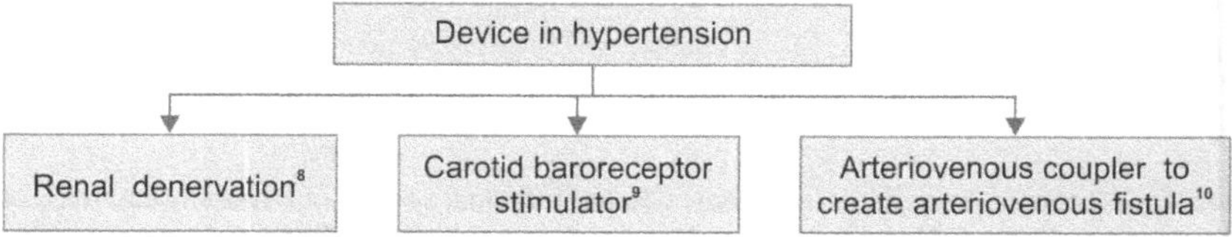

REFERENCES

1. Whelton PK, Carey RM, Aronow WS, Casey DE Jr, Collins KJ, Dennison Himmelfarb C, et al. 2017 ACC/AHA/AAPA/ABC/ ACPM/AGS/APhA/ASH/ASPC/NMA/PCNA Guideline for the Prevention, Detection, Evaluation, and Management of High Blood Pressure in Adults: Executive Summary: a report of the American College of Cardiology/American Heart Association Task Force on Clinical Practice Guidelines. J Am Coll Cardiol. 2018;71:2199-269.

2. Williams B, Mancia G, Spiering W, Agabiti Rosei E, Azizi M, Burnier M, et al. 2018 ESC/ESH Guidelines for the management of arterial hypertension. Eur Heart J. 2018;39:3021-104.

3. NICE (2019). Hypertension in adults: diagnosis and management. NICE guideline [NG136]. [online] Available from https://www.nice.org.uk/guidance/ng136 [Last accessed July, 2022].

4. Unger T, Borghi C, Charchar F, Khan NA, Poulter NR, Prabhakaran D, et al. 2020 International Society of Hypertension Global Hypertension Practice Guidelines. Hypertens. 2020;75(6):1334-57.

5. Jeemon P, Amodeo C, Balabanova D, Campbell NRC, Gaita D, Kario K, et al. World Heart Federation Roadmap for Hypertension – A 2021 update. Global Heart. 2021;16(1):63.

6. Lee HY, Shin J, Kim GH, Park S, Ihm SH, Kim HC, et al. 2018 Korean Society of Hypertension Guidelines for the management of hypertension. part II. Diagnosis and treatment of hypertension. Clin Hypertens. 2019;25:20.

7. Stergiou GS, Palatini P, Parati G, O'Brien E, Januszewicz A, Lurbe E, et al. 2021 European Society of Hypertension practice guidelines for office and out-of-office blood pressure measurement. J Hypertens. 2021;39:1293-302.

8. Bhatt DL, Kandzari DE, O'Neill WW, D'Agostino R, Flack JM, Katzen BT, et al; SYMPLICITY HTN-3 Investigators. A controlled trial of renal denervation for resistant hypertension. N Engl J Med. 2014;370:1393-401.

9. Bisognano JD, Kaufman CL, Bach DS, Lovett EG, de Leeuw P; DEBuT-HT and Rheos Feasibility Trial Investigators. Improved cardiac structure and function with chronic treatment using an implantable device in resistant hypertension: results from European and United States trials of the Rheos system. J Am Coll Cardiol. 2011;57(17):1787-88.

10. obo MD, Sobotka PA, Stanton A, Cockcroft JR, Sulke N, Dolan E, et al; ROX CONTROL HTN Investigators. Central arteriovenous anastomosis for the treatment of patients with uncontrolled hypertension (the ROX CONTROL HTN study): a randomised controlled trial. Lancet. 2015;385:1634-41.

CHAPTER 5

Secondary Hypertension: General Approach

INTRODUCTION

Secondary hypertension is defined as hypertension secondary to an identifiable etiology. The prevalence of secondary hypertension is around 5–15% of hypertensive population.[1] The etiology should be tried to diagnose at early age and corrected. Diagnosis at later age with long-standing hypertension leads to irreversible vascular change and target organ damage.

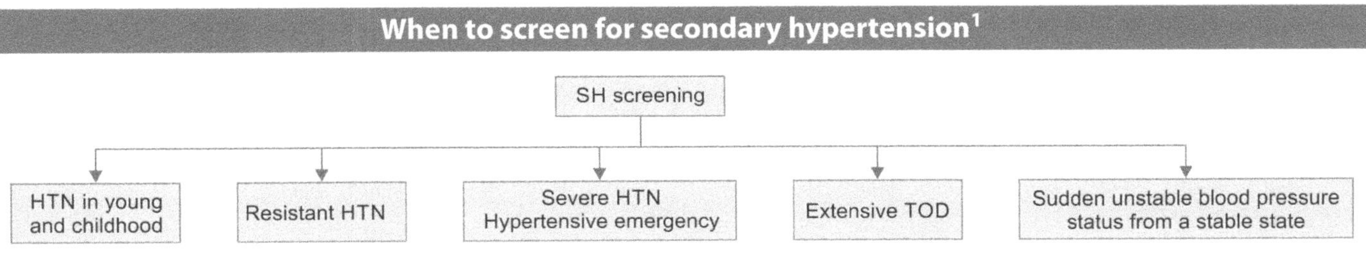

(SH: secondary hypertension; HTN: hypertension; TOD: target organ damage)

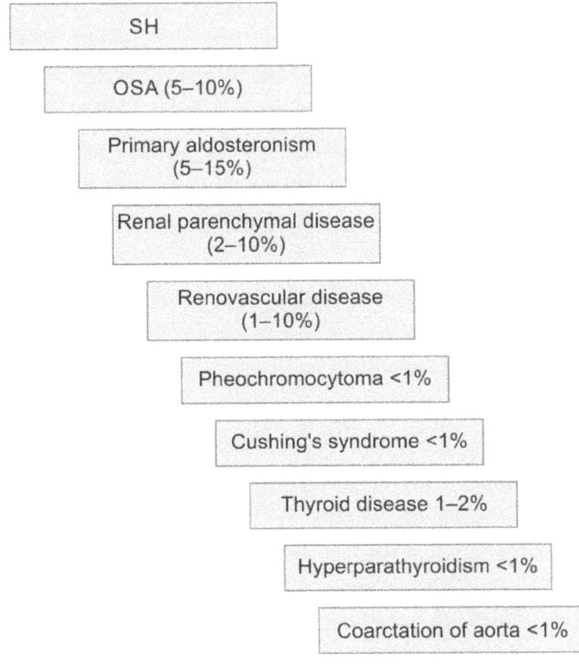

(SH: secondary hypertension; OSA: obstructive sleep apnea)

REFERENCES

1. Rivoli SF, Scherrer U, Messerli FH. Secondary arterial hypertension: when, who, and how to screen? Eur Heart J. 2014;35(19):1245-54.
2. Williams B, Mancia G, Spiering W, Agabiti Rosei E, Azizi M, Burnier M, et al.; ESC Scientific Document Group. 2018 ESC/ESH Guidelines for the management of arterial hypertension. Eur Heart J. 2018;39:3021-104.

CHAPTER 6

Secondary Hypertension: Obstructive Sleep Apnea

INTRODUCTION

Sleep-disordered breathing is defined as upper airway obstruction during sleep and includes obstructive sleep apnea syndrome (OSAS), central sleep apnea, and obesity hyperventilation syndrome. Out of these the most common is OSAS, which is characterized by pharyngeal collapse during sleep. Up to 50% of the patients with OSAS develop hypertension which may become resistant. The most effective management of OSAS is continuous positive airway pressure (CPAP), which does not have any dramatic effect on blood pressure control. There is a modest reduction in 24-hour blood pressure, of which night-time pressure responds most.

Diagnosis of obstructive sleep apnea syndrome: American Academy of Sleep Medicine[1]

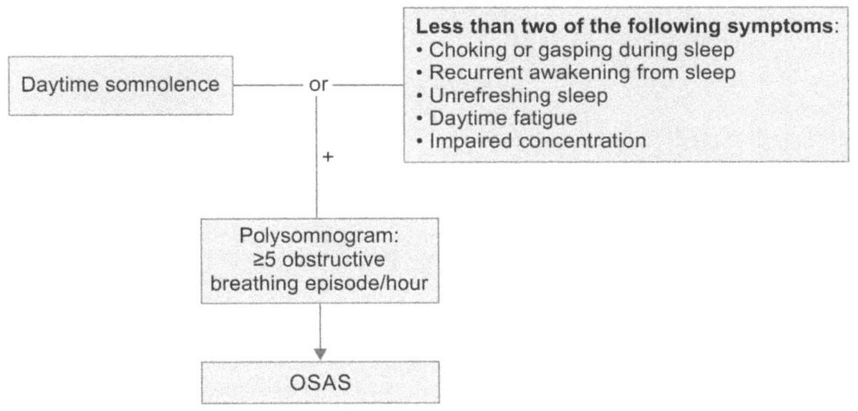

(OSAS: obstructive sleep apnea syndrome)

Pathophysiology of hypertension in obstructive sleep apnea syndrome[2]

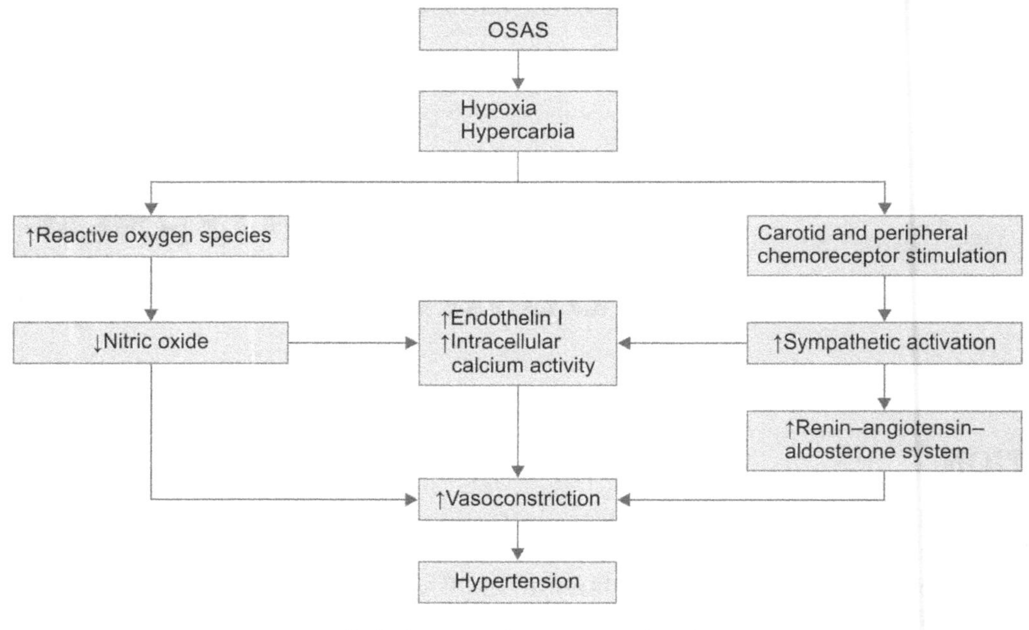

(OSAS: obstructive sleep apnea syndrome)

Initial assessment of obstructive sleep apnea syndrome and hypertension[2]

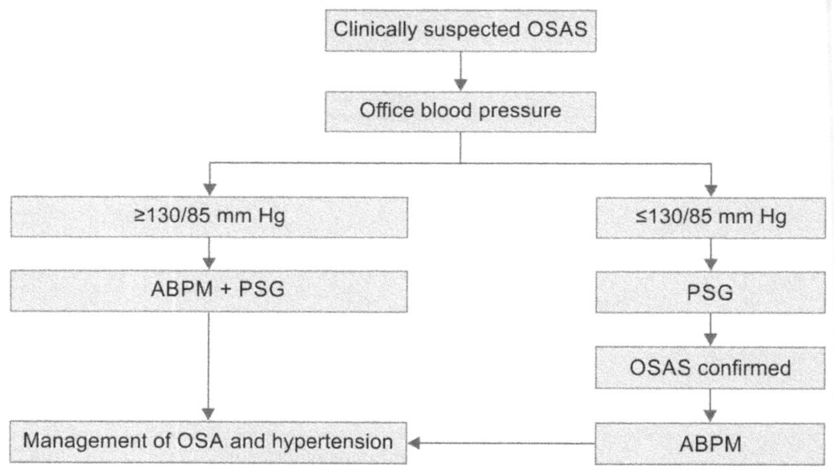

(ABPM: ambulatory blood pressure monitoring; OSAS: obstructive sleep apnea syndrome; PSG: polysomnography)

Management of obstructive sleep apnea syndrome and hypertension

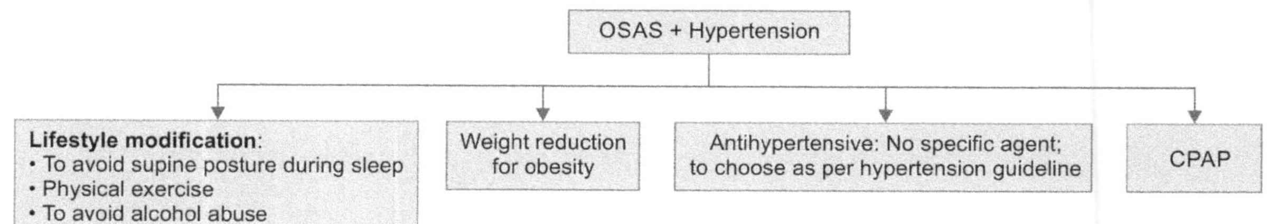

(CPAP: continuous positive airway pressure; OSAS: obstructive sleep apnea syndrome)

REFERENCES

1. Sleep-related breathing disorders in adults: recommendations for syndrome definition and measurement techniques in clinical research. The Report of an American Academy of Sleep Medicine Task Force. Sleep. 1999;22:667-89.
2. Parati G, Lombardi C, Hedner J, Bonsignore MR, Grote L, Tkacova R, et al. Recommendations for the management of patients with obstructive sleep apnoea and hypertension. Eur Respir J. 2013;41:523-38.

CHAPTER 7

Renal Hypertension: Chronic Kidney Disease

INTRODUCTION

Prevalence of hypertension in chronic kidney disease (CKD) is 60–90%. The grade of hypertension depends on the grade of CKD. The mechanism of hypertension is multifactorial including salt retention, volume expansion, sympathoadrenal overactivation, renin–angiotensin system (RAS) overactivation, endothelial dysfunction, and others. RAS inhibitor, angiotensin converting enzyme (ACE) inhibitor or angiotensin receptor blocker (ARB), is the first-line therapy for hypertension in CKD, specifically with proteinuria. ACE inhibitor or ARB causes glomerular efferent arteriolar vasodilation by counteracting the effect of angiotensin II, leading to fall in intraglomerular filtration pressure and glomerular filtration rate (GFR), which suppresses proteinuria and induces hyperkalemia. As CKD patients are salt sensitive and have reduced capacity of salt excretion, salt restriction plays a very important issue in hypertension management. Physiological nocturnal dip of blood pressure is lost in CKD patients. Bedtime dose of at least one hypertensive may maintain this dip and make better control of blood pressure.

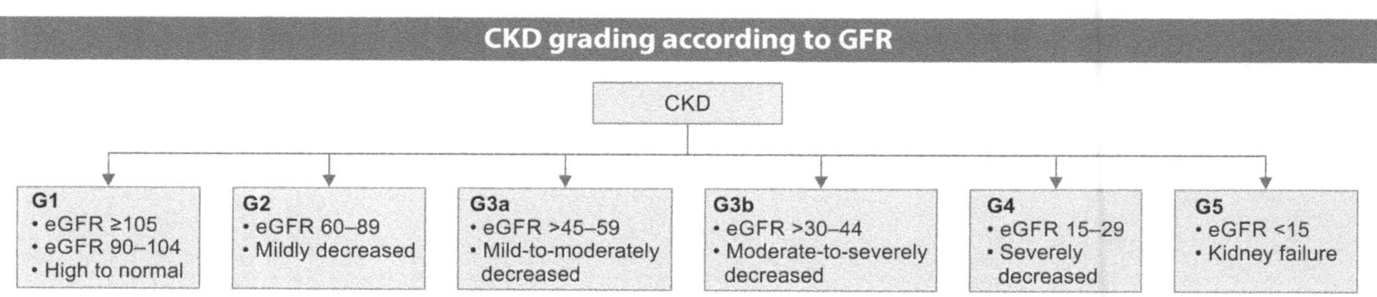

(CKD: chronic kidney disease; eGFR: estimated glomerular filtration rate–mL/min/1.73 m^2; GFR: glomerular filtration rate)

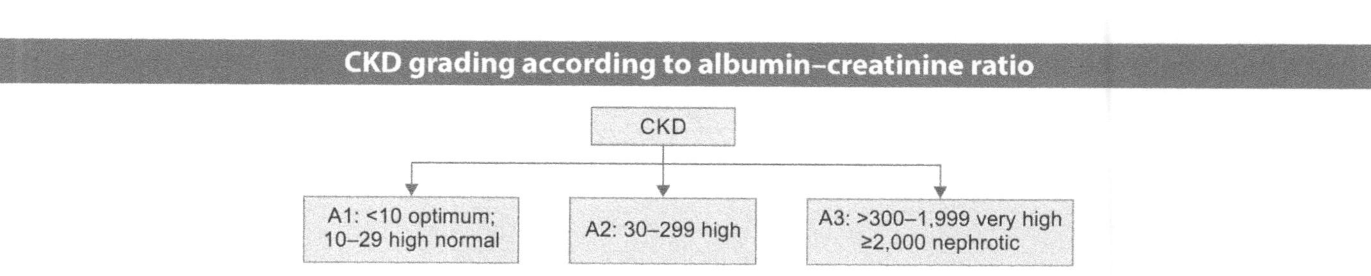

Note: ACR is given in mg/g or µg/mg.
(CKD: chronic kidney disease)

Pathophysiology of hypertension in CKD

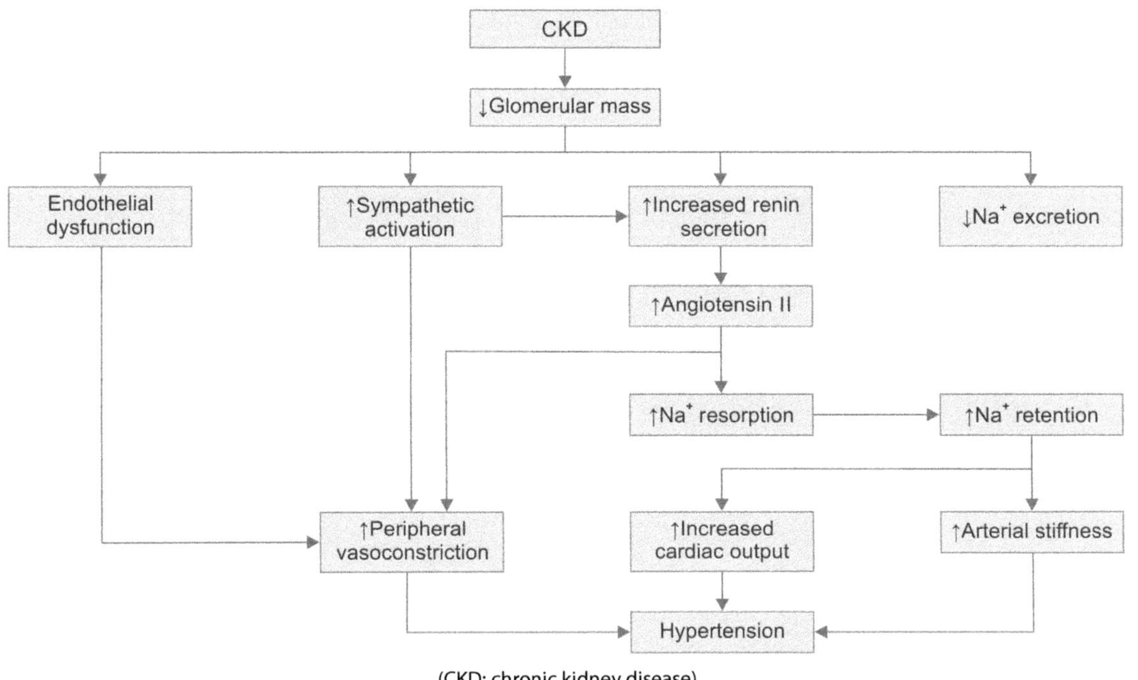

(CKD: chronic kidney disease)

Medical management of hypertension in CKD: First-line drug[1]

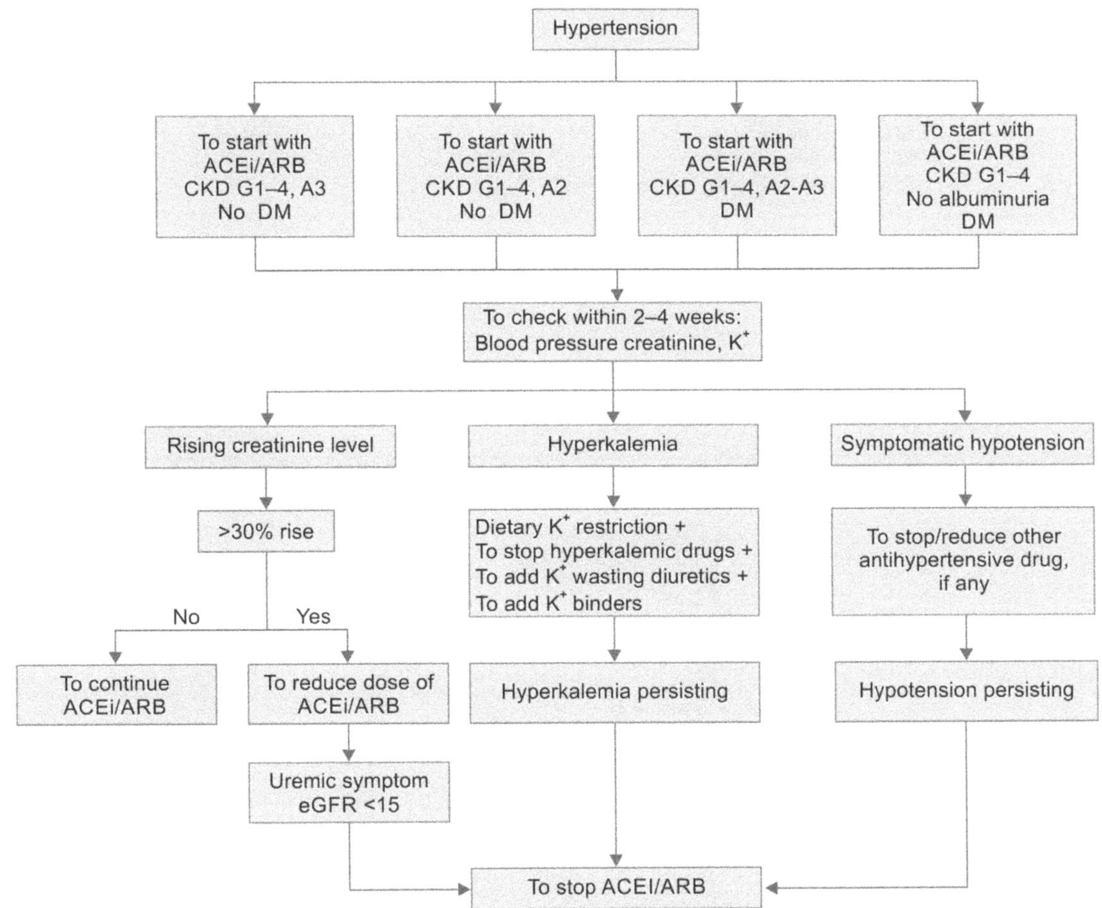

(ACEi: angiotensin converting enzyme inhibitor; ARB: angiotensin receptor blocker; CKD: chronic kidney disease; DM: diabetes mellitus; eGFR: estimated glomerular filtration rate)

Medical management of hypertension in CKD: Second-line drug[1]

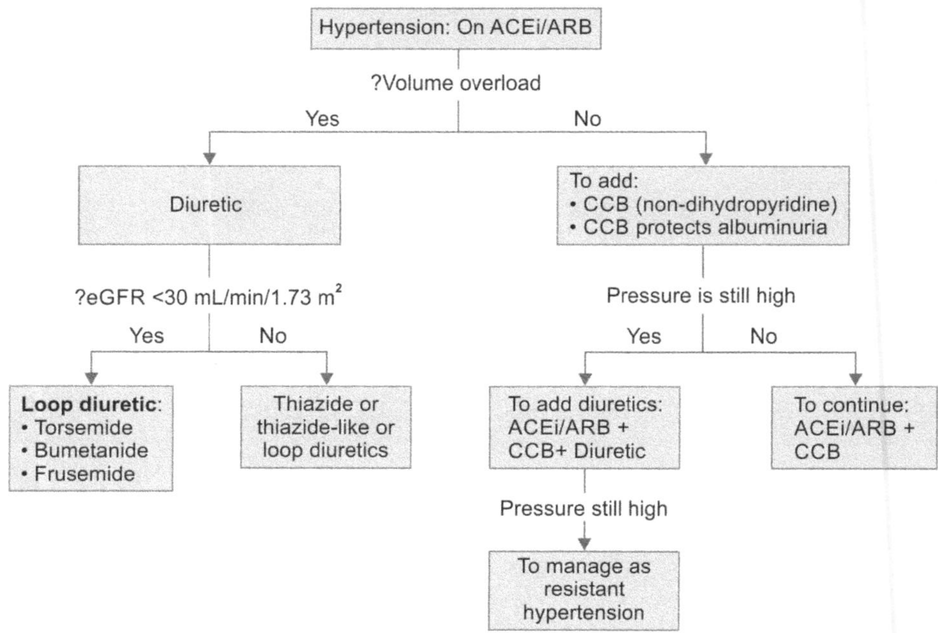

(ACEi: angiotensin converting enzyme inhibitor; ARB: angiotensin receptor blocker; CCB: calcium channel blockers; CKD: chronic kidney disease; eGFR: estimated glomerular filtration rate)

Medical management of hypertension in patients on dialysis

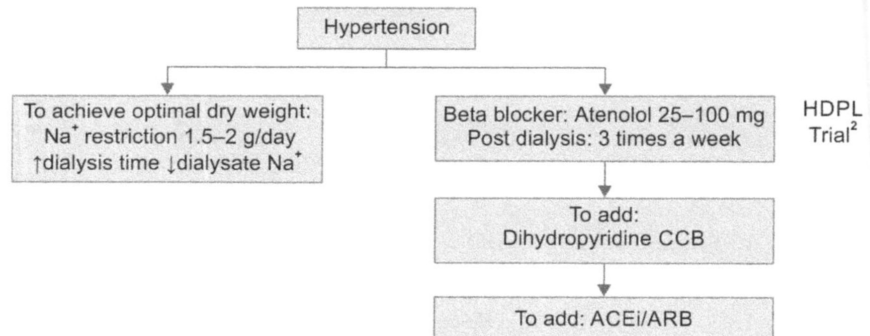

(ACEi: angiotensin converting enzyme inhibitor; ARB: angiotensin receptor blocker; CCB: calcium channel blocker)

Medical management of hypertension in kidney transplant recipient

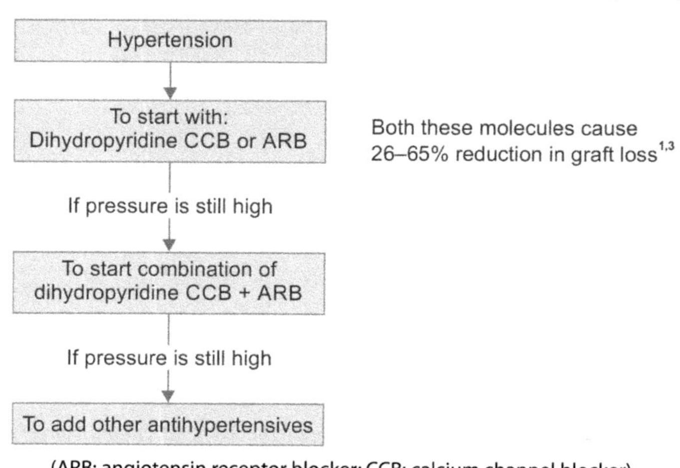

(ARB: angiotensin receptor blocker; CCB: calcium channel blocker)

REFERENCES

1. Kidney Disease: Improving Global Outcomes (KDIGO) Blood Pressure Work Group. KDIGO 2021 clinical practice guideline for the management of blood pressure in chronic kidney disease. Kidney Int. 2021;99(3S):S1-S87.
2. Agarwal R, Sinha AD, Pappas MK, Abraham TN, Tegegne GG. Hypertension in hemodialysis patients treated with atenolol or lisinopril: a randomized controlled trial. Nephrol Dial Transplant. 2014; 29(3):672-81.
3. van der Schaaf MR, Hene RJ, Floor M, Blankestijn PJ, Koomans HA. Hypertension after renal transplantation. Calcium channel or converting enzyme blockade? Hypertension. 1995;25:77-81.

CHAPTER 8

Renal Hypertension: Renovascular Hypertension

INTRODUCTION

Renovascular hypertension (RVH) is one of the most common causes of both secondary hypertension and resistant hypertension. RVH accounts for 1–2% of all causes of general population with hypertension, whereas its prevalence is 6.5% in hypertensive population above 65 years of age and 5.8% in younger population with secondary hypertension.[1] Fibromuscular dysplasia (FMD) and atherosclerotic renal artery stenosis (ARAS) are the two most common causes for renal artery stenosis.

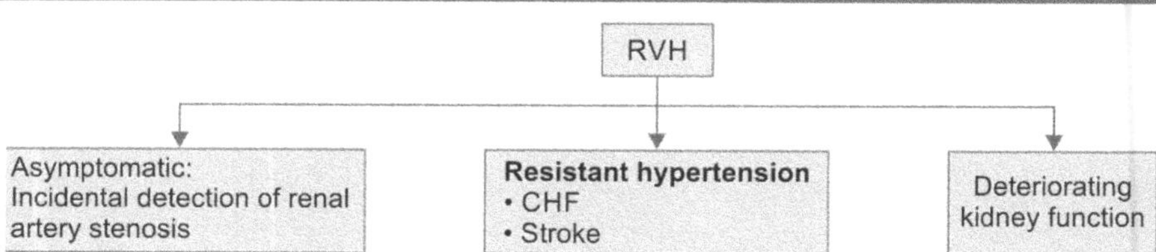

(ARAS: atherosclerotic renal artery stenosis; FMD: fibromuscular dysplasia; RVH: renovascular hypertension)

(CHF: congestive heart failure; RVH: renovascular hypertension)

Pathophysiology of hypertension in renovascular hypertension

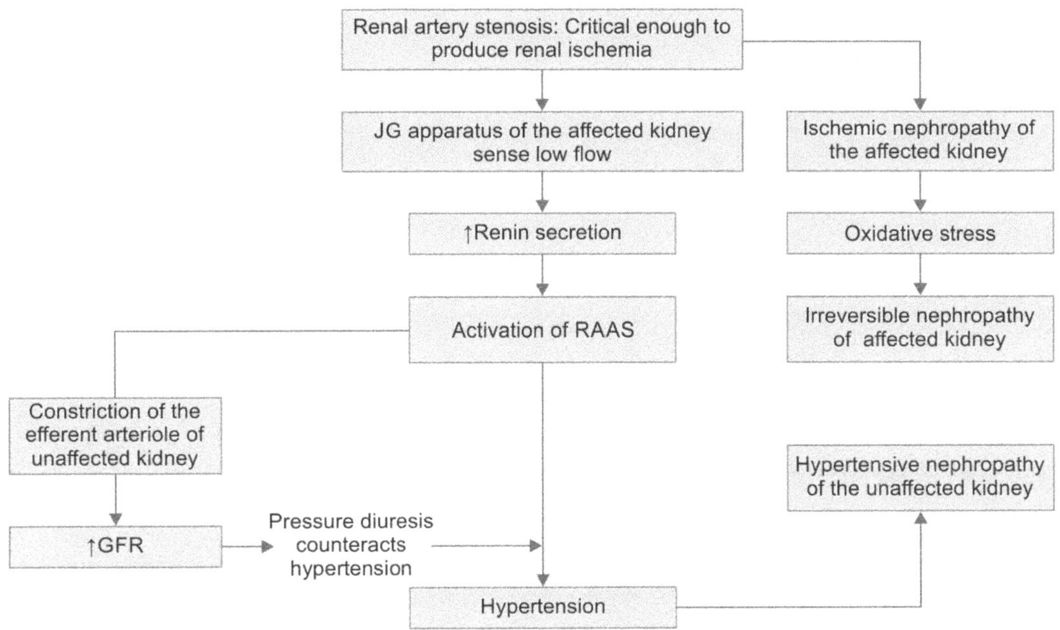

(GFR: glomerular filtration rate; JG: juxtaglomerular; RAAS: renin–angiotensin–aldosterone axis; RVH: renovascular hypertension)

Imaging for renovascular hypertension[1]

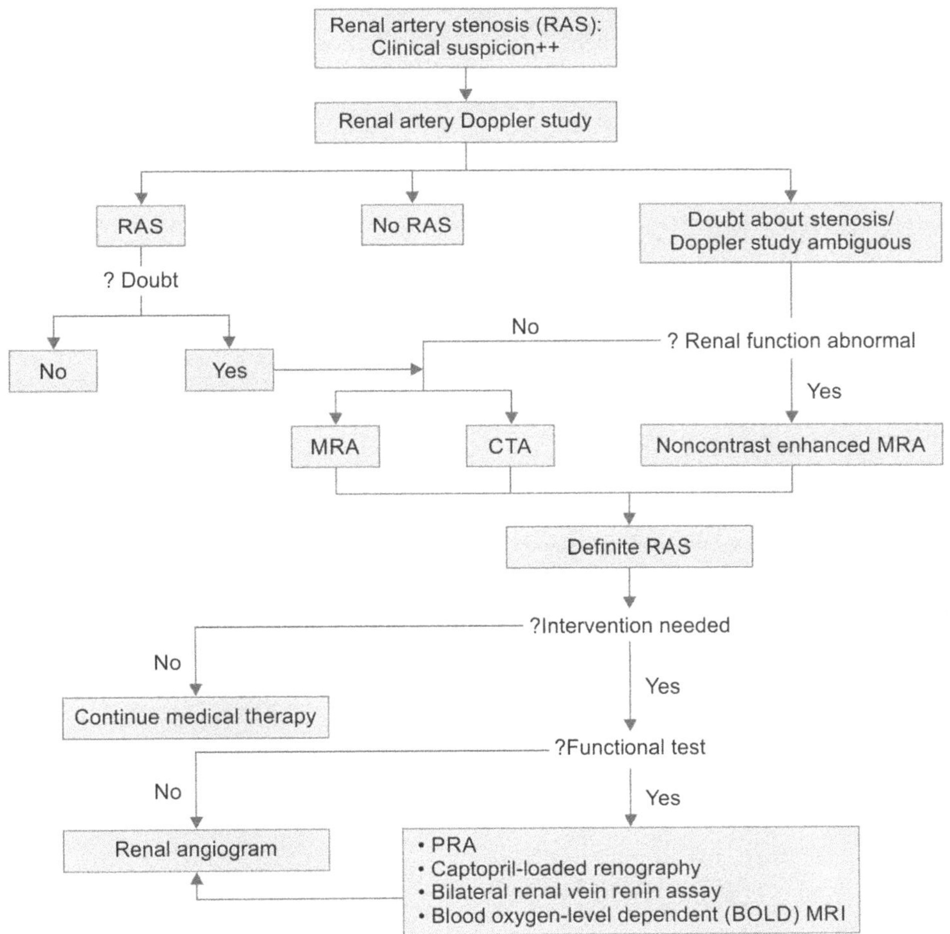

(CTA: computed tomography angiogram; MRA: magnetic resonance angiogram; MRI: magnetic resonance imaging; PRA: plasma renin activity)

Medical management of atherosclerotic renal artery stenosis[2]

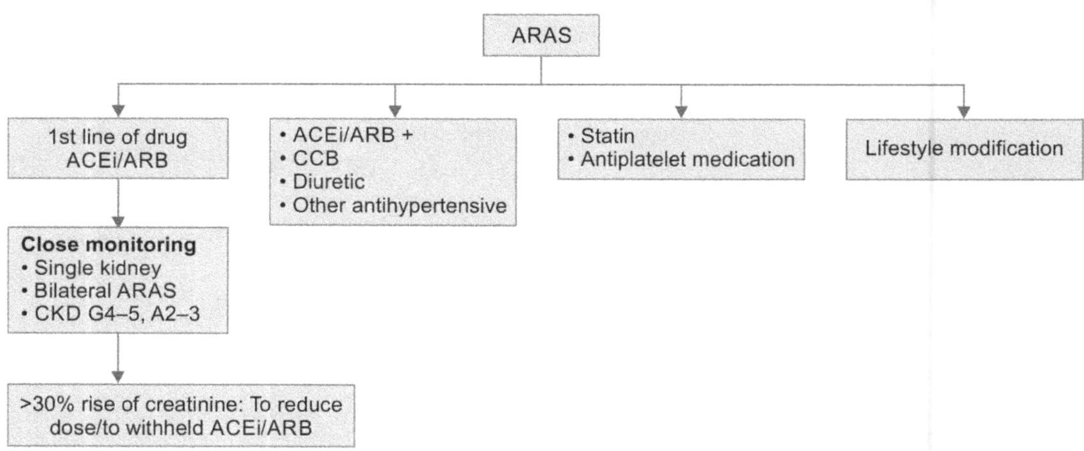

(ACEi: angiotensin converting enzyme inhibitor; ARAS: atherosclerotic renal artery stenosis; ARB: angiotensin receptor blocker; CCB: calcium channel blocker)

Management of atherosclerotic renal artery stenosis: Revascularization[3]

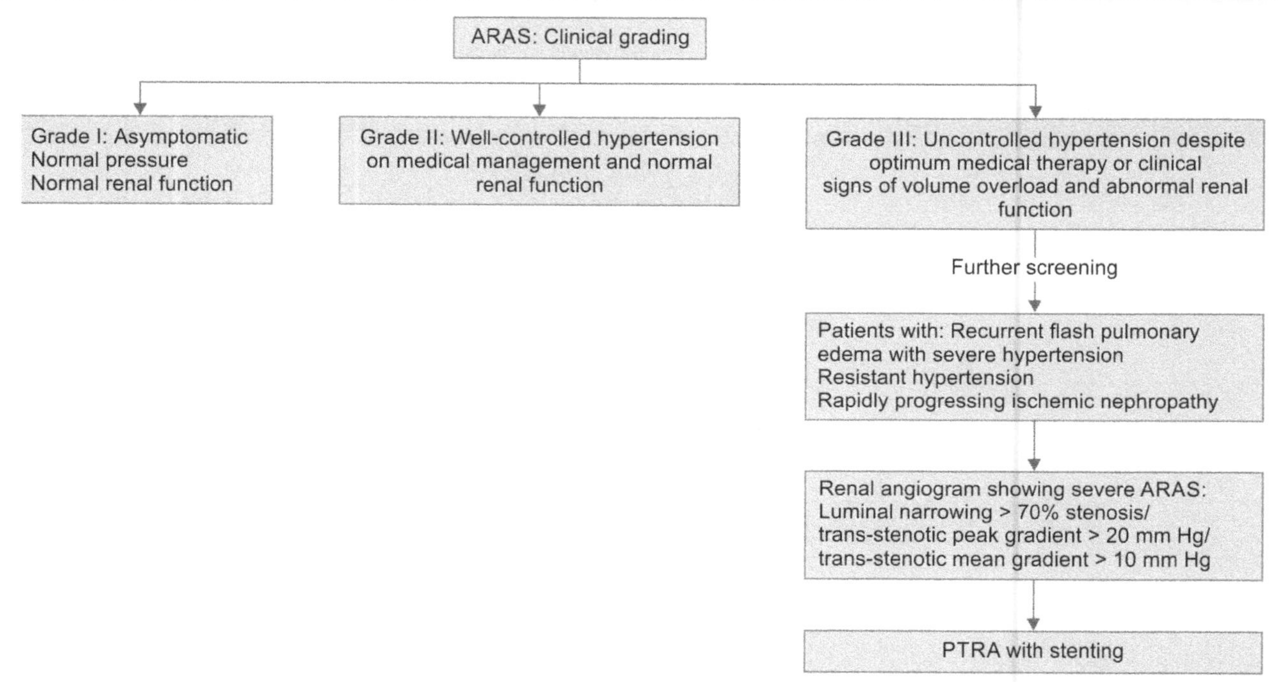

(ARAS: atherosclerotic renal artery stenosis; PTRA: percutaneous transluminal renal angioplasty)

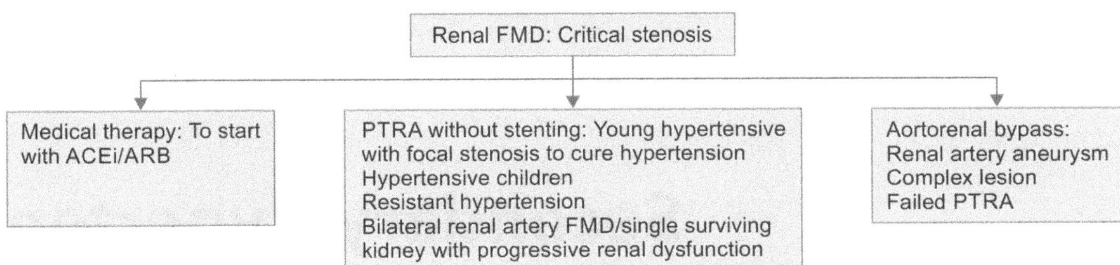

(ACEi: angiotensin converting enzyme inhibitor; ARB: angiotensin receptor blocker; FMD: fibromuscular dysplasia; PTRA: percutaneous transluminal renal angioplasty)

REFERENCES

1. Derkx FH, Schalekamp MA. Renal artery stenosis and hypertension. Lancet 1994;344(8917):237-9.
2. Badila E, Tintea E. How to manage renovascular hypertension. An article from the e-journal of the ESC council for cardiology practice. ESC. 2014;13:8-9.
3. Bailey SR, Beckman JA, Dao TD, Misra S, Sobieszczyk PS, White CJ, et al. ACC/AHA/SCAI/SIR/SVM 2018 appropriate use criteria for peripheral artery intervention: a report of the American college of cardiology appropriate use criteria task force, American heart association, society for cardiovascular angiography and interventions, society of interventional radiology, and society for vascular medicine. J Am Coll Cardiol. 2019;73(2):214-37.
4. Klein AJ, Jaff MR, Gray BH, Aronow HD, Bersin RM, Diaz-Sandoval LJ, et al. SCAI appropriate use criteria for peripheral arterial interventions: an update. Catheter Cardiovasc Interv. 2017;90(4):E90-E110.

CHAPTER 9

Secondary Hypertension: Primary Aldosteronism

INTRODUCTION

Primary aldosteronism (PA) or Conn's syndrome is characterized by high aldosterone production inappropriate for sodium status. This inappropriate aldosterone production leads to suppressed plasma renin activity, sodium retention, increased potassium excretion, and hypertension. Its prevalence is more than 5–10% in hypertensive population[1] and approximately 20% in resistant hypertensive population. The importance of PA, other than its higher prevalence and treatability, is its higher association with cardiovascular morbidity and mortality, higher stroke rate, higher incidence of target organ damage, and higher incidence of hypertension getting resistant. PA is commonly diagnosed between 20 and 60 years of age. Polyuria and nocturia due to hypokalemia-induced concentration defect may occasionally be the presenting symptoms.

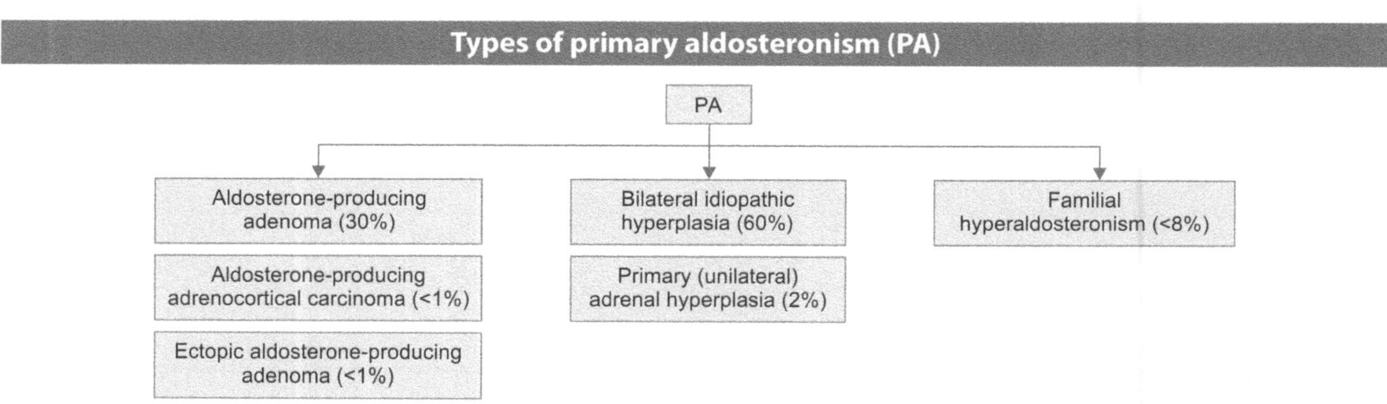

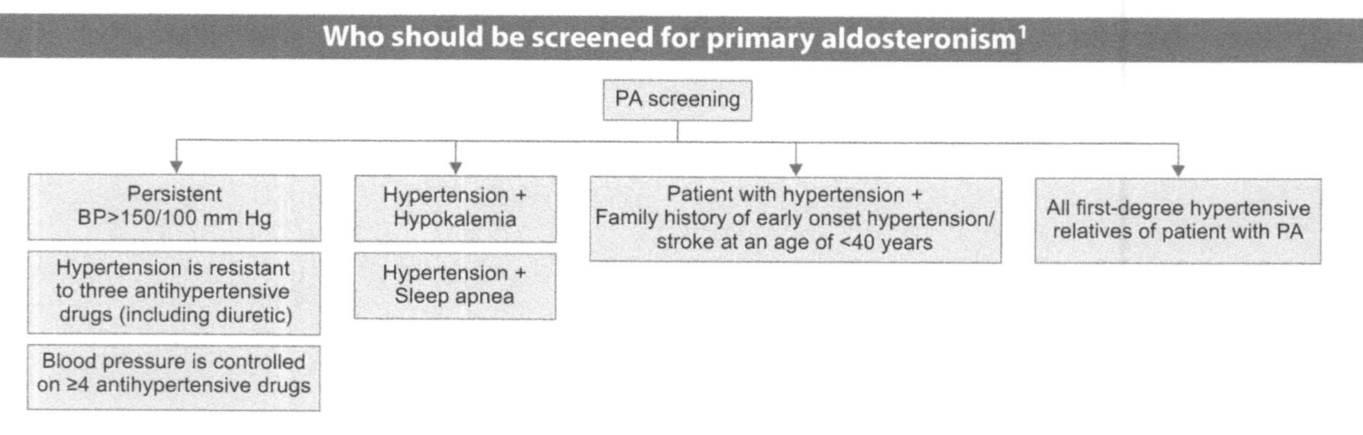

How to diagnose primary aldosteronism[1]

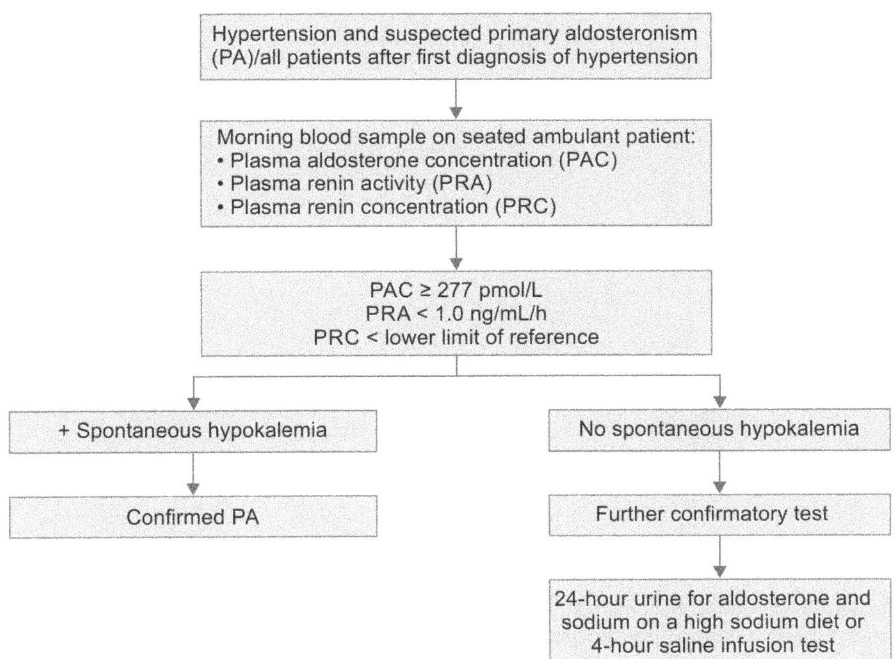

Management of primary aldosteronism[1,2]

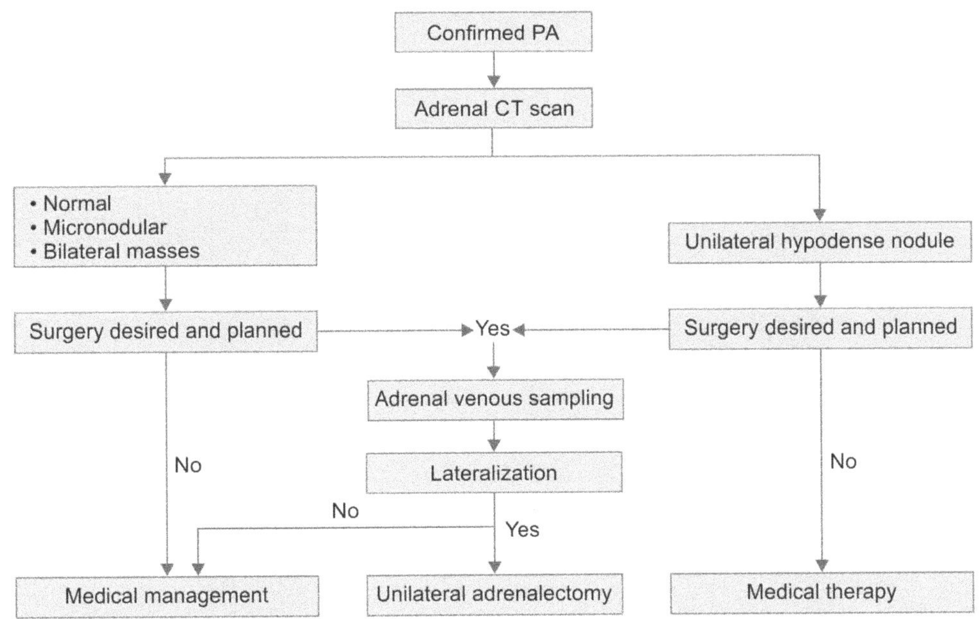

(CT: computed tomography; PA: primary aldosteronism)

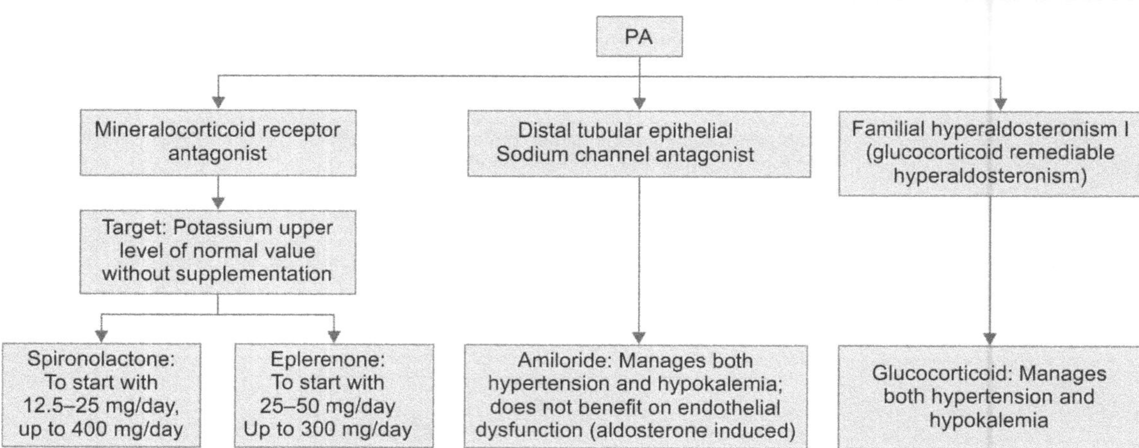

REFERENCES

1. Funder JW, Carey RM, Mantero F, Murad MH, Reincke M, Shibata H, et al. The management of primary aldosteronism: case detection, diagnosis, and treatment: an endocrine society clinical practice guideline. J Clin Endocrinol Metab. 2016;101(5):1889-916.
2. Carey RM. Diagnosing and managing primary aldosteronism in hypertensive patients: a case-based approach. Curr Cardiol Rep. 2016;18(10):97.

CHAPTER 10

Secondary Hypertension: Pheochromocytoma

INTRODUCTION

Pheochromocytoma is a neuroendocrine tumor. In 85% of cases, the tumor arises from adrenal medulla.[1] In 15–20% of cases, the tumor arises from sympathetic ganglia in thorax, abdomen, and pelvis when it is named as paraganglioma. Pheochromocytoma and paraganglioma (PPGL) are tumors that arise from chromaffin cells and cause hypertension in 90% of cases. PPGL present with the classic triad of symptoms of episodic headache, palpitation, and sweating. In 80% of cases, all PPGL can be explained by genetic alteration.

Different types of pheochromocytoma and paraganglioma

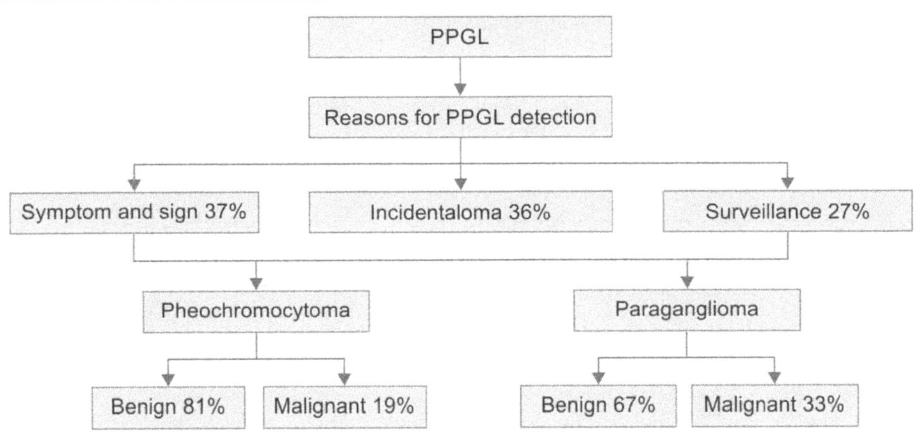

(PPGL: pheochromocytoma and paraganglioma)

Who should be screened for pheochromocytoma and paraganglioma[1]

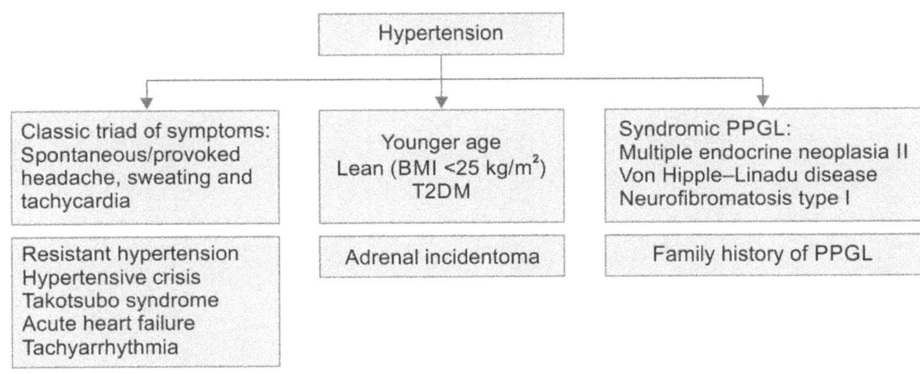

(PPGL: pheochromocytoma and paraganglioma; T2DM: type 2 diabetes mellitus)

How to diagnose pheochromocytoma and paraganglioma[2,3]

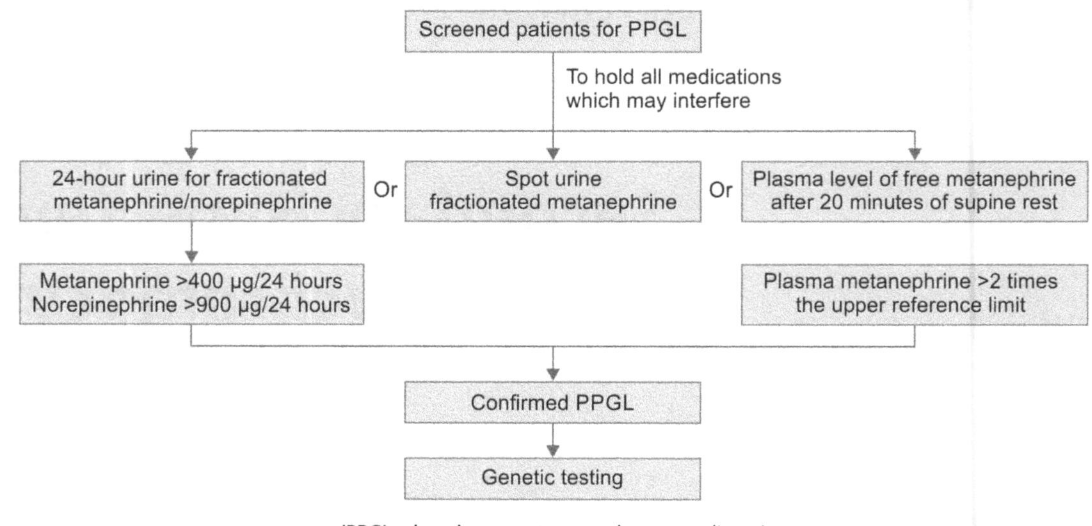

(PPGL: pheochromocytoma and paraganglioma)

Pheochromocytoma and paraganglioma localization[2,3]

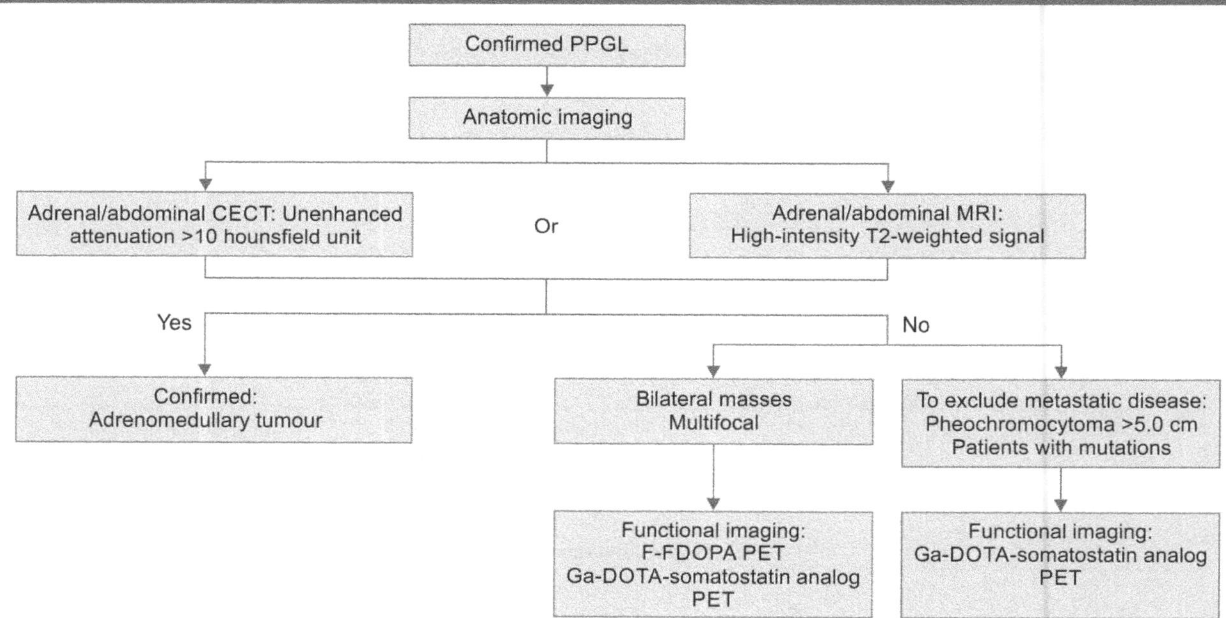

(CECT: contrast-enhanced computed tomography; MRI: magnetic resonance imaging; PET: positron emission tomography; PPGL: pheochromocytoma and paraganglioma)

Management of pheochromocytoma and paraganglioma[1,2,3]

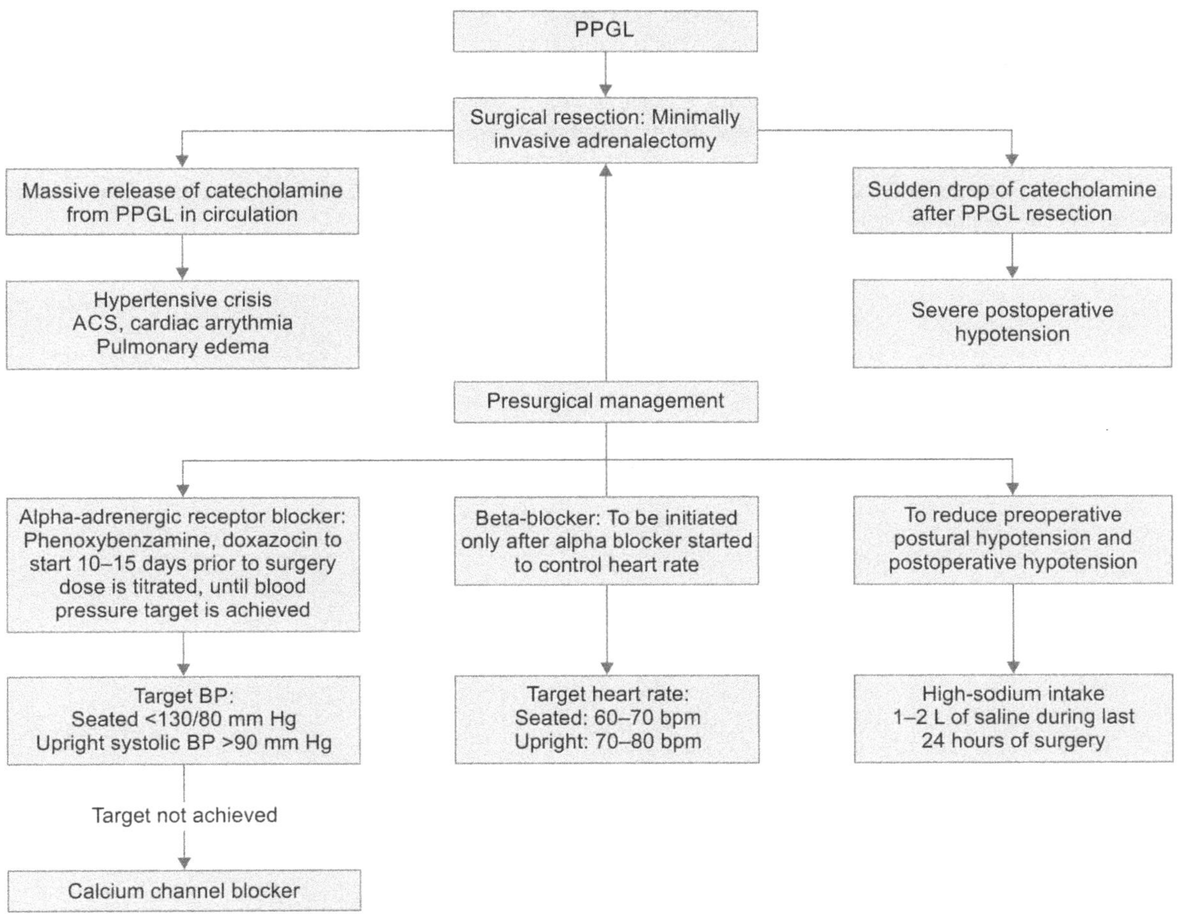

(ACS: acute coronary syndrome; BP: blood pressure; PPGL: pheochromocytoma and paraganglioma)

Follow-up of pheochromocytoma and paraganglioma after surgical resection[1,2,3]

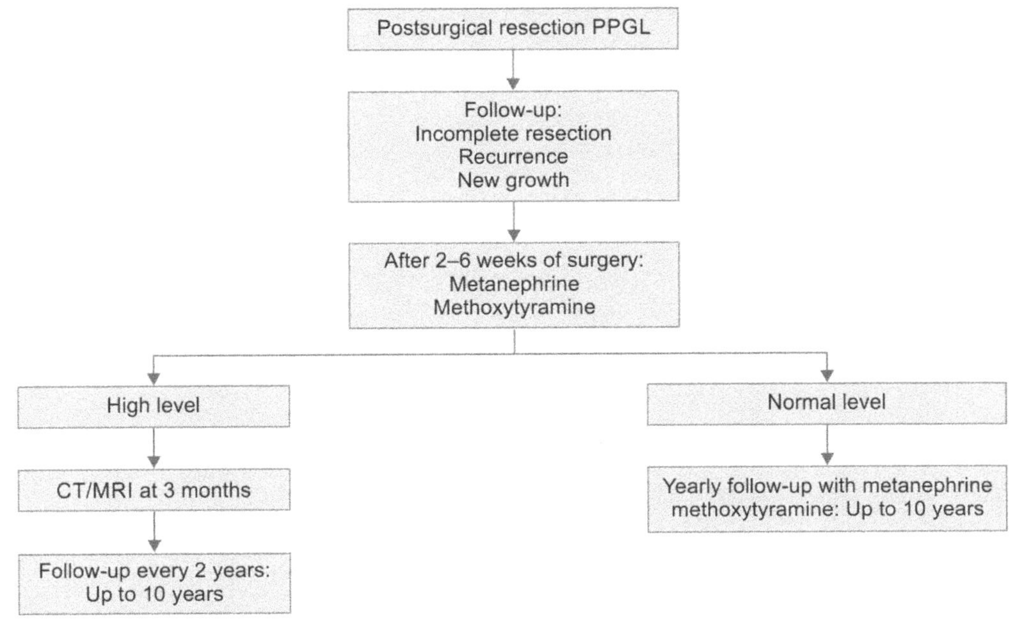

(CT: computed tomography; MRI: magnetic resonance imaging; PPGL: pheochromocytoma and paraganglioma)

REFERENCES

1. Lender JWM, Kerstens MN, Amar L, Prejbisz A, Robledo M, Taieb D, et al. Genetics, diagnosis, management and future directions of research of phaeochromocytoma and paraganglioma: a position statement and consensus of the Working Group on Endocrine Hypertension of the European Society of Hypertension. J Hypertens. 2020;38:1443-56.
2. Takekoshi K, Satoh F, Tanabe A, Okamoto T, Ichihara A, Tsuiki M, et al. Correlation between urinary fractionated metanephrines in 24-hour and spot urine samples for evaluating the therapeutic effect of metyrosine: a subanalysis of a multicenter, open-label phase I/II study. Endocr J. 2019;66:1063-72.
3. Lenders JW, Duh QY, Eisenhofer G, Gimenez-Roqueplo AP, Grebe SK, Murad MH, et al. Pheochromocytoma and paraganglioma: an endocrine society clinical practice guideline. J Clin Endocrinol Metab. 2014; 99:1915-42.

CHAPTER 11

Secondary Hypertension: Cushing's Syndrome

INTRODUCTION

Cushing's syndrome (CS), also known as hypercortisolism, is an endocrine disorder due to prolonged effect of glucocorticoid excess. The effect produces major morbidities including systemic hypertension, morbid obesity, glucose impairment, dyslipidemia, and osteoporosis and 2–5-fold increase in mortality,[1] mainly due to cardiovascular complication.

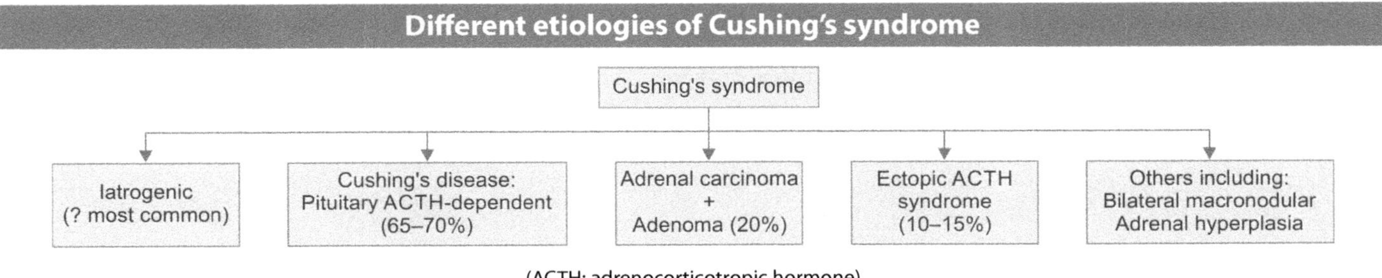

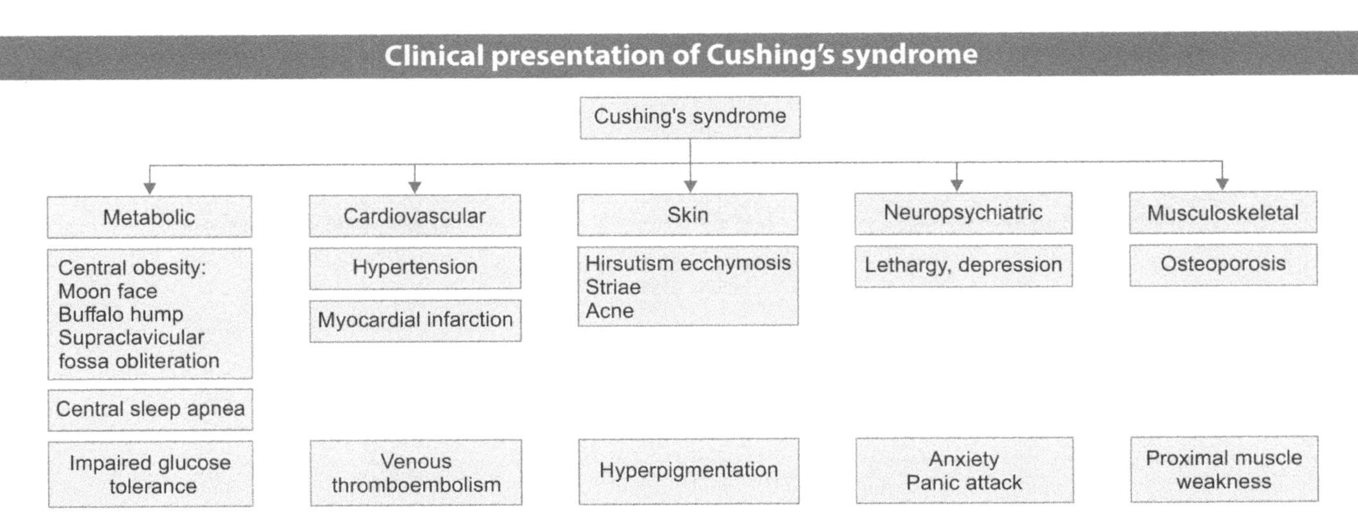

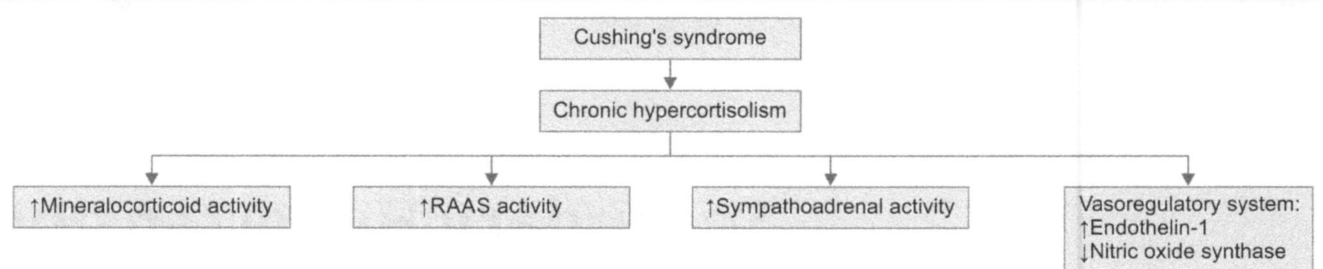

Pathogenesis of hypertension in Cushing's syndrome[2]

(RAAS: renin–angiotensin–aldosterone system)

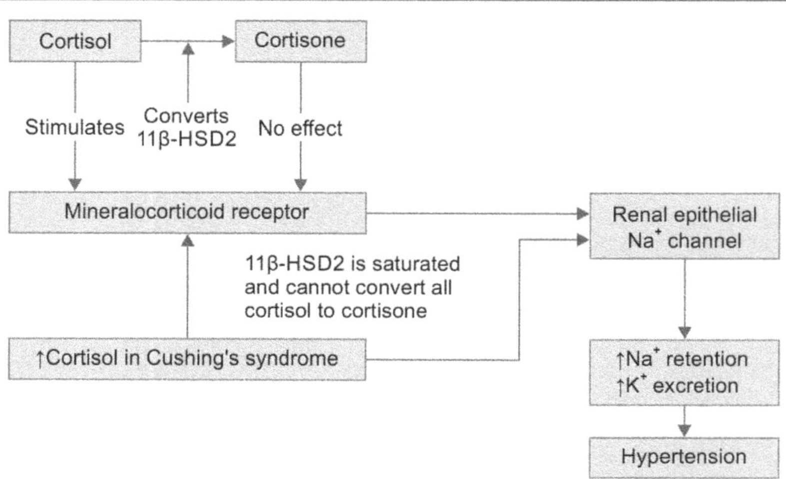

Mechanism of hypertension due to mineralocorticoid activity

(11β-HSD2: 11β-hydroxysteroid dehydrogenase type 2)

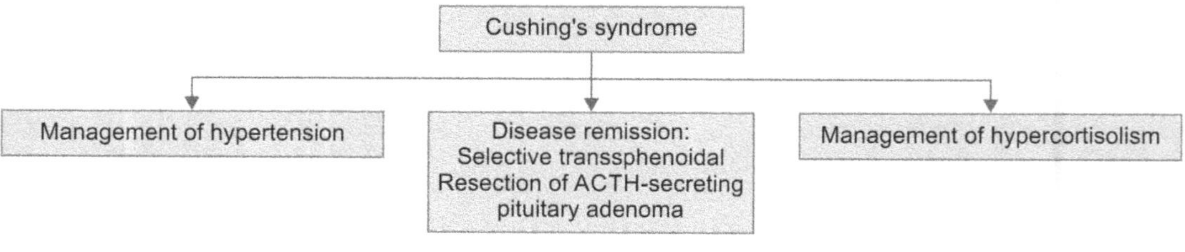

Management of Cushing's syndrome[3]

(ACTH: adrenocorticotropic hormone)

Management of hypertension in Cushing's syndrome[3]

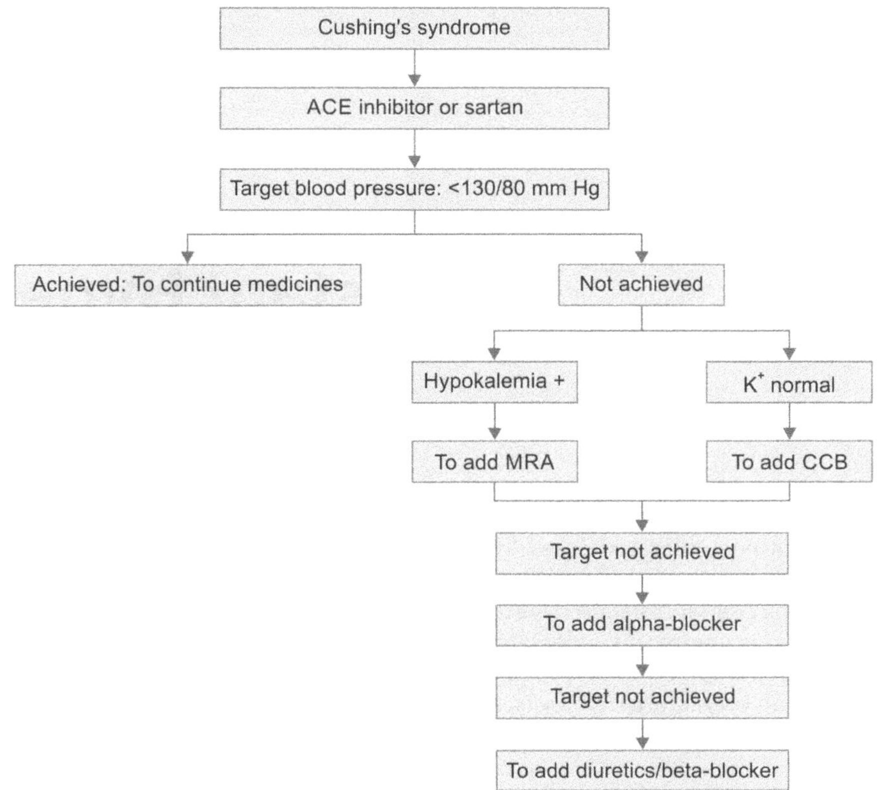

(ACE: angiotensin-converting enzyme; CCB: calcium channel blocker; MRA: mineralocorticoid receptor antagonist)

Management of hypercortisolism in Cushing's syndrome[3,4]

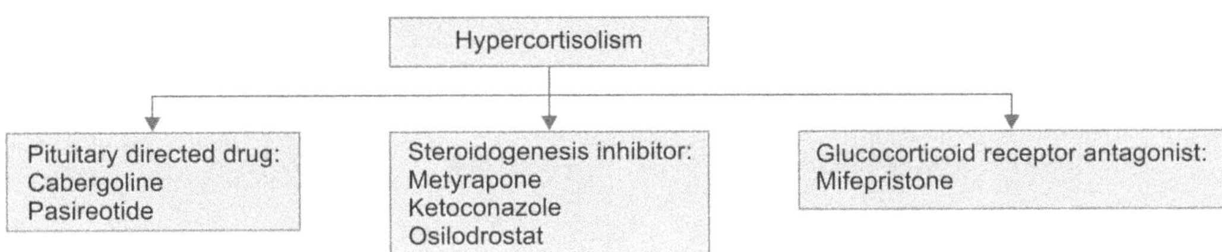

REFERENCES

1. Graversen D, Vestergaard P, Stochholm K, Gravholt CH, Jorgensen JO. Mortality in Cushing's syndrome: a systematic review and meta-analysis. Eur J Intern Med. 2012;23(3):278-82.
2. Nieman LK, Biller BM, Findling JW, Newell-Price J, Savage MO, Stewart PM, et al. The diagnosis of Cushing's syndrome: an Endocrine Society clinical practice guideline. J Clin Endocrinol Metab. 2008;93:1526-40.
3. Nieman LK, Biller BM, Findling JW, Murad MH, Newell-Price J, Savage MO, et al; Endocrine Society. Treatment of Cushing's syndrome: an Endocrine Society clinical practice guideline. J Clin Endocrinol Metab. 2015;100(8):2807-31.
4. Isidori AM, Graziadio C, Paragliola RM, Cozzolino A, Ambrogio AG, Colao A, et al. The hypertension of Cushing's syndrome: controversies in the pathophysiology and focus on cardiovascular complications. J Hypertens. 2015;33(1):44-60.

CHAPTER 12

Resistant Hypertension

INTRODUCTION

Resistant hypertension is defined as the state when blood pressure remains uncontrolled despite three BP-lowering drugs, including diuretics in optimal or best-tolerated doses. The state should be confirmed by home blood pressure monitoring (HBPM) or ambulatory blood pressure monitoring (ABPM). Prevalence of resistant hypertension in treated patient may be 5–30%.[1] However, after excluding pseudoresistant hypertension, the prevalence may come down to less than 10% of treated patients. Resistant hypertension is commonly associated with obesity, albuminuria, diabetes mellitus, obstructive sleep apnea, and loss of nocturnal dip pattern of blood pressure. Patients with resistant hypertension are associated with higher risk of chronic kidney disease and premature cardiovascular events and stroke.

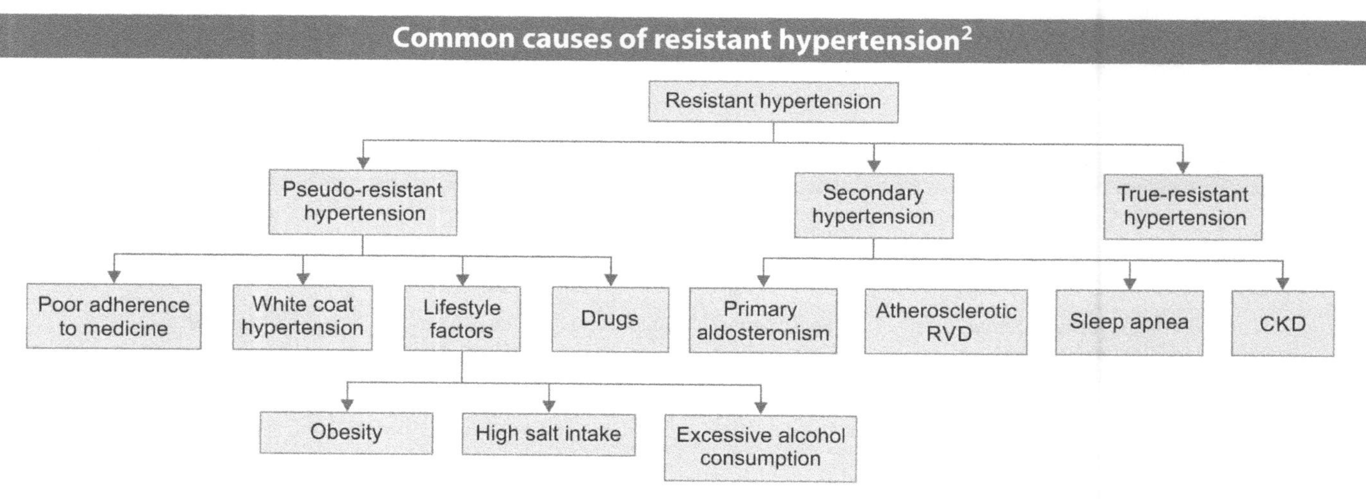

Evaluation of patient with resistant hypertension[1,3]

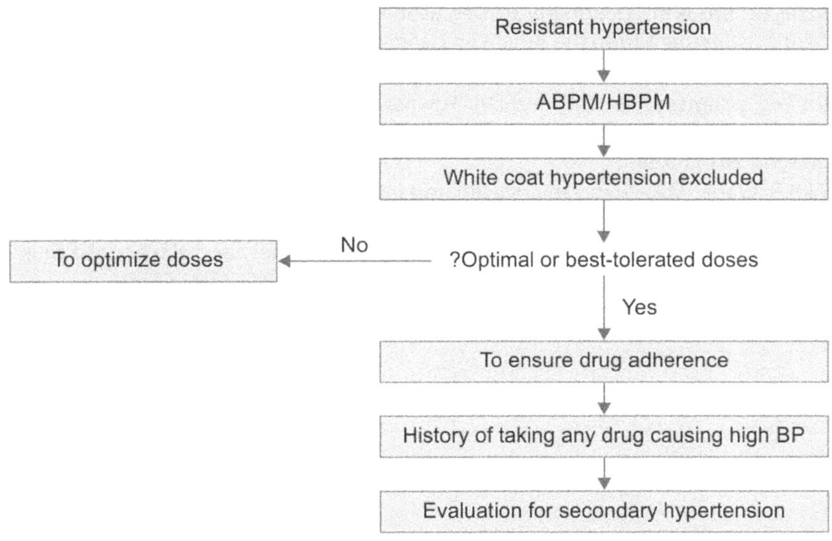

(ABPM: ambulatory blood pressure monitoring; HBPM: home blood pressure monitoring)

Management of resistant hypertension[1,4,5]

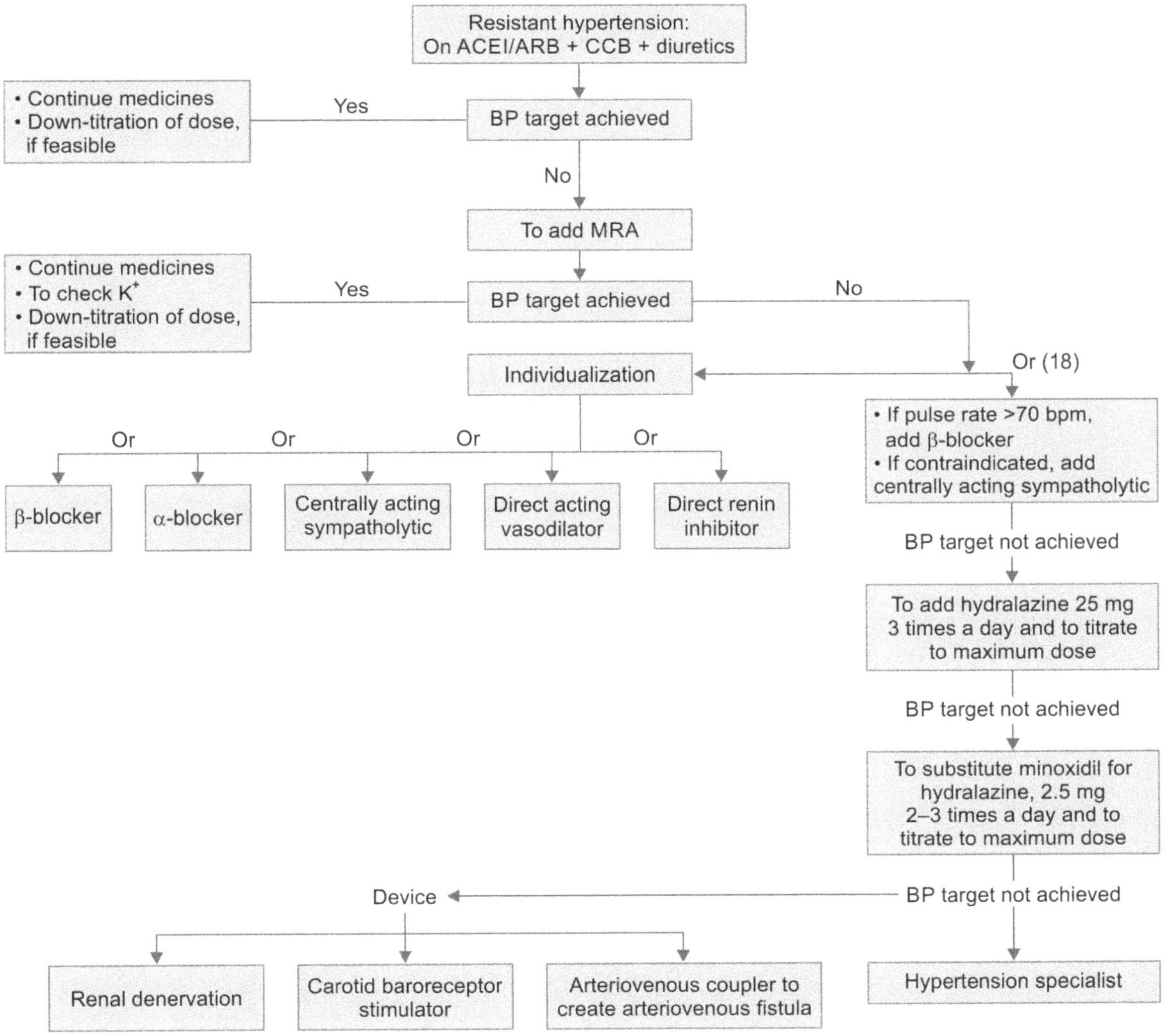

REFERENCES

1. Carey RM, Calhoun DA, Bakris GL, Brook RD, Daugherty SL, Dennison-Himmelfarb CR, et al. Resistant hypertension: detection, evaluation, and management—A scientific statement from the American Heart Association. Hypertension. 2018;72:e53-e90.
2. Hyman DJ, Pavlik V. Medication adherence and resistant hypertension. J Hum Hypertens. 2015;29:213-8.
3. White WB, Turner JR, Sica DA, Bisognano JD, Calhoun DA, Townsend RR, et al. Detection, evaluation, and treatment of severe and resistant hypertension: proceedings from an American Society of Hypertension Interactive Forum held in Bethesda, MD, USA, October 10th 2013. J Am Soc Hypertens. 2014;8:743-57.
4. Kjeldsen SE, Julius S, Dahlöf B, Weber MA. Physician (investigator) inertia in apparent treatment-resistant hypertension—insights from large randomized clinical trials. Lennart Hansson Memorial Lecture. Blood Press. 2015;24:1-6.
5. Worthley SG, Tsioufis CP, Worthley MI, Sinhal A, Chew DP, Meredith IT, et al. Safety and efficacy of a multi-electrode renal sympathetic denervation system in resistant hypertension: the EnligHTN I trial. Eur Heart J. 2013;34:2132-40.

Dyslipidemia

CHAPTER 13

Dyslipidemia: General Approach

INTRODUCTION

Fasting versus nonfasting testing issues: The present trend is to advise a nonfasting lipid panel. There is not much difference in level in two states. Nonfasting triglyceride (TG) is usually equal to fasting TG + 26 mg/dL, whereas total cholesterol, low-density lipoprotein cholesterol (LDL-C), and non-high-density lipoprotein cholesterol (non-HDL-C) are 8 mg/dL less than the fasting level; HDL-C, lipoprotein (Lp)(a), and apolipoprotein-B (ApoB) levels are same in two states. In fasting state, plasma contains atherogenic lipoproteins of hepatic origin, whereas in nonfasting state, serum contains in addition, intestinal origin. Hence, a nonfasting lipid panel may better capture atherogenic lipoproteins.

Non-HDL and ApoB issues: When TG level is high, TG replaces some part of cholesterol in LDL particles. TG induces more production of atherogenic small dense LDL particles. Thus, LDL-C becomes an unreliable estimation of cholesterol in LDL particle number. On the other hand, remnants of chylomicrons, very-low-density lipoprotein cholesterol (VLDL-C) and Lp(a) also accumulate in arterial wall and promote aerogenesis. All these atherogenic factors are reflected by non-HDL-C and ApoB but not by LDL-C alone.

Lp(a) issue: ApoB is covalently bound to plasminogen in Lp(a) which is a LDL-like particle. Lp(a) is not influenced by lifestyle factors, because it is controlled by gene locus on chromosome 6 and heritable in 90% of the cases. Its blood level remains same throughout life; hence, single estimation in lifetime is enough for its assessment. A high level of Lp(a) is associated with high risk of atherosclerotic heart disease and recurrent events.

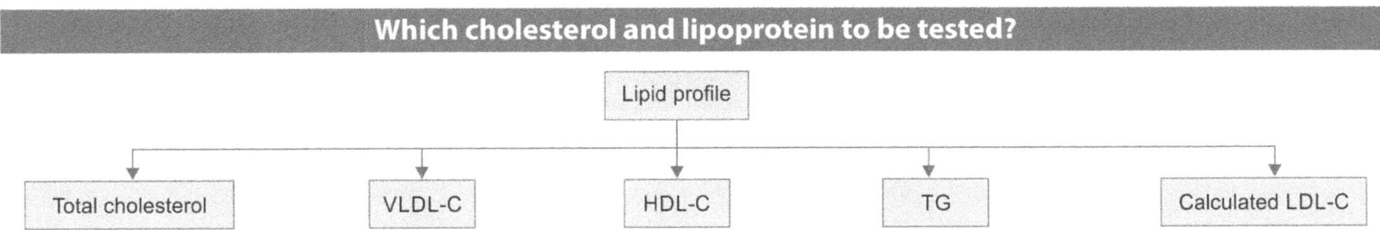

(HDL-C: high-density lipoprotein cholesterol; LDL-C: low-density lipoprotein cholesterol; VLDL-C: very-low-density lipoprotein cholesterol; TG: triglyceride)

How to calculate LDL-C?

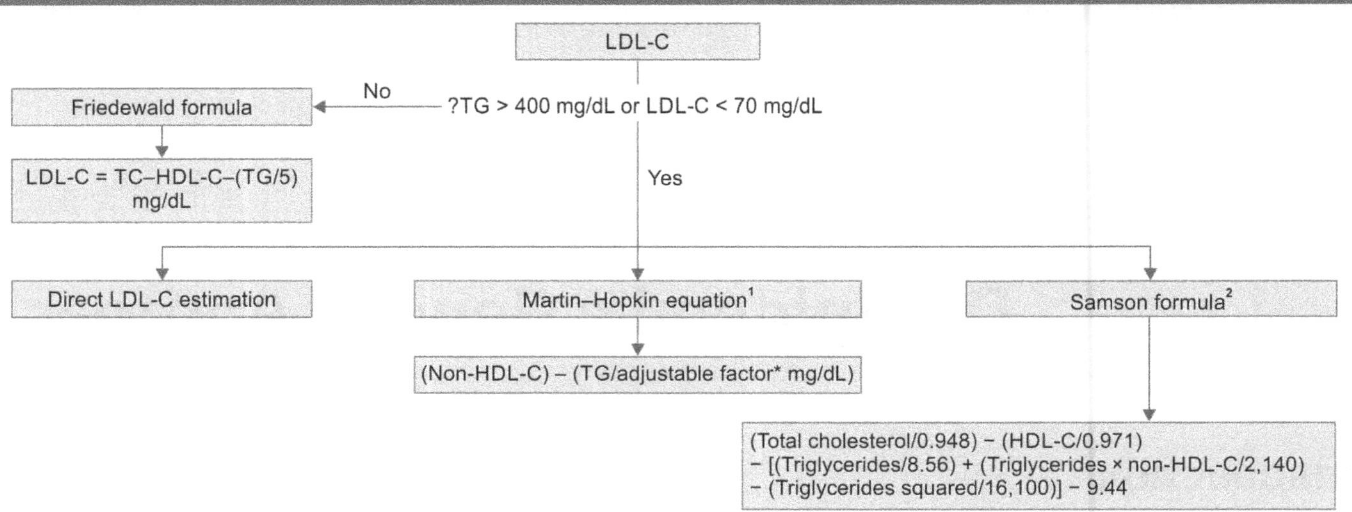

*Adjustable factor is determined as the strata-specific median TG:VLDL-C ratio
(HDL-C: high-density lipoprotein cholesterol; LDL-C: low-density lipoprotein cholesterol; TG: triglyceride; VLDL-C: very-low-density lipoprotein cholesterol)

Additional parameters to be tested in specific situations

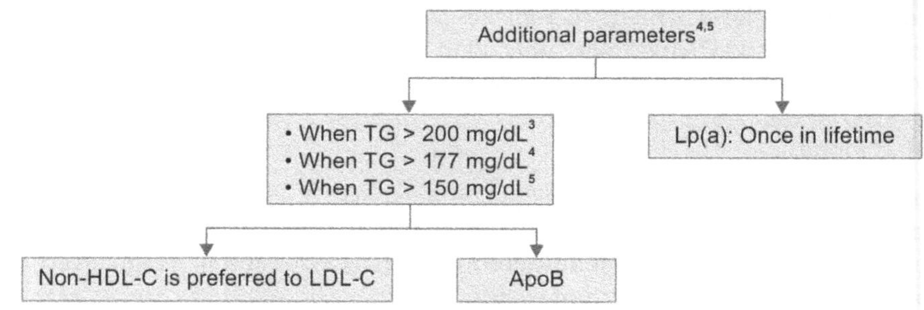

(HDL-C: high-density lipoprotein cholesterol; LDL-C: low-density lipoprotein cholesterol; TG: triglyceride)

Fasting versus nonfasting lipid profile estimation

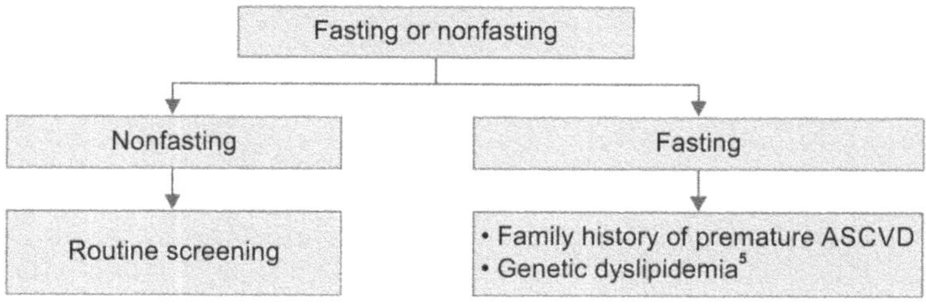

(AVCSD: atherosclerotic cardiovascular disease)

Primary prevention: Who to screen?[6]

Primary prevention

Any person ≥40 years of age

Any person associated with any of the following conditions irrespective of age

- Clinical evidence of ASCVD
- Abdominal aortic aneurysm
- DM
- Hypertension

- Smoker
- F/H of premature CVD
- F/H of dyslipidemia
- CKD

- Obesity
- Inflammatory disease
- HIV infection
- Erectile dysfunction

- COPD
- H/o pregnancy-induced hypertension
- Stigmata of dyslipidemia*

*Corneal arcus, xanthelasma, xanthoma
(ASCVD: atherosclerotic cardiovascular disease; CKD: chronic kidney disease; COPD: chronic obstructive pulmonary disease;
DM: diabetes mellitus; HIV: human immunodeficiency virus; H/o: History of; F/H: family history)

Different atherosclerotic cardiovascular risk calculators: Framingham Risk Score

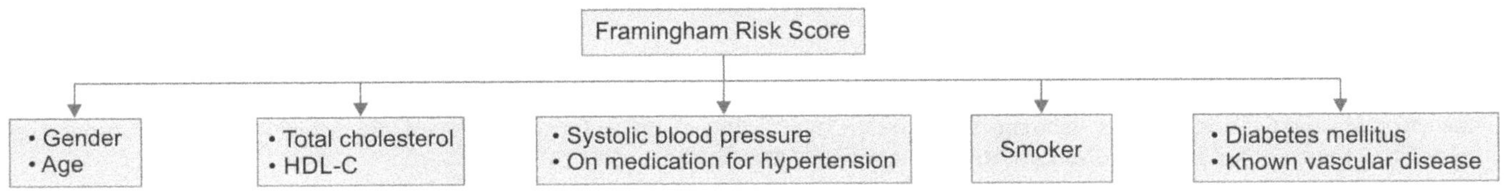

Framingham Risk Score

- Gender
- Age

- Total cholesterol
- HDL-C

- Systolic blood pressure
- On medication for hypertension

Smoker

- Diabetes mellitus
- Known vascular disease

Note: Low risk: <10%, intermediate risk: 10–19.9%, high risk: ≥20%
(HDL-C: high-density lipoprotein cholesterol)

Different atherosclerotic cardiovascular risk calculators: ASCVD risk score

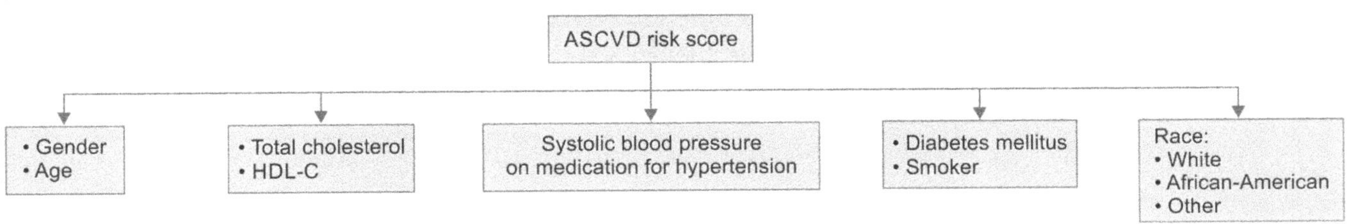

ASCVD risk score

- Gender
- Age

- Total cholesterol
- HDL-C

Systolic blood pressure on medication for hypertension

- Diabetes mellitus
- Smoker

Race:
- White
- African-American
- Other

Note: 10-year ASCVD risk: Low risk: <5%, borderline risk: 5–7.4%, intermediate risk: 7.5–19.9%, high risk: ≥20%
(ASCVD: atherosclerotic cardiovascular disease)

Different atherosclerotic cardiovascular risk calculators: Systematic Coronary Risk Evaluation (SCORE)[7]

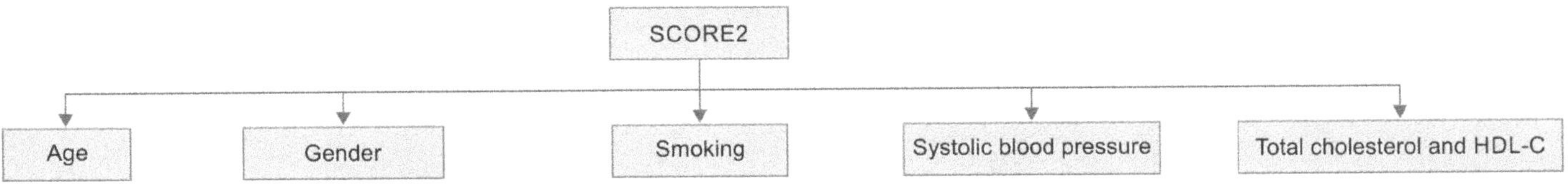

SCORE2

Age

Gender

Smoking

Systolic blood pressure

Total cholesterol and HDL-C

Note: 10-year ASCVD risk: Low risk: <1%, moderate risk: ≥1–<5%, high risk: ≥5–<10%, very high risk: ≥10%
(SCORE2: Systematic Coronary Risk Evaluation 2)

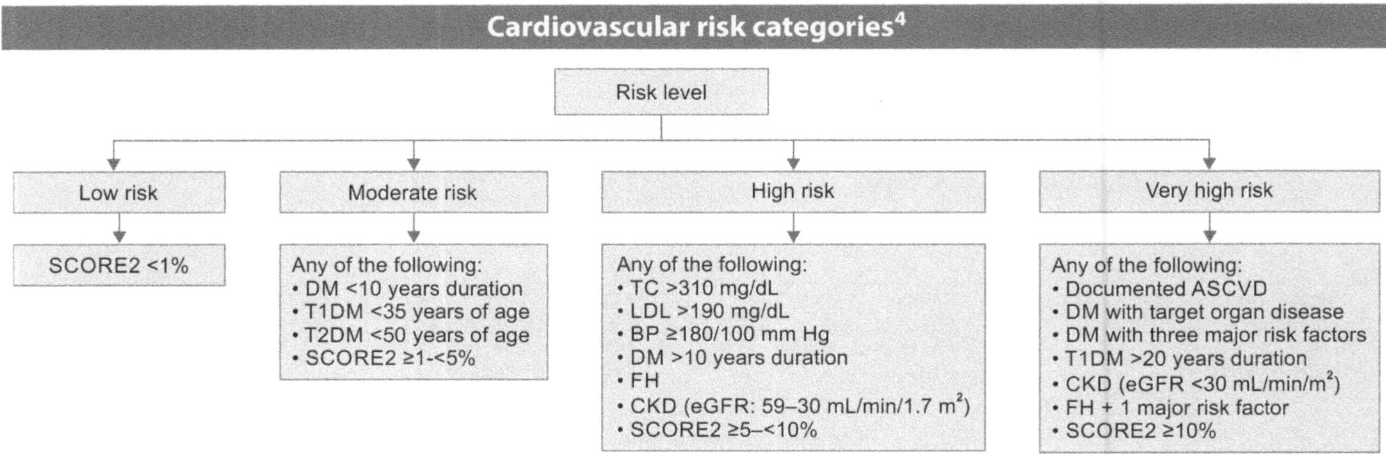

(ASCVD: atherosclerotic cardiovascular disease; CKD: chronic kidney disease; DM: diabetes mellitus; ESC: European Society of Cardiology; eGFR: estimated glomerular filtration rate; FH: familial hypercholesterolemia; LDL: low-density lipoprotein; SCORE2: Systematic Coronary Risk Evaluation 2; T1DM: type 1 diabetes mellitus; T2DM: type 2 diabetes mellitus; TC: total cholesterol)

REFERENCES

1. Martin SS, Blaha MJ, Elshazly MB, Michos ED, McEvoy JW, Blaha MJ, et al. Comparison of a novel method vs the Friedewald equation for estimating low-density lipoprotein cholesterol levels from the standard lipid profile. JAMA. 2013;310(19):2061-68.

2. Sampson M, Ling C, Sun Q, Harb R, Ashmaig M, Warnick R, et al. A new equation for calculation of low-density lipoprotein cholesterol in patients with normolipidemia and/or hypertriglyceridemia. JAMA Cardiol. 2020;5(5):540-8.

3. Grundy SM, Stone NJ, Bailey AL, Beam C, Birtcher KK, Blumenthal RS, et al. 2018AHA/ACC/AACVPR/AAPA/ABC/ACPM/ADA/AGS/APhA/ASPC/NLA/PCNA Guideline on the Management of Blood Cholesterol: A Report of the American College of Cardiology/American Heart Association Task Force on Clinical Practice Guidelines. J Am Coll Cardiol. 2018.

4. Mach F, Baigent C, Catapano AL, Koskinas KC, Casula M, Badimon L, et al. 2019 ESC/EAS Guidelines for the management of dyslipidaemias: lipid modification to reduce cardiovascular risk: The Task Force for the management of dyslipidaemias of the European Society of Cardiology (ESC) and European Atherosclerosis Society (EAS). Eur Heart J. 2019;41(1):111-88.

5. Newman CB, Blaha MJ, Boord JB, Cariou B, Chait A, Fein HG, et al. Lipid management in patients with endocrine disorders: An endocrine society clinical practice guideline. J Clin Endocrinol Metab. 2020;105(12):3613-82.

6. Pearson GJ, Thanassoulis G, Anderson TJ, Barry AR, Couture P, Dayan N, et al. 2021 Canadian Cardiovascular Society guidelines for the management of dyslipidemia for the prevention of cardiovascular disease in adults. Can J Cardiol. 2021;37:1129-50.

7. SCORE2 risk prediction algorithm: new models to estimate 10-year risk of cardiovascular disease in Europe Eur Heart J. 2021;42:2439-54.

CHAPTER 14

Dyslipidemia: Management

INTRODUCTION

The major target of lipid-lowering therapy is low-density lipoprotein (LDL) cholesterol. Once the target is achieved, then triglyceride is addressed. Dyslipidemia in homozygous familial hypercholesterolemia is the most difficult situation for lipid management. Statin is still the mainstay of therapy. However, over decades, several other molecules are now available in the lipid management armamentarium.

Prevention strategy in relation to LDL-C level: ESC risk scoring followed[1]

LDL-C level (mg/dL)

	<55	55 to <70	70 to <100	100 to <116	116 to <190	≥190
Low risk: <1%	Lifestyle	Lifestyle	Lifestyle	Lifestyle	Lifestyle ± drug	Lifestyle + drug
Moderate risk: ≥1 to <5%	Lifestyle	Lifestyle	Lifestyle	Lifestyle ± drug	Lifestyle ± drug	Lifestyle + drug
High risk: ≥5 to <10%	Lifestyle	Lifestyle	Lifestyle ± drug	Lifestyle + drug	Lifestyle + drug	Lifestyle + drug
Very high risk: ≥10%	Lifestyle	Lifestyle ± drug	Lifestyle + drug	Lifestyle + drug	Lifestyle + drug	Lifestyle + drug
Secondary prevention	Lifestyle + drug	Lifestyle + drug	Lifestyle + drug	Lifestyle + drug	Lifestyle + drug	Lifestyle + drug

(LDL-C: low-density lipoprotein cholesterol)

Low-to-moderate risk: Further critical assessment to decide drug treatment[1-3]

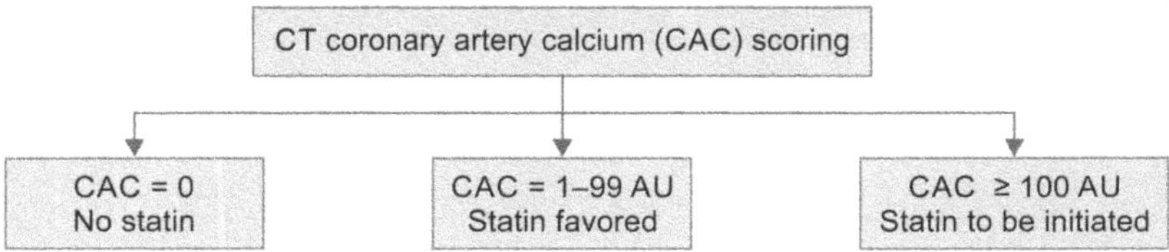

Treatment target of different lipoprotein and cholesterol[1]

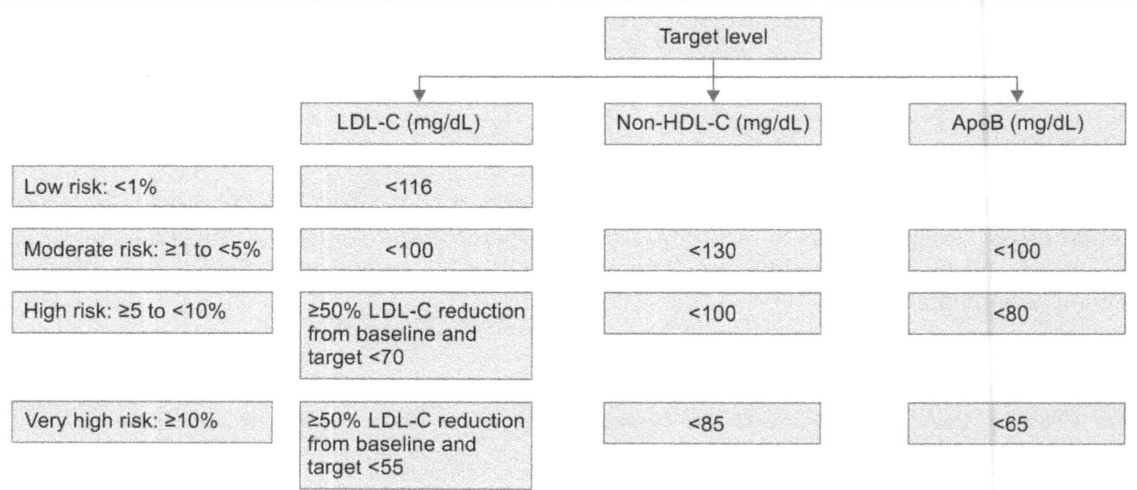

Molecules other than statin for management of dyslipidemia

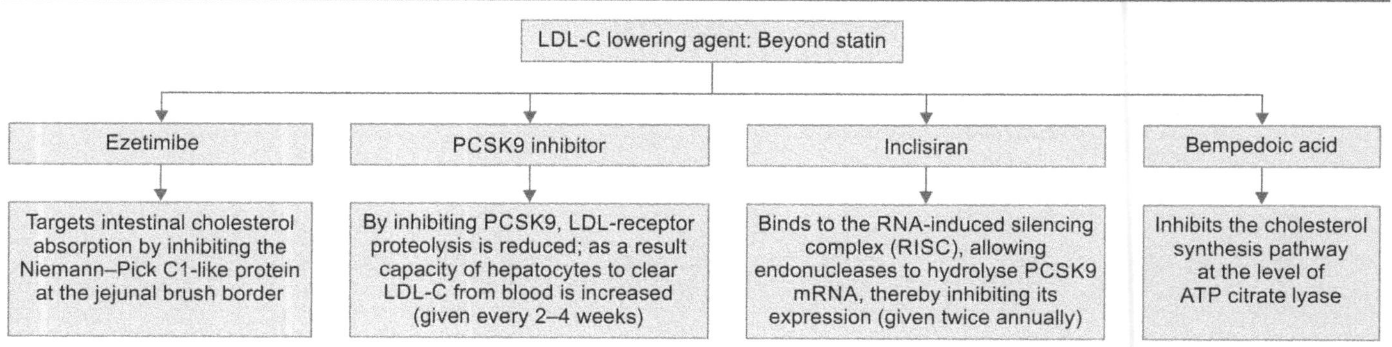

(ATP: adenosine triphosphate; LDL-C: low-density lipoprotein cholesterol; mRNA: messenger ribonucleic acid; PCSK9: proprotein convertase subtilisin/kexin type 9; RNA: ribonucleic acid)

Pharmacological management to achieve LDL-C target[1-3]

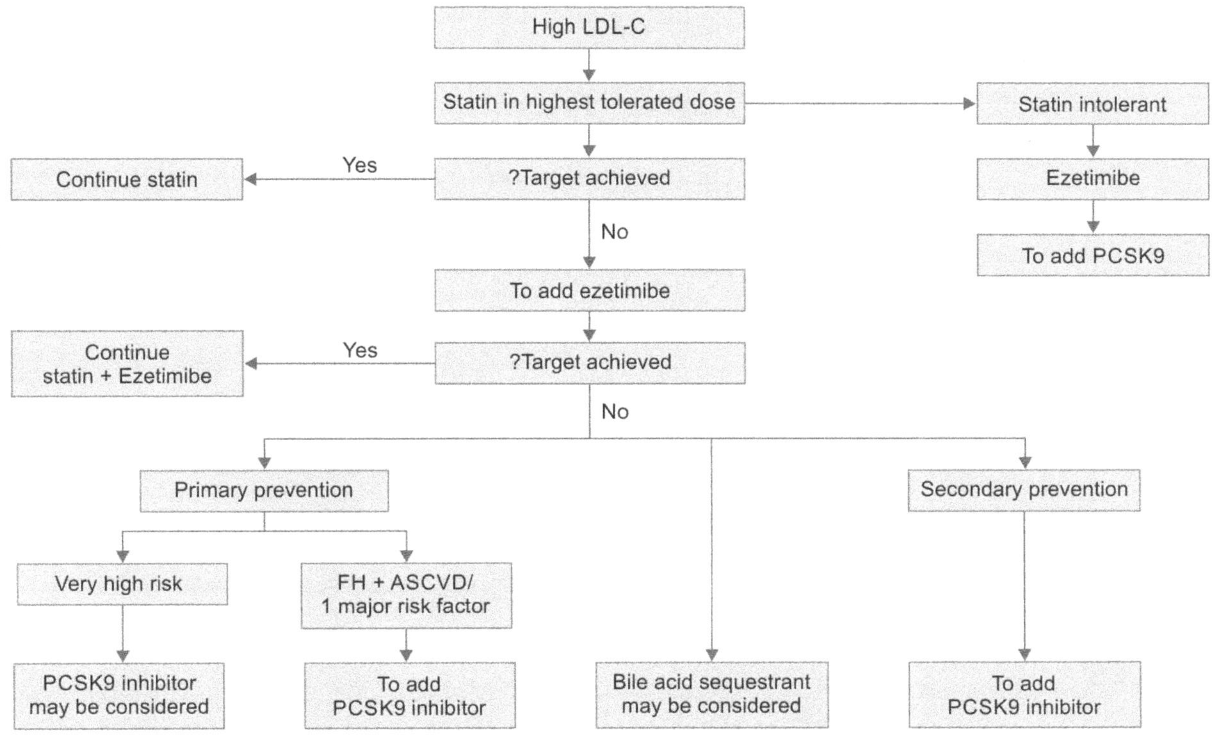

(ASCVD: atherosclerotic cardiovascular disease; FH: familial hypercholesterolemia; LDL-C: low-density lipoprotein cholesterol; PCSK9: proprotein convertase subtilisin/kexin type 9)

Pharmacological management of hypertriglyceridemia[1]

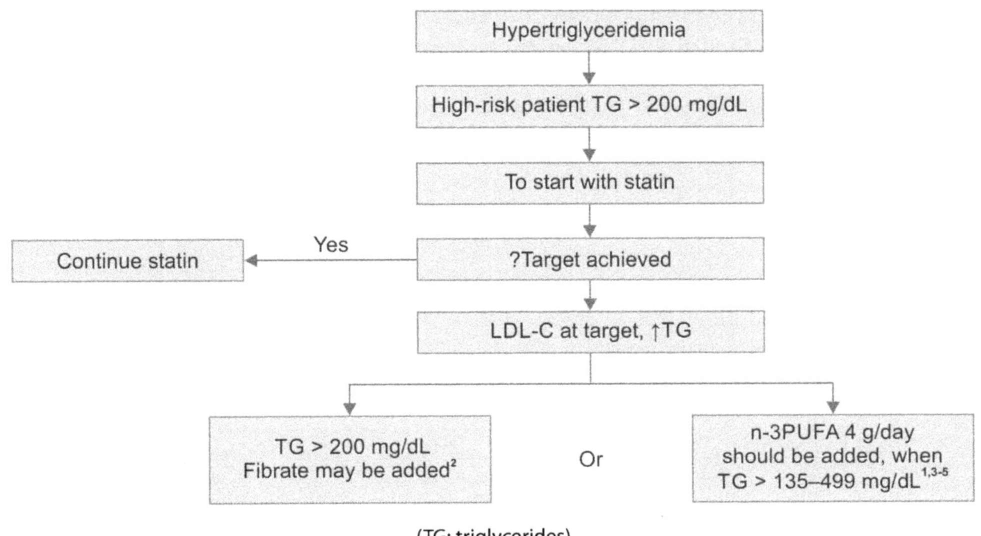

(TG: triglycerides)

Management of homozygous familial hypercholesterolemia (HoFH)

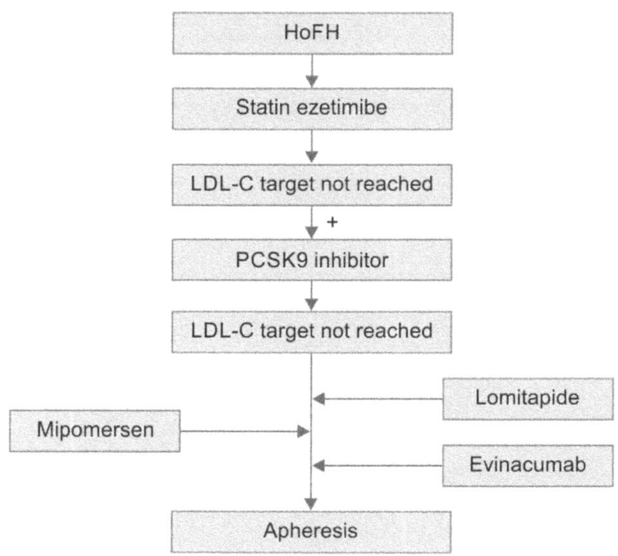

(LDL-C: low-density lipoprotein cholesterol; PCSK9: proprotein convertase subtilisin/kexin type 9)

REFERENCES

1. Mach F, Baigent C, Catapano AL, Kosikinas KC, Casula M, Badimon L, et al. 2019 ESC/EAS Guidelines for the management of dyslipidaemias: lipid modification to reduce cardiovascular risk: The task force for the management of dyslipidaemias of the European Society of Cardiology (ESC) and European Atherosclerosis Society (EAS). Eur Heart J. 2019;41(1):111-88.

2. Grundy SM, Stone NJ, Bailey AL, Beam C, Birtcher KK, Blumenthal RS, et al. 2018 AHA/ACC/AACVPR/AAPA/ABC/ACPM/ADA/AGS/APhA/ASPC/NLA/PCNA guideline on the management of blood cholesterol: A report of the American College of Cardiology/American Heart Association task force on clinical practice guidelines. J Am Coll Cardiol. 2018.

3. Newman CB, Blaha MJ, Boord JB, Cariou B, Chait A, Fein HG, et al. Lipid Management in Patients with Endocrine Disorders: An Endocrine Society Clinical Practice Guideline. J Clin Endocrinol Metab. 2020;105(12):3613-82.

4. Pearson GJ, Thanassoulis G, Anderson TJ, et al. 2021 Canadian Cardiovascular Society Guidelines for the Management of Dyslipidemia for the Prevention of Cardiovascular Disease in Adults. Can J Cardiol. 2021;37:1129.

5. Bhatt DL, Steg PG, Miller M, Brinton EA, Jacobson TA, Ketchum SB, et al; REDUCE-IT Investigators. Cardiovascular risk reduction with icosapent ethyl for hypertriglyceridemia. N Engl J Med. 2019;380:11-22.

Coronary Artery Disease

CHAPTER 15

Atherosclerotic Coronary Artery Disease: Definition

INTRODUCTION

Atherosclerotic coronary artery disease (CAD) is a disease process in which atheromatous plaque is deposited in the epicardial coronary artery. The plaque may be nonobstructive, obstructive, or occlusive. The disease process is chronic, progressive, and stable punctuated by an acute or unstable period due to plaque rupture or erosion. Depending on the mode of presentation, CAD is categorized into acute and chronic coronary syndrome.

In 1971, World Health Organization (WHO) defined acute myocardial infarction (MI) as typical ischemic pain, ECG changes in the form of development of new Q-wave and initial rise and subsequent fall of biomarkers of myocardial necrosis.[1] In the same year, Fowler introduced the term unstable angina (UA). Subsequently, another subset, non-Q-wave MI was described where the typical chest pain and rise and fall of biomarkers were associated without any new Q-wave in ECG. The term acute coronary syndrome (ACS) first appeared in 1986.[2] However, the term was formally described by Valentin Fuster in 1992 where he described ACS as MI, UA, or ischemic sudden death.[3] In the early part of this century, three groups were included in ACS, namely UA, ST-segment-elevation myocardial infarction (STEMI), and non-ST-segment-elevation myocardial infarction (NSTEMI). The term non-Q-wave MI was replaced by NSTEMI. This evolution set a new definition of MI. Latest is the fourth[4] universal definition of MI.

Along with the evolution of terminology, a significant evolution happened in the field of myocardial injury biomarker. Creatine phosphokinase (CPK) and creatine phosphokinase-myocardial band (CPK-MB) were gradually replaced by troponin followed by high-sensitivity troponin. Using high-sensitivity cardiac troponin (hs-cTn), which shows a raised level within the first hour of MI, there has been a 4% absolute and 24% relative rise in the detection of type I MI. As cTn can detect even minor myocyte necrosis in the spectrum of ACS, UA is getting marginalized and NSTEMI is becoming the most common entity.

The normal range of these biomarkers and the cutoff value show wide variation according to different assays, age, sex, physical activity, and many other factors. 99th percentile upper reference limit (URL) for hs-cTnI is 40 ng/L according to The Beckman Coulter Access AccuTnI+3 assay.[5] Coefficiency of variation of the assay is less than 10% at 40 ng/L; the limit of detection is 8 ng/L, and the limit of blank is 5 ng/L. Similarly, 99th percentile URL for hs-cTnT is 14 ng/L.[6] cTn is elevated in cardiac condition other than MI. Thus, interpretation of these biomarkers should be done in pari passu to clinical features.

Classification of coronary syndrome

Coronary syndrome
- Acute coronary syndrome
  - STEMI
  - NSTEMI
  - Unstable angina
- Chronic coronary syndrome

(NSTEMI: non-ST-segment-elevation myocardial infarction; STEMI: ST-segment-elevation myocardial infarction)

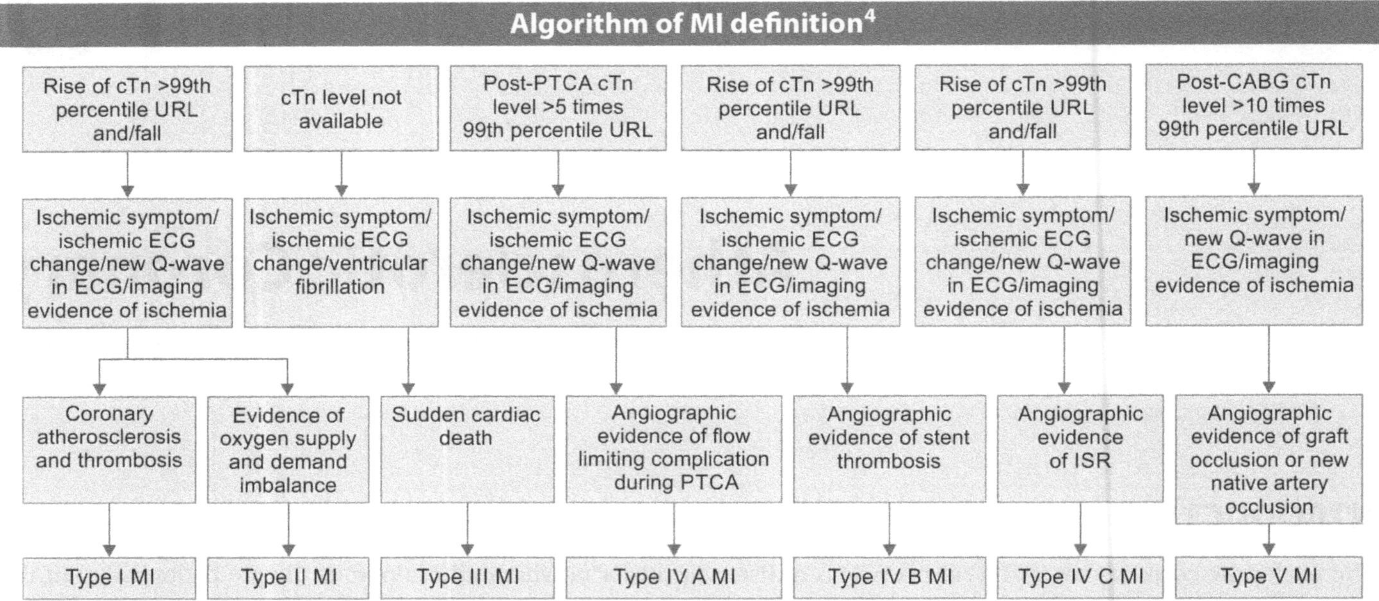

(CABG: coronary artery bypass graft; cTn: cardiac troponin; ECG: electrocardiogram; ISR: in-stent restenosis; MI: myocardial infarction; PTCA: percutaneous transluminal coronary angioplasty; URL: upper rate limit)

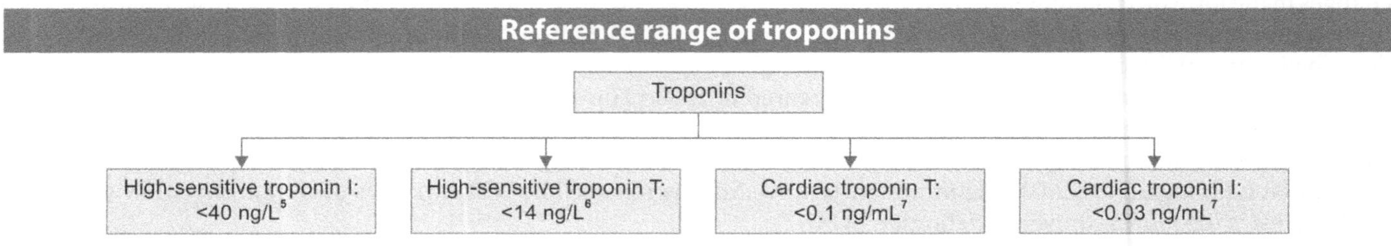

REFERENCES

1. World Health Organization. Working Group on the Establishment of Ischemic Heart Disease Registers. Report of the Fifth Working Group, Copenhagen. In: Report No. Eur 8201 (5). Geneva: World Health Organization; 1971.
2. Angelini P, Leachman R, Heibig J. Flow characteristics of coronary balloon catheters. Tex Heart Inst J. 1986;13:213-5.
3. Fuster V, Badimon L, Badimon JJ, Chesebro JH. The pathogenesis of coronary artery disease and the acute coronary syndromes (2). N Engl J Med. 1992;326:242-50.
4. Thygesen K, Alpert JS, Jaffe AS, Chaitman BR, Bax JJ, Morrow DA, White HD; ESC Scientific Document Group. Fourth universal definition of myocardial infarction (2018). Eur Heart J. 2019;40:237-69.
5. Mariathas M, Allan R, Ramamoorthy A, Olechowski B, Hinton J, Azor M, et al. True 99th centile of high sensitivity cardiac troponin for hospital patients: prospective, observational cohort study. BMJ. 2019;364:1729.
6. Eggers KM, Jernberg T, Lindahl B. Unstable Angina in the Era of Cardiac Troponin Assays with Improved Sensitivity: A Clinical Dilemma. Am J Med. 2017;130(12):1423-30.
7. Pagana KD, Pagana TJ, Pagana TN. Mosby's Diagnostic and Laboratory Test Reference, 14th edition. St. Louis: Elsevier; 2019.

Non-ST-segment Elevation Myocardial Infarction: Approach

INTRODUCTION

Non-ST-segment elevation myocardial infarction (NSTEMI) is a clinical syndrome defined by characteristic symptoms of myocardial ischemia without being associated with any persistent electrocardiographic (ECG) ST elevation and subsequent release of biomarkers of myocardial necrosis. ECG changes may include transient ST-segment elevation, transient, or persistent ST-segment depression, and T-wave changes (flattening, inversion, or pseudonormalization). Presenting ECG may be even normal in 30% of cases.

As mentioned earlier, the incidence of NSTEMI in the spectrum of acute coronary syndrome (ACS) has been increased rapidly over decades, from one-third in 1995 to more than half in 2015.[1] The approach to NSTEMI has also changed drastically. Early angiography and percutaneous coronary intervention (PCI) have increased from 9% and 12.5% in 1995 to 60% and 67% in 2015, respectively.[1]

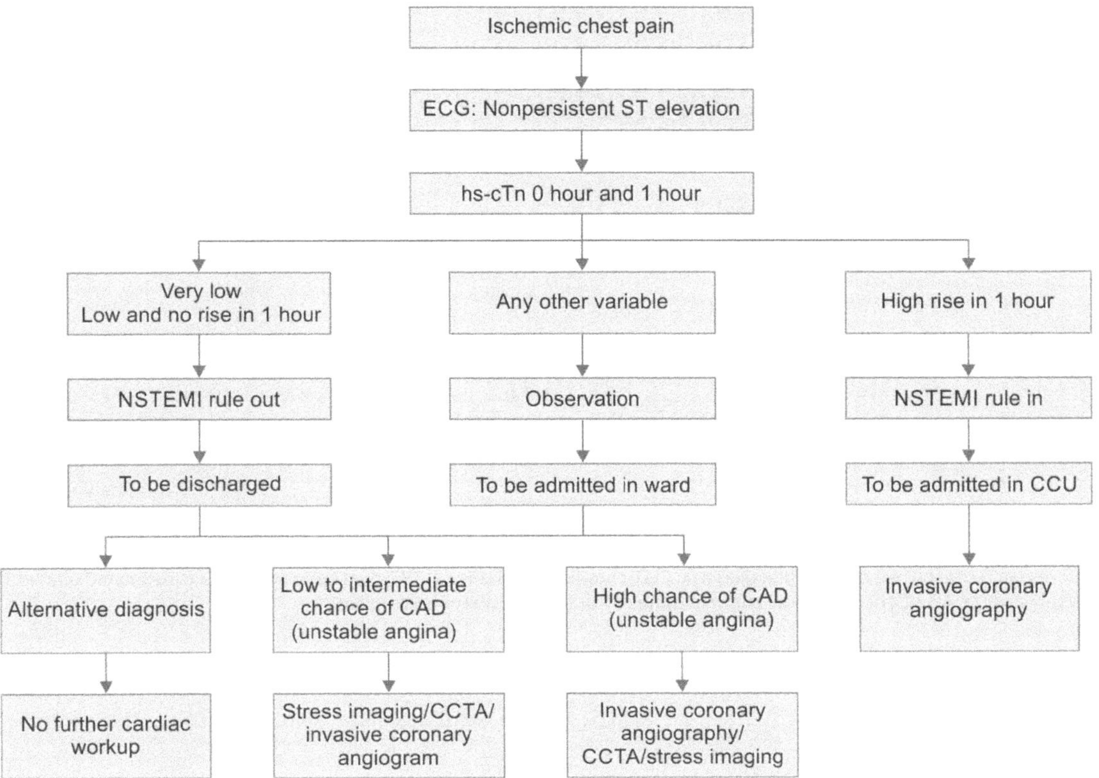

(hs-cTn: high-sensitivity cardiac troponin; 0h: cTn tested on arrival; 1h: cTn tested at 1 hour; CAD: coronary artery disease; CCU: coronary care unit; CCTA: coronary computed tomography angiography; NSTEMI: Non-ST-segment elevation myocardial infarction)

NSTEMI risk stratification strategy

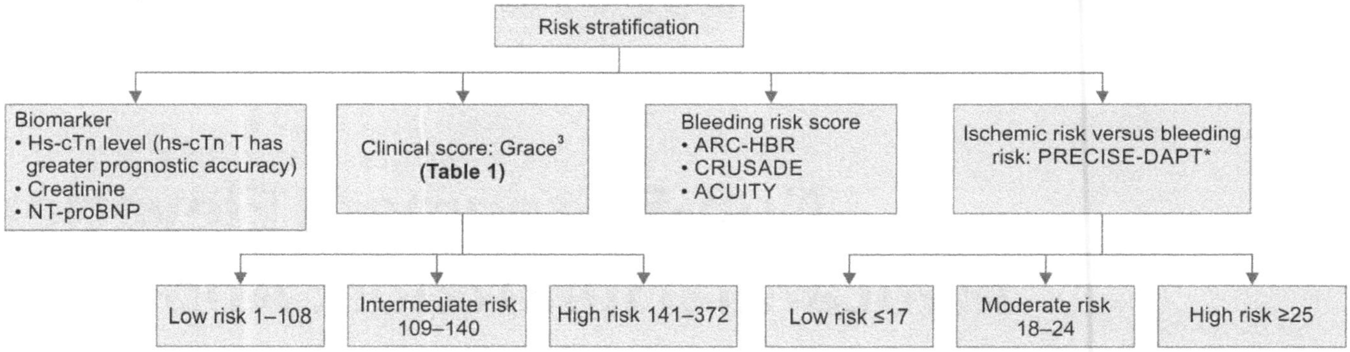

Risk stratification

Biomarker
- Hs-cTn level (hs-cTn T has greater prognostic accuracy)
- Creatinine
- NT-proBNP

Clinical score: Grace[3] **(Table 1)**

Bleeding risk score
- ARC-HBR
- CRUSADE
- ACUITY

Ischemic risk versus bleeding risk: PRECISE-DAPT*

Low risk 1–108 | Intermediate risk 109–140 | High risk 141–372

Low risk ≤17 | Moderate risk 18–24 | High risk ≥25

*PRECISE-DAPT **(Fig. 1)** determines the duration of dual antiplatelets (DAPT), balancing the ischemic and bleeding risk; in a patient with a score >25 prolonged DAPT is associate with no ischemic benefit but a large bleeding burden, whereas in a patient with a score <25 a prolonged DAPT duration is associated with marked ischemic benefit without any increase in bleeding burden.

TABLE 1: GRACE ischemic risk score.[3]

Age (years)	S	HR (bpm)	S	SBP (mm Hg)	S	Creatinine	S	Killip class	S
<39	0	<70	0	<80	40	<0.4	1	I	0
40–49	18	70–89	5	80–89	37	0.4–0.79	4	II	15
50–59	36	90–109	10	100–119	30	0.8–1.19	7	III	29
60–69	55	110–149	17	120–139	23	1.2–1.59	10	IV	44
70–79	73	150–199	26	140–159	17	1.6–1.99	13	Cardiac arrest	30
80–89	91	>200	34	160–199	7	2–3.99	21	Cardiac markers	13
>90	100			>200	0	>4	28	ST-segment deviation	17

(HR: heart rate; S: score; SBP: systolic blood pressure; GRACE: Global Registry of Acute Coronary Events)

Criteria* for high-bleeding risk during PCI as per academic research consortium

ARC-HBR[4]

Major
- On long-term OAC
- eGFR <30 mL/min
- Hb: <11 g/dL
- Spontaneous bleeding requiring admission/transfusion in past 6 months

- Chronic bleeding diastasis
- CLD
- Active malignancy
- H/o intracranial hemorrhage
- Platelet count <100 × 10⁹/L

- Moderate-to-severe ischemic stroke/6 months
- Recent major surgery/trauma by 30 days
- Nondeferable major surgery on DAPT

Minor
- Age ≥75 years eGFR 30–59 mL/min
- Hb: 11–12.9 (man); 11–11.9 (woman)
- Spontaneous bleeding requiring admission/transfusion in past 12 months On NSAID/steroid

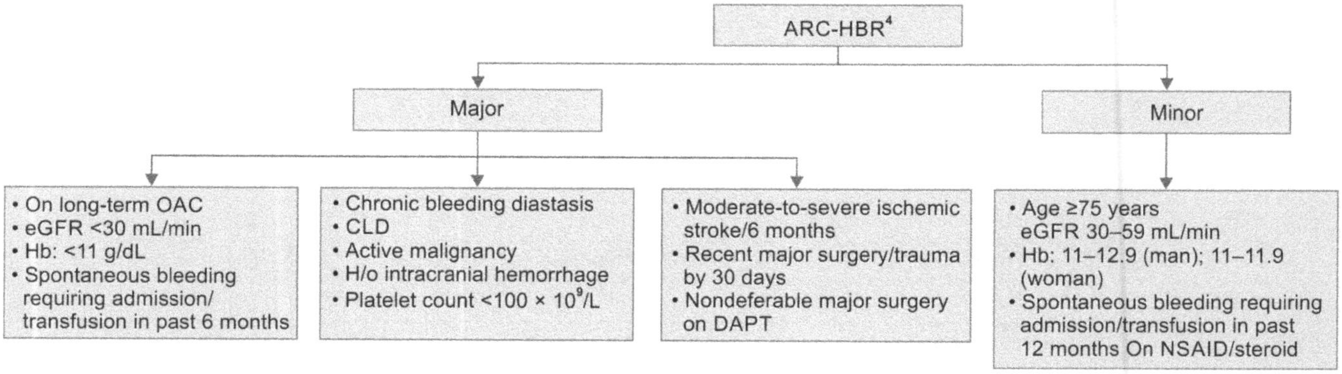

*High-bleeding risk: If at least one major or two minor criteria are met at the time of percutaneous coronary intervention.

(ARC-HBR: academic research consortium for high bleeding risk; CLD: chronic liver disease; DAPT: dual antiplatelet; eGFR: estimated glomerular filtration rate; Hb: hemoglobin; H/o: history of; NSAID: non-steroidal anti-inflammatory drug; OAC: oral anticoagulant)

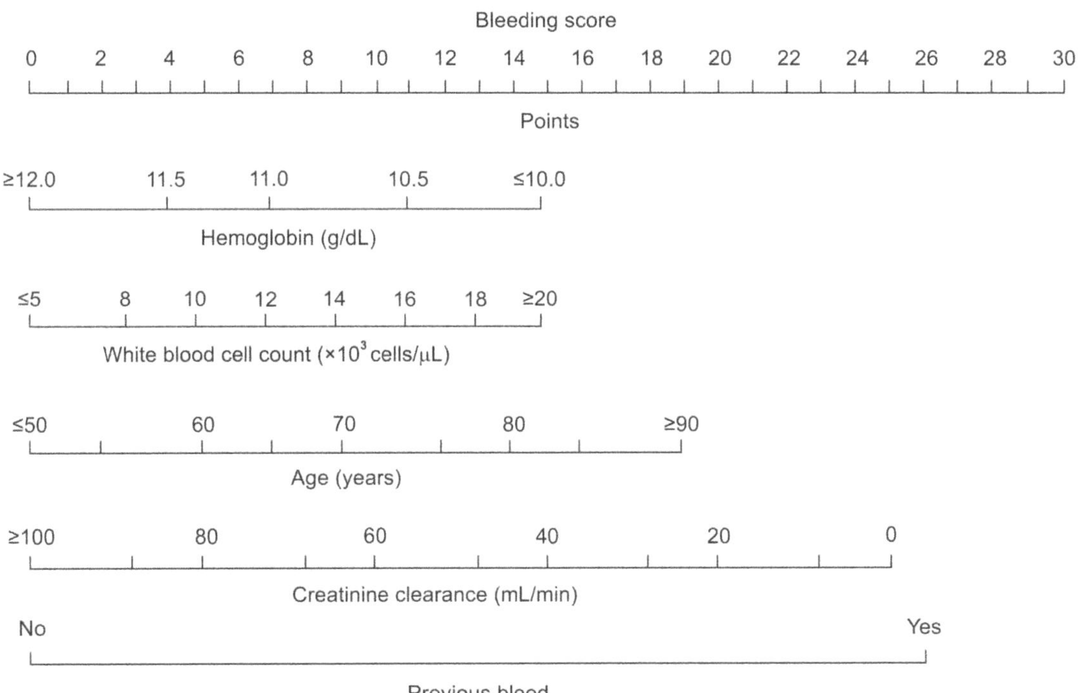

FIG. 1: PRECISE-DAPT integrated ischemic/bleeding risk score and nomogram.[5]

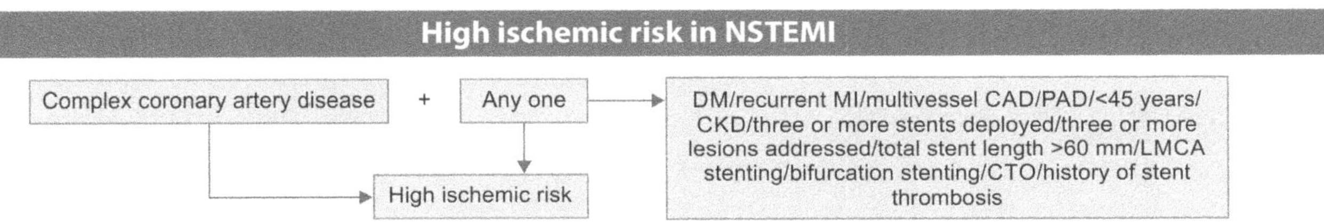

(CAD: coronary artery disease; CKD: chronic kidney disease; CTO: chronic total occlusion; DM: diabetes mellitus; LMCA: left main coronary artery; MI: myocardial infarction; PAD: peripheral artery disease)

REFERENCES

1. Puymirat E, Simon T, Cayla G, Cottin Y, Elbaz M, Coste P et al., USIK, USIC 2000, and FAST-MI investigators. Acute myocardial infarction: changes in patient characteristics, management, and 6-month outcomes over a period of 20 years in the FAST-MI program (French Registry of Acute ST-Elevation or Non-ST-Elevation Myocardial Infarction) 1995 to 2015. Circulation. 2017;136:1908-19.
2. Collet JP, Thiele H, Barbato E, Barthélémy O, Bauersachs J, Bhatt DL, et al. ESC Scientific Document Group. 2020 ESC Guidelines for the management of acute coronary syndromes in patients presenting without persistent ST-segment elevation Eur Heart J. 2021;42:1289-1367.
3. D'Ascenzo F, Biondi-Zoccai G, Moretti C, Bollati M, Omede P, Sciuto F, et al. TIMI, GRACE and alternative risk scores in acute coronary syndromes: a meta-analysis of 40 derivation studies on 216,552 patients and of 42 validation studies on 31,625 patients. Contemp Clin Trials. 2012;33(3):507-14.
4. Urban P, Mehran R, Colleran R, Angiolillo DJ, Byrne RA, Capodanno D, et al. Defining high bleeding risk in patients undergoing percutaneous coronary intervention: a consensus document from the Academic Research Consortium for High Bleeding Risk. Eur Heart J. 2019;40:2632-53.
5. Costa F, van Klaveren D, James S, Heg D, Raber L, Feres F, et al; PRECISE-DAPT Study Investigators. Derivation and validation of the predicting bleeding complications in patients undergoing stent implantation and subsequent dual antiplatelet therapy (PRECISE-DAPT) score: a pooled analysis of individual-patient datasets from clinical trials. Lancet. 2017;389:1025-34.

CHAPTER 17

Non-ST Elevated Myocardial Infarction: Medical Management

INTRODUCTION

There has been a major evolution in non-ST-elevated myocardial infarction (NSTEMI) management over the last 3 decades, in terms of diagnosis, medical management, and transcatheter intervention.[1] The most important change in medical management is the evolution of antithrombotic therapy. Transcatheter intervention plays a major role.Revision of anti-platelet and anticoagulant before surgical management is very important (**Box 1**).

Anti-ischemic medications in NSTEMI management

Anti-ischemic medications

Sublingual/IV nitrate: Recommended

Early initiation of beta-blocker: Recommended

(IV: intravenous)

Antiplatelet strategy in NSTEMI before taking patient to CathLab

Anti-platelet therapy (pretreatment)

Aspirin: At presentation loading dose followed by maintenance dose

P2Y12 inhibitor: When to load—When angiography is not delayed, P2Y12 inhibitor is loaded after knowing coronary anatomy

- Which P2Y12 inhibitor: Prasugrel or ticagrelor (in case of intolerance or contraindication, clopidogrel can be used)
- Between prasugrel/ticagrelor: Prasugrel may have an edge, when patients proceed to intervention

---

BOX 1: Anticoagulant strategy before CABG.

- On VKA, when CABG is urgent prothrombin complex concentrate of four inactivated factors and oral vitamin K are used to restore hemostasis
- On NOAC, when CABG is urgent prothrombin complex concentrate of activated factors or reversal agent can be used to restore hemostasis
- When CABG is planned, NOAC is held for 48 hours before surgery and resumed as soon as the bleeding is controlled. Single antiplatelet agent is added

Anticoagulant strategy in NSTEMI prior, in, and out of CathLab

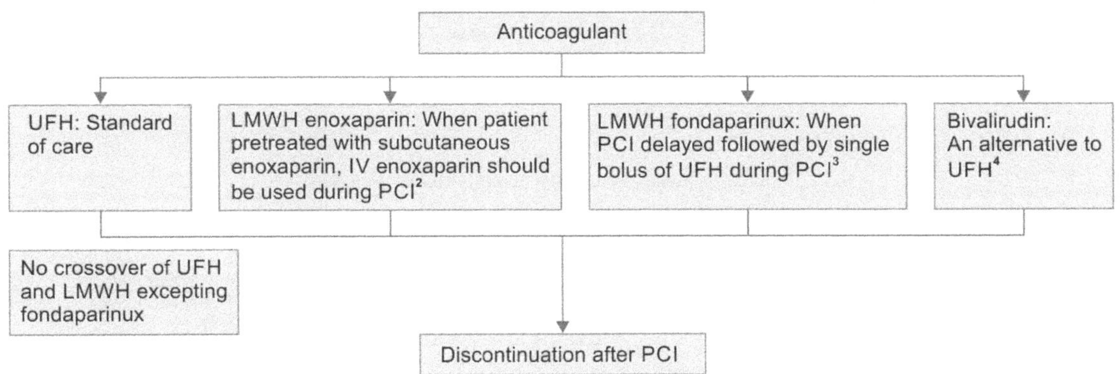

(IV: intravenous; LMWH: low-molecular weight heparin; PCI: percutaneous coronary intervention; UFH: unfractionated heparin)

Further antiplatelet strategy in NSTEMI in CathLab

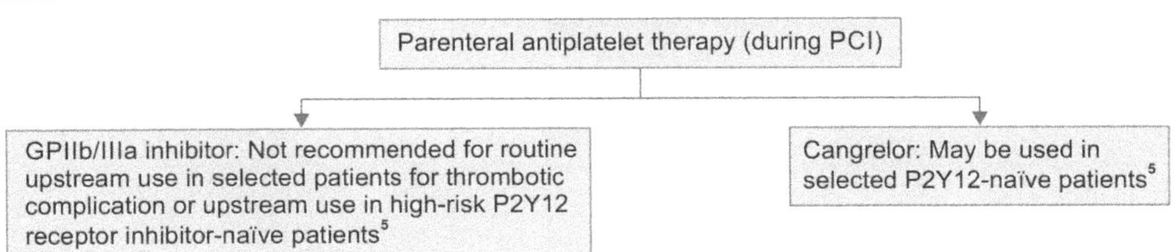

(GP: glycoprotein; PCI: percutaneous coronary intervention)

Post-PCI antiplatelet strategy

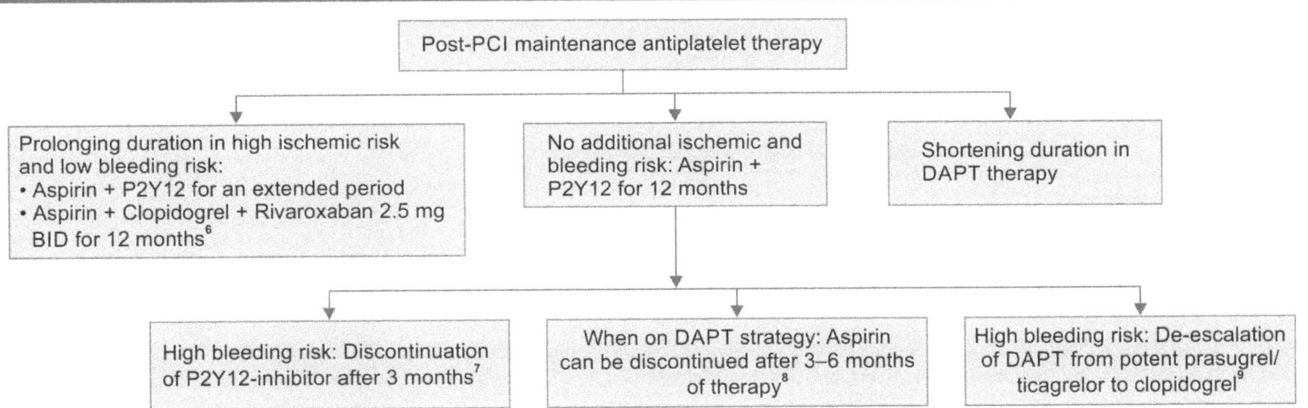

(DAPT: double antiplatelet therapy; PCI: percutaneous coronary intervention)

Antithrombotic strategy for AF patient on oral anticoagulant and posted for PCI for NSTEMI

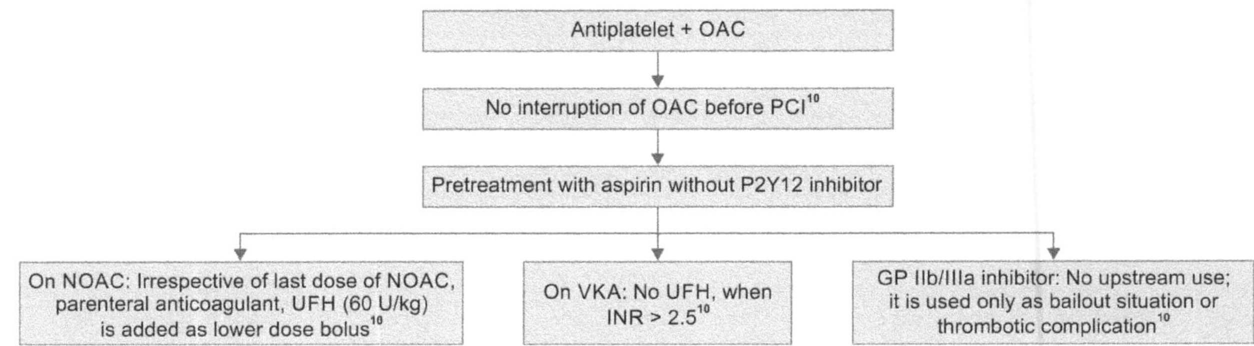

(AF: atrial fibrillation; INR: international normalized ratio; NOAC: novel oral anticoagulant; OAC: oral anticoagulant; NOAC: novel oral anticoagulant; UFH: unfractionated heparin; VKA: vitamin-K antagonist)

Antiplatelet strategy for AF patient on oral anticoagulant post-PCI[10]

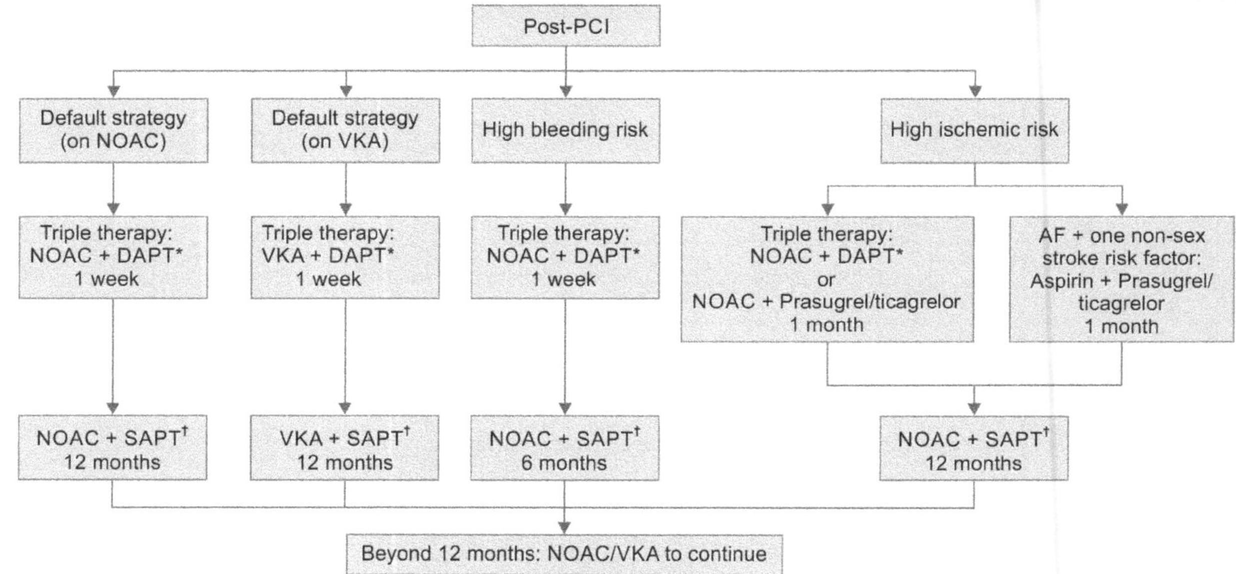

*Aspirin + preferably clopidogrel
[†]Preferably clopidogrel

(AF: atrial fibrillation; INR: international normalized ratio; NOAC: novel oral anticoagulant; OAC: oral anticoagulant; UFH: unfractionated heparin; VKA: vitamin-K antagonist)

Major bleeding management strategy in an anticoagulated patient

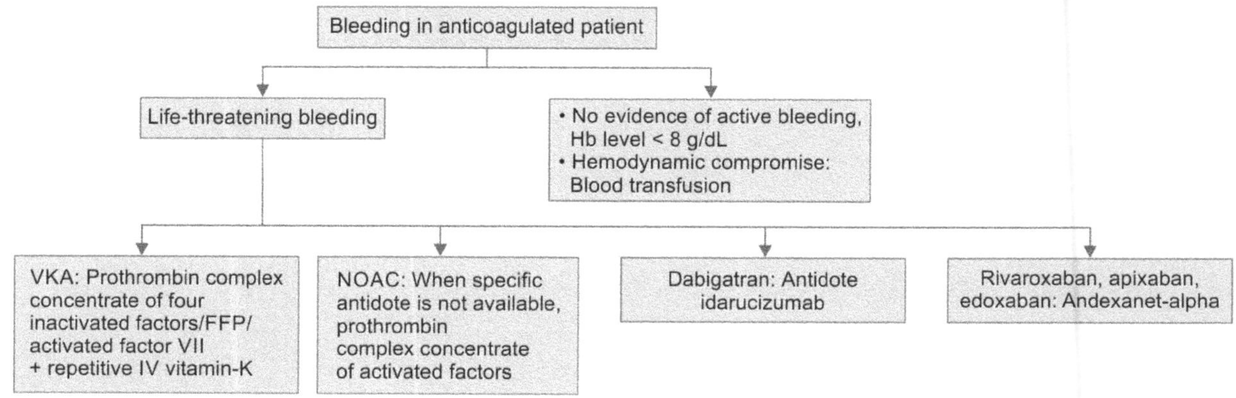

(FFP: fresh frozen plasma; IV: intravenous; NOAC: novel oral anticoagulant; VKA: vitamin-K antagonist)

REFERENCES

1. Puymirat E, Simon T, Cayla G, Cottin Y, Elbaz M, Coste P, et al; USIK, USIC 2000, and FAST-MI investigators. Acute myocardial infarction: changes in patient characteristics, management, and 6-month outcomes over a period of 20 years in the FAST-MI program (French Registry of Acute ST-Elevation or Non-ST-Elevation Myocardial Infarction) 1995 to 2015. Circulation. 2017;136:1908-19.
2. Silvain J, Beygui F, Barthelemy O, Pollack C Jr, Cohen M, Zeymer U, et al. Efficacy and safety of enoxaparin versus unfractionated heparin during percutaneous coronary intervention: systematic review and meta-analysis. BMJ. 2012;344:e553.
3. Steg PG, Jolly SS, Mehta SR, Afzal R, Xavier D, Rupprecht HJ, et al; FUTURA/OASIS-8 Trial Group. Low-dose vs standard-dose unfractionated heparin for percutaneous coronary intervention in acute coronary syndromes treated with fondaparinux: the FUTURA/OASIS-8 randomized trial. JAMA. 2010;304:1339-49.
4. Kastrati A, Neumann FJ, Schulz S, Massberg S, Byrne RA, Ferenc M, et al; ISAR-REACT 4 Trial Investigators. Abciximab and heparin versus bivalirudin for non-ST-elevation myocardial infarction. N Engl J Med. 2011;365:1980-9.
5. Neumann FJ, Sousa-Uva M, Ahlsson A, Alfonso F, Banning AP, Benedetto U, et al; ESC Scientific Document Group. 2018 ESC/EACTS Guidelines on myocardial revascularization. Eur Heart J. 2019;40:87-165.
6. Mega JL, Braunwald E, Wiviott SD, Bassand JP, Bhatt DL, Bode C, et al; Gibson CM, ATLAS ACS 2-TIMI 51 Investigators. Rivaroxaban in patients with a recent acute coronary syndrome. N Engl J Med. 2012;366:9-19.
7. Palmerini T, Della Riva D, Benedetto U, Bacchi Reggiani L, Feres F, Abizaid A, et al. Three, six, or twelve months of dual antiplatelet therapy after DES implantation in patients with or without acute coronary syndromes: an individual patient data pairwise and network meta-analysis of six randomized trialsand 11,473 patients. Eur Heart J. 2017;38:1034-43.
8. Mehran R, Baber U, Sharma SK, Cohen DJ, Angiolillo DJ, Briguori C, et al. Ticagrelor with or without aspirin in high-risk patients after PCI. N Engl J Med. 2019;381:2032-42.
9. Claassens DMF, Vos GJA, Bergmeijer TO, Hermanides RS, van't Hof AWJ, et al. A genotype-guided strategy for oral P2Y12 inhibitors in primary PCI. N Engl J Med. 2019;381:1621-31.
10. Collet JP, Thiele H, Barbato E, Barthélémy O, Bauersachs J, Bhatt DL, et al. ESC Scientific Document Group. 2020 ESC Guidelines for the management of acute coronary syndromes in patients presenting without persistent ST-segment elevation. Eur Heart J. 2021;42(14):1289-367.

CHAPTER 18

Non-ST Elevated Myocardial Infarction: Invasive Management

INTRODUCTION

There has been a major evolution in non-ST-elevated myocardial infarction (NSTEMI) management over the last three decades which is clearly reflected in the following data of French registry.[1] In patients with NSTEMI, percutaneous coronary intervention ≤72 hours from admission increased from 9 (1995) to 60% (2015). 6-month mortality consistently decreased in patients with NSTEMI from 17.2 to 6.9% in 2010 and 6.3% in 2015.

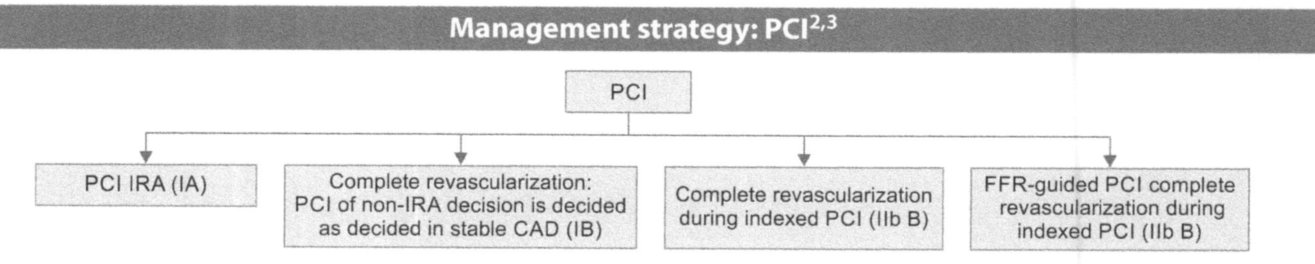

(aVR: augmented vector right; CCTA: coronary computed tomography angiography; NSTEMI: non-ST-elevated myocardial infarction)

(CAD: coronary artery disease; FFR: fractional flow reserve; IRA: infarct-related artery; PCI: percutaneous coronary intervention)

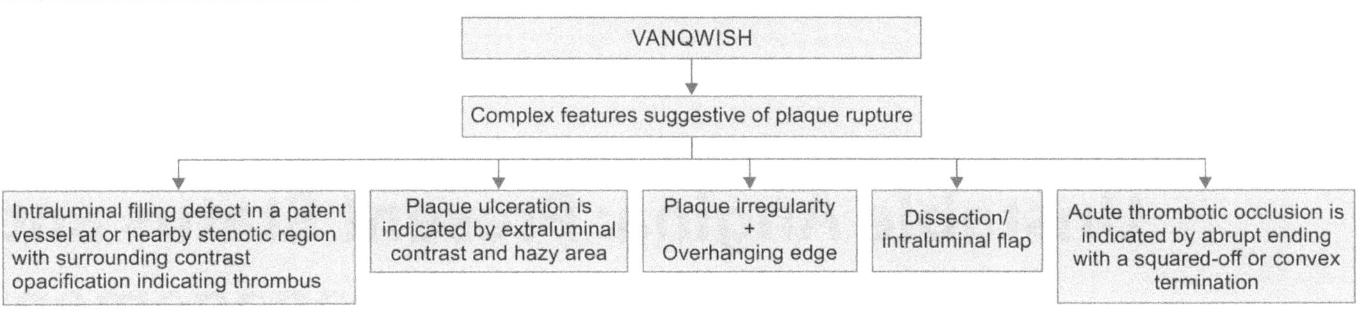

(VANQWISH: Veterans Affairs Non-Q-Wave Infarction Strategies in Hospital)

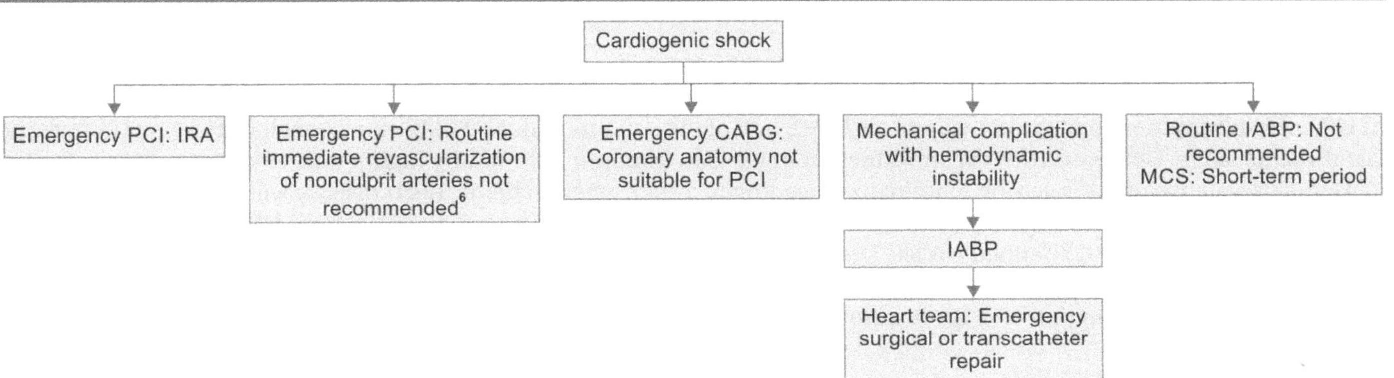

(CABG: coronary artery bypass graft; IABP: intra-aortic balloon pump; IRA: infarct-related artery; MCS: mechanical circulatory support; PCI: percutaneous coronary intervention)

REFERENCES

1. Puymirat E, Simon T, Cayla G, Cottin Y, Elbaz M, Coste P, et al; USIK, USIC 2000, and FAST-MI investigators. Acute myocardial infarction: changes in patient characteristics, management, and 6-month outcomes over a period of 20 years in the FAST-MI program (French Registry of Acute ST-Elevation or Non-ST-Elevation Myocardial Infarction) 1995 to 2015. Circulation. 2017;136:1908-19.
2. Collet JP, Thiele H, Barbato E, Barthélémy O, Bauersachs J, Bhatt DL, et al. ESC Scientific Document Group. 2020 ESC Guidelines for the management of acute coronary syndromes in patients presenting without persistent ST-segment elevation Eur Heart J. 2020;42(14):1289-367.
3. Lawton JS, Tamis-Holland JE, Bangalore S, Bates ER, Beckie TM, Bischoff JM, et al. 2021 ACC/AHA/SCAI Guideline for Coronary Artery Revascularization J Am Coll Cardiol. 2022;79:e21-e29.
4. Kerensky RA, Wade M, Deedwania P, Boden WE, Pepine CJ; Veterans Affairs Non-Q-Wave Infarction Stategies in-Hospital (VANQWISH) Trial Investigators. Revisiting the culprit lesion in non-Q-wave myocardial infarction. Results from the VANQWISH trial angiographic core laboratory. J Am Coll Cardiol. 2002;39(9):1456-3.
5. Neumann FJ, Sousa-Uva M, Ahlsson A, Alfonso F, Banning AP, Benedetto U, et al; ESC Scientific Document Group. 2018 ESC/EACTS Guidelines on myocardial revascularization. Eur Heart J. 2019;40:87-165.
6. Thiele H, Akin I, Sandri M, Fuernau G, de Waha S, Meyer-Saraei R, et al; CULPRIT-SHOCK Investigators. PCI strategies in patients with acute myocardial infarction and cardiogenic shock. N Engl J Med. 2017;377:2419-32.

Unstable Angina: Present Status and Management

INTRODUCTION

Eugene Braunwald said regarding unstable angina (UA)—"Is it time for a requiem?"[1] Before 1930, ischemic heart disease had two presentations: stable angina and acute myocardial infarction (AMI). The concept of UA was first introduced by Fowler[2] in 1971. After introduction of the concept of NSTEMI, half of the patients with NSTEMI were considered having UA over the last three decades. However, with the introduction of cardiac troponin followed by high-sensitivity cardiac troponin (hs-cTn), the prevalence of UA is getting marginalized leading to a state when ischemic heart disease will again have two sets of presentation, namely stable angina (chronic coronary syndrome) and AMI (including STEMI and NSTEMI). In 2008, World Health Organization (WHO) defined UA as "Unstable angina is diagnosed when there are new or worsening symptoms of ischemia (or changing symptom pattern) and ischemic ECG changes...with normal biomarkers. The distinction between new angina, worsening angina and UA is notoriously difficult and based on a clinical assessment and a careful and full clinical history."[3]

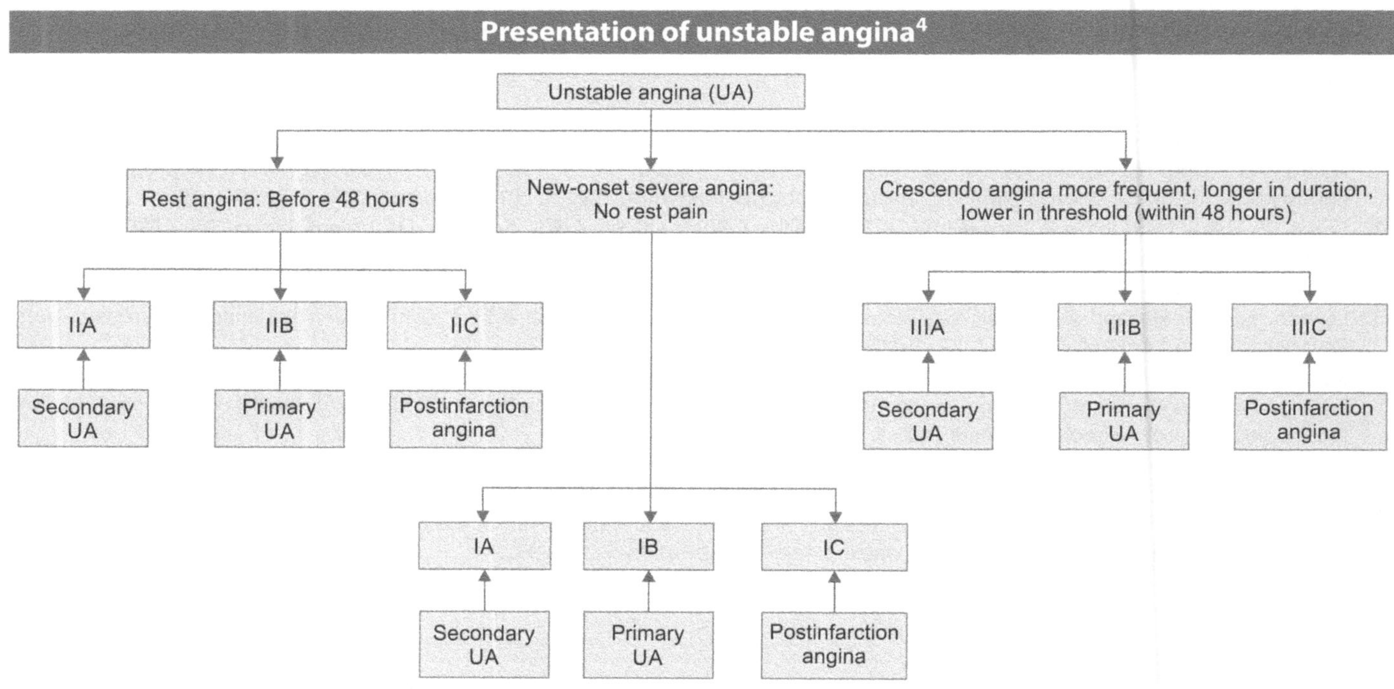

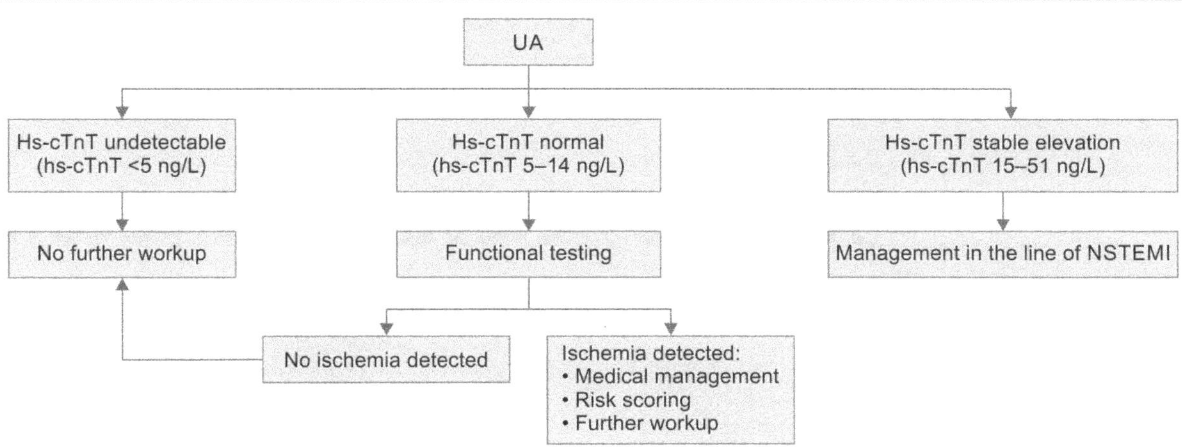

(hs-cTnT: high-sensitivity cardiac troponin T; NSTEMI: non-ST-elevated myocardial infarction; UA: unstable angina)

REFERENCES

1. Braunwald E, Morrow DA. Unstable angina Is it time for requiem? Circulation. 2013;127:2452-7.
2. Fowler NO. "Preinfarctional" angina: a need for an objective definition and for a controlled clinical trial of its management. Circulation. 1971;44:755-8.
3. Mendis S, Thygesen K, Kuulasmaa K, Giampaoli S, Mahonen M, Blackett KN, et al. World Health Organization definition of myocardial infarction: 2008–09 revision. Int J Epidemiol. 2011;40:139-46.
4. Braunwald E. Unstable angina. A classification. Circulation. 1989;80:410-4.
5. Collet JP, Thiele H, Barbato E, et al; ESC Scientific Document Group. 2020 ESC Guidelines for the management of acute coronary syndromes in patients presenting without persistent ST-segment elevation Eur Heart J. 2020;42(14):1289-367.

CHAPTER 20

Acute ST-elevation Myocardial Infarction: Reperfusion

INTRODUCTION

ST-elevation myocardial infarction (STEMI) is a type I myocardial infarction (MI) presenting with persistent (>20 minute) ST elevation in ECG. As defined in American Heart Association (AHA)/American College of Cardiology (ACC) guideline,[1] "STEMI is a clinical syndrome defined by characteristic symptoms of myocardial ischemia in association with persistent electrocardiographic (ECG) ST elevation and subsequent release of biomarkers of myocardial necrosis."

Persistent ECG ST-segment elevation **(Box 1)** is the hallmark of STEMI and dictates the decision of immediate thrombolysis. However, in certain situations ST-segment elevation may not be looking classical **(Box 2)**. The incidence of STEMI is gradually decreasing over decades, replaced by NSTEMI. In Europe, the incidence ranged from 43 to 144 per 100,000 per year, whereas in USA, the incidence came down from 1999 to 2008 as 133 to 50 per 100,000 per year.[2,3] The incidence is more common in younger and male population.

Reperfusion without unnecessary time loss is the most important issue in the management of STEMI **(Table 1)**. Time loss must be shortened at first physical contact, at non-PCI-capable center, and at PCI-capable center. Cardiac biomarkers should be sent at earliest. However, the test or any other routine imaging should not delay reperfusion strategy.[2,3]

BOX 1: ECG criteria of ST-elevation myocardial infarction (STEMI).[2]

ST elevation at J point: At least two contiguous leads in V_2–V_3

- ≥2.5 mm (0.2 mV) in men < 40 years
- 2 mm (0.2 mV) in men
- 1.5 mm (0.15 mV) in women

and/or

- ≥1 mm (0.1 mV) in other contiguous chest leads or limb leads

---

BOX 2: Atypical ECG change in ST-elevation myocardial infarction (STEMI).

- New-onset or presumably new-onset LBBB
- ST depression ≥ 0.5 mm in V_1–V_3 and ST-segment elevation in V_7–V_9 indicates true posterior wall MI due to LCX involvement
- ST depression ≥ 1 mm in eight or more surface leads and ST-segment elevation in aVR indicates left main or left main equivalent occlusion

(aVR: augmented vector right; LBBB: left bundle branch block; LCX: left circumflex coronary artery; MI: myocardial infarction)

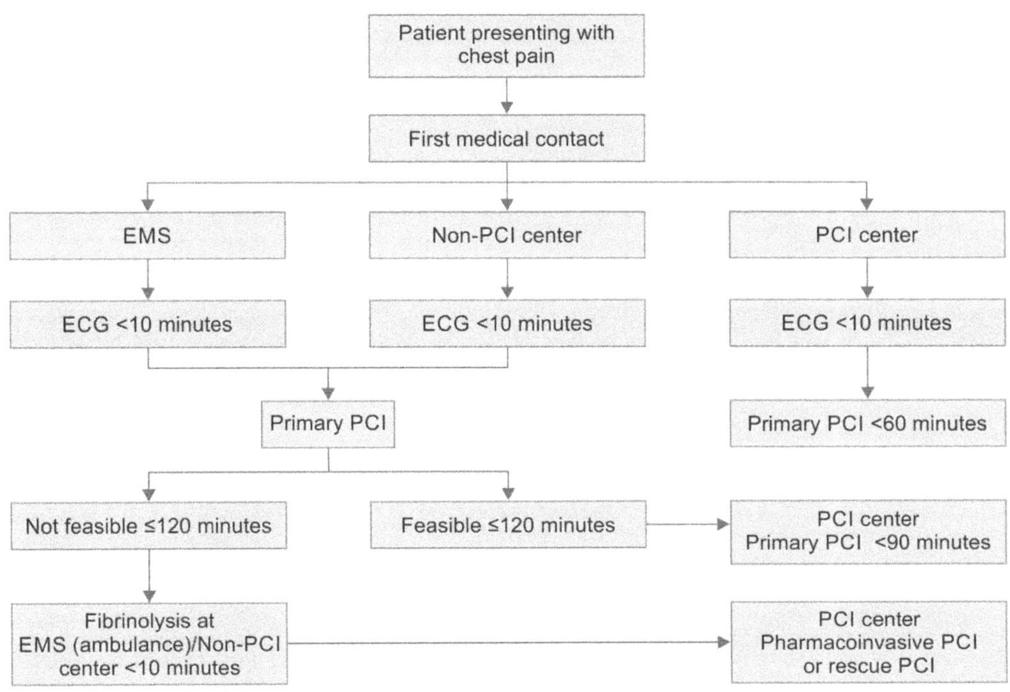

(EMS: emergency medical services; PCI: percutaneous coronary intervention)

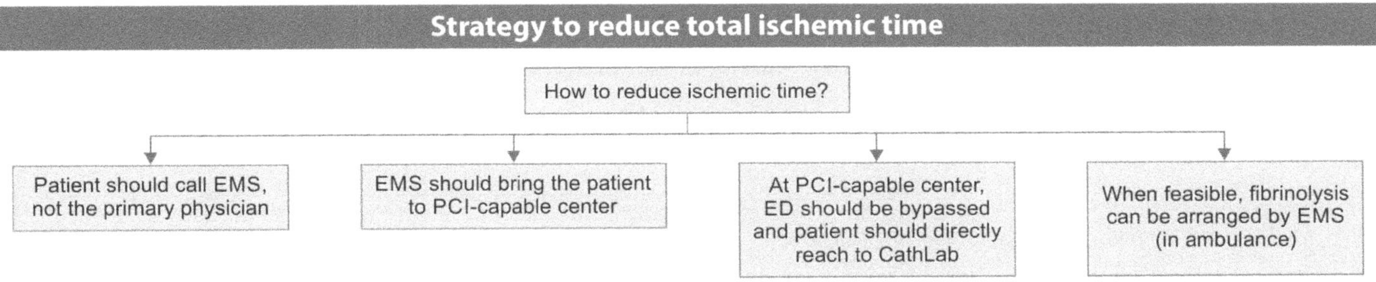

(ED: emergency department; EMS: emergency medical service; PCI: percutaneous coronary intervention)

TABLE 1: Reperfusion strategy.[2]

	Reperfusion	PPCI	Fibrinolysis	Others	Class
≤12 hour ischemic symptom, persistent ↑ST	+	+			IA
≤12 hour ischemic symptom, persistent ↑ST, timely PPCI not available	+		+		IA
>12 hour of onset of symptom: Ischemic symptom/hemodynamic instability/life-threatening arrhythmia	+	+			IC
Ongoing ischemic symptom suggestive of MI, absent ST elevation associated with cardiogenic shock/recurrent chest pain/gross arrhythmia or cardiac arrest/mechanical complication/heart failure/recurrent dynamic ST-T changes	+	+			IC
Presenting late (12–48 hours) after onset of symptoms	+	+			IIaB
Symptoms relieved, ↑ST resolved				Early angiography (within 24 hours)	IC

(MI: myocardial infarction; PPCI: primary percutaneous coronary intervention)

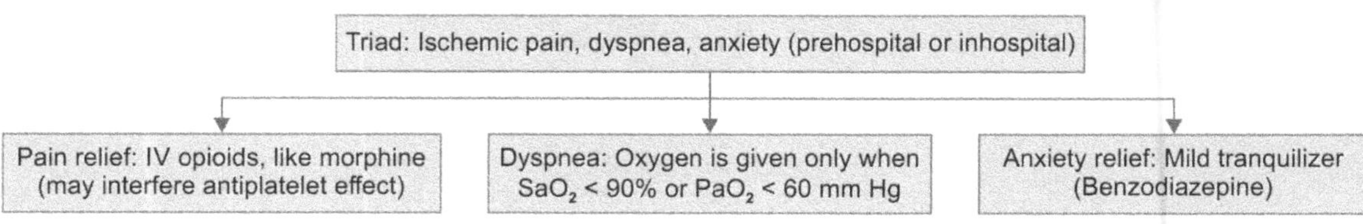
Management of presenting symptoms in STEMI
Triad: Ischemic pain, dyspnea, anxiety (prehospital or inhospital)
Pain relief: IV opioids, like morphine (may interfere antiplatelet effect)
Dyspnea: Oxygen is given only when SaO₂ < 90% or PaO₂ < 60 mm Hg
Anxiety relief: Mild tranquilizer (Benzodiazepine)
(IV: intravenous; PaO₂: pressure of oxygen; SaO₂: oxygen saturation)

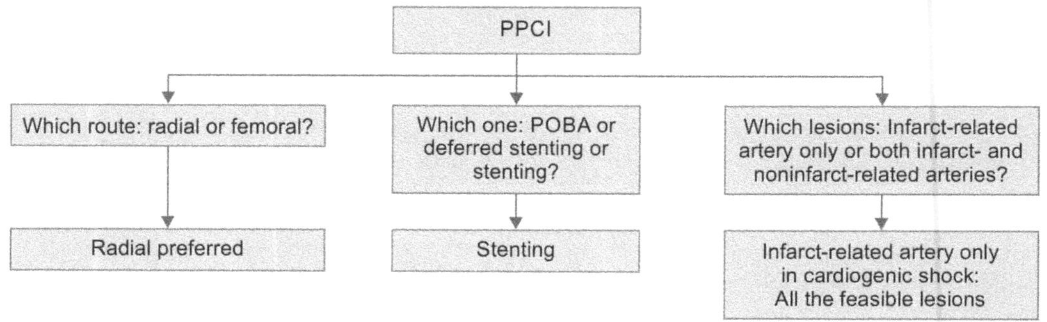
Primary percutaneous coronary intervention strategy[2,4]
PPCI
Which route: radial or femoral?
Which one: POBA or deferred stenting or stenting?
Which lesions: Infarct-related artery only or both infarct- and noninfarct-related arteries?
Radial preferred
Stenting
Infarct-related artery only in cardiogenic shock: All the feasible lesions
(POBA: plain old balloon angioplasty; PPCI: primary percutaneous coronary intervention)

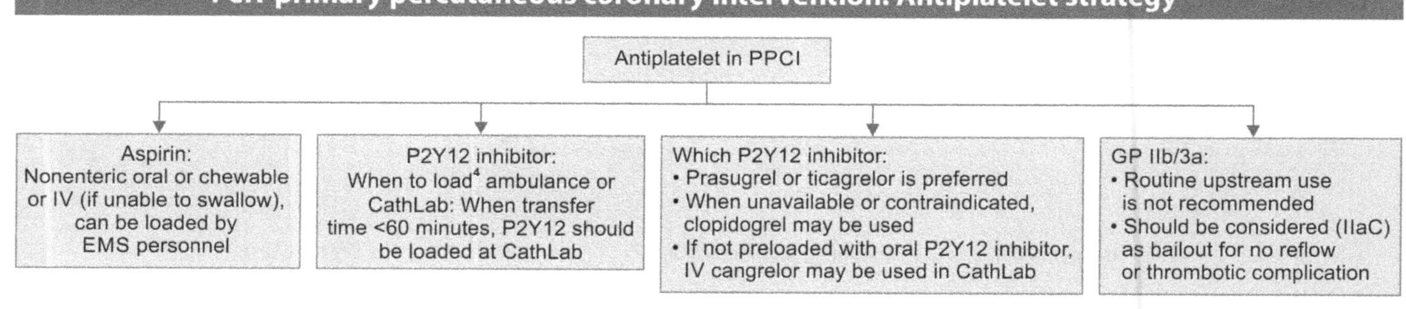
Peri-primary percutaneous coronary intervention: Antiplatelet strategy[2,4]
Antiplatelet in PPCI
Aspirin: Nonenteric oral or chewable or IV (if unable to swallow), can be loaded by EMS personnel
P2Y12 inhibitor: When to load ambulance or CathLab: When transfer time <60 minutes, P2Y12 should be loaded at CathLab
Which P2Y12 inhibitor:
• Prasugrel or ticagrelor is preferred
• When unavailable or contraindicated, clopidogrel may be used
• If not preloaded with oral P2Y12 inhibitor, IV cangrelor may be used in CathLab
GP IIb/3a:
• Routine upstream use is not recommended
• Should be considered (IIaC) as bailout for no reflow or thrombotic complication
(EMS: emergency medical service; GP: glycoprotein; IV: intravenous; PPCI: primary percutaneous coronary intervention)

Peri-primary percutaneous coronary intervention: Anticoagulant strategy[2,4]
Anticoagulant in PPCI
UFH:
• Preferred agent (IC)
• Benefit of ACT to tailor dose is not established
• Routine postprocedural UFH is not indicated
Enoxaparin (IIA): Can be routinely used (IIA)
Bivalirudin:
• Can be used in place of UFH in HIT
• Can be routinely used (IIA)
• Less bleeding, more chance of AST
Fondaparinux (IIIB): Not recommended
(ACT: activated clotting time; AST: acute stent thrombosis; HIT: heparin induced thrombocytopenia; UFH: unfractionated heparin)

Fibrinolysis strategy in STEMI

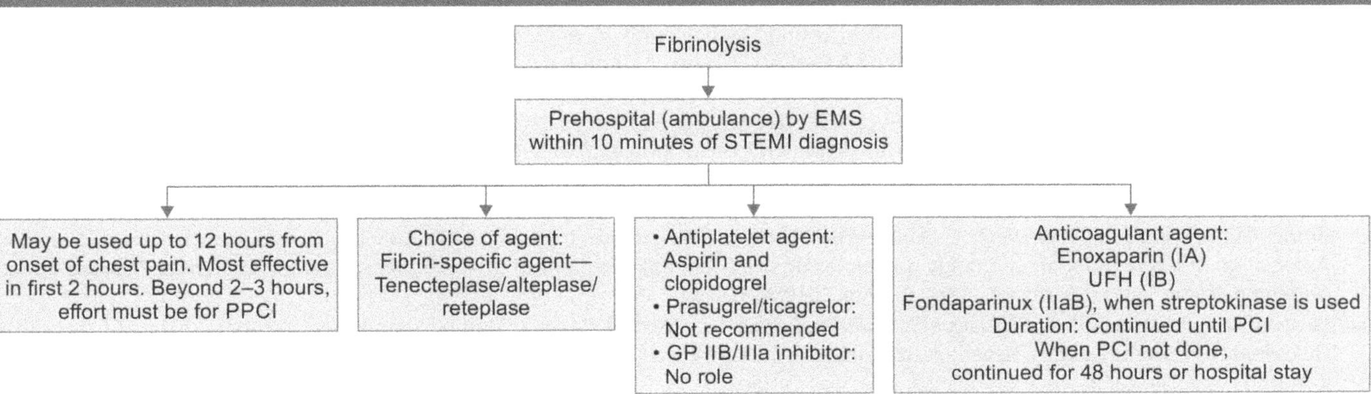

(EMS: emergency medical service; GP: glycoprotein; PCI: percutaneous coronary intervention; PPCI: primary percutaneous coronary intervention; UFH: unfractionated heparin)

Contraindication to fibrinolysis in STEMI[2]

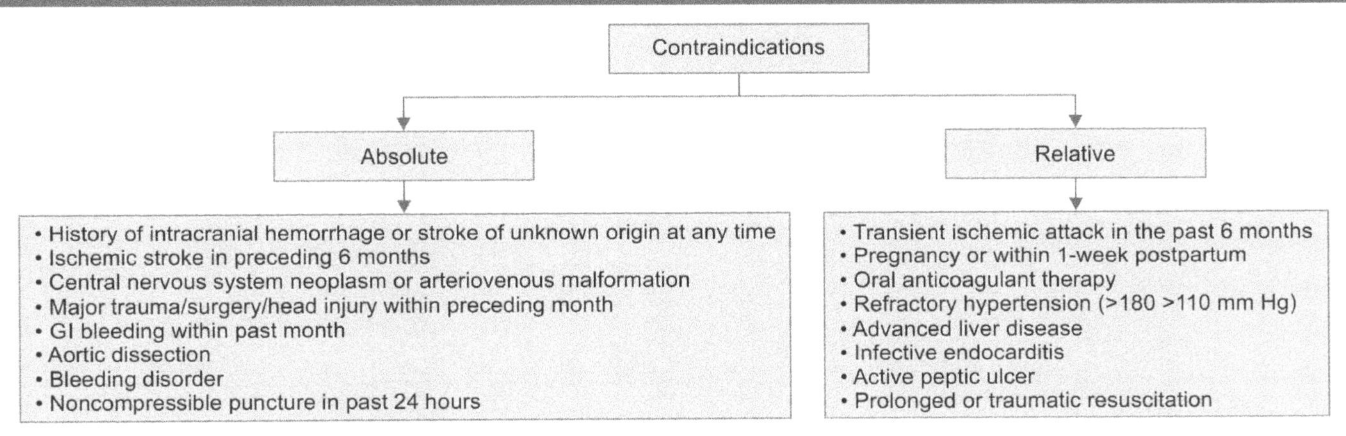

(GI: gastrointestinal)

Strategy for pharmacoinvasive intervention[2,4]

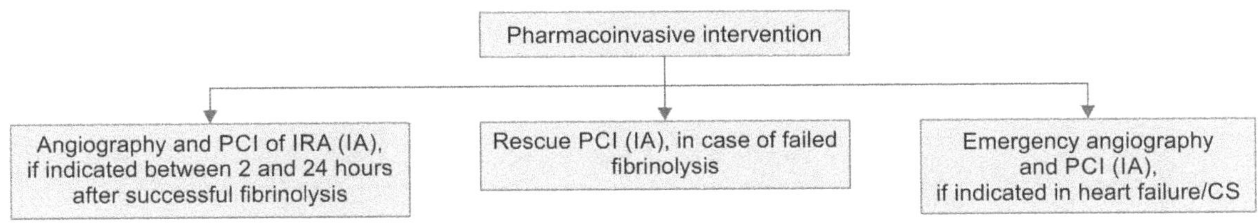

(CS: cardiogenic shock; IRA: infarct-related artery; PCI: percutaneous coronary intervention)

Strategy for management for STEMI with multivessel coronary artery disease[5]

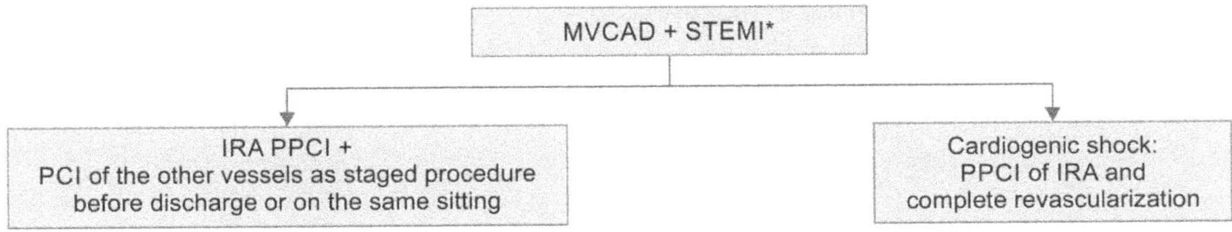

*STEMI is associated with multivessel coronary artery disease (MVCAD) in 50% of cases.[5]
(IRA: infarct-related artery; MVCAD: multivessel coronary artery disease; PCI: percutaneous coronary intervention; PPCI: primary percutaneous coronary intervention; STEMI: ST-elevation myocardial infarction)

REFERENCES

1. O'Gara PT, Kushner FG, Ascheim DD, Casey DE Jr, Chung MK, de Lemos JA, et al. 2013 ACCF/AHA guideline for the management of ST-elevation myocardial infarction. A report of the American College of Cardiology Foundation/American Heart Association task force on practice guidelines. Circulation. 2013;127(4):e362-e425.

2. Ibanez B, James S, Agewall S, Antunes MJ, Bucciarelli-Ducci C, Bueno H, et al; ESC Scientific Document Group. 2017 ESC Guidelines for the management of acute myocardial infarction in patients presenting with ST-segment elevation: The Task Force for the management of acute myocardial infarction in patients presenting with ST-segment elevation of the European Society of Cardiology (ESC). Eur Heart J. 2018;39(2):119-77.

3. Wong GC, Welsford M, Ainsworth C, Abuzeid W, Fordyce CB, Greene J, et al. 2019 Canadian Cardiovascular Society/Canadian Association of Interventional Cardiology guidelines on the acute management of ST-elevation myocardial infarction: Focused update on regionalization and reperfusion. Can J Cardiol. 2019;35:107-32.

4. Lawton JS, Tamis-Holland JE, Bangalore S, Bates ER, Beckie TM, Bischoff JM, et al; Writing Committee Members. 2021 ACC/AHA/SCAI Guideline for Coronary Artery Revascularization: A Report of the American College of Cardiology/American Heart Association Joint Committee on Clinical Practice Guidelines. J Am Coll Cardiol. 2022;79:e21-e29.

5. Dziewierz A, Siudak Z, Rakowski T, Zasada W, Dubiel JS, Dudek D. Impact of multivessel coronary artery disease and noninfarct-related artery revascularization on outcome of patients with ST-elevation myocardial infarction transferred for primary percutaneous coronary intervention (from the EUROTRANSFER registry). Am J Cardiol. 2010;106(3):342-7.

CHAPTER 21

ST-elevation Myocardial Infarction: Predischarge and Postdischarge Program

INTRODUCTION

All patients with ST-elevated myocardial infarction (STEMI) should be kept in coronary care unit following reperfusion. Early transfer to ward and discharge from hospital after successful revascularization are not associated with any increased morbidity or mortality.[1]

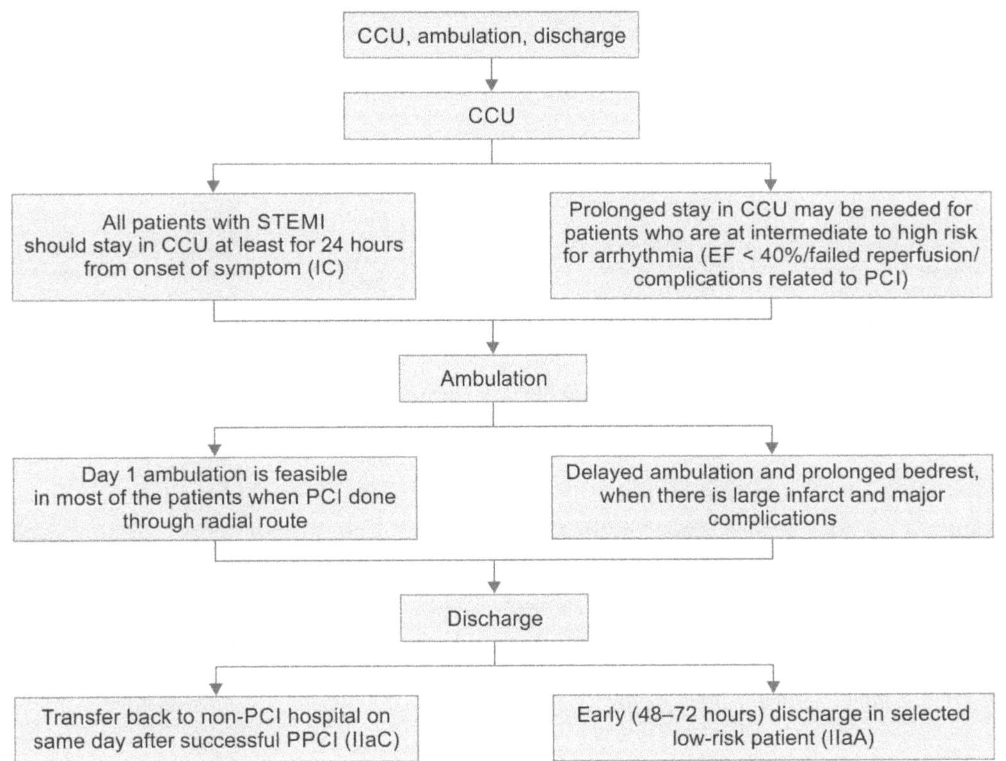

(CCU: coronary care unit; EF: ejection fraction; PCI: percutaneous coronary intervention; PPCI: primary percutaneous coronary intervention; STEMI: ST-elevated myocardial infarction)

Low-risk patients for early discharge in STEMI

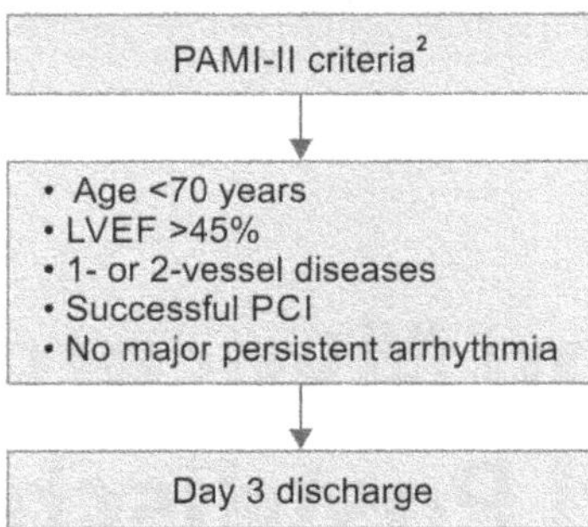

(LVEF: left ventricular ejection fraction; PAMI-II: primary angioplasty in myocardial infarction; PCI: percutaneous coronary intervention)

Acute and late-risk stratification in STEMI

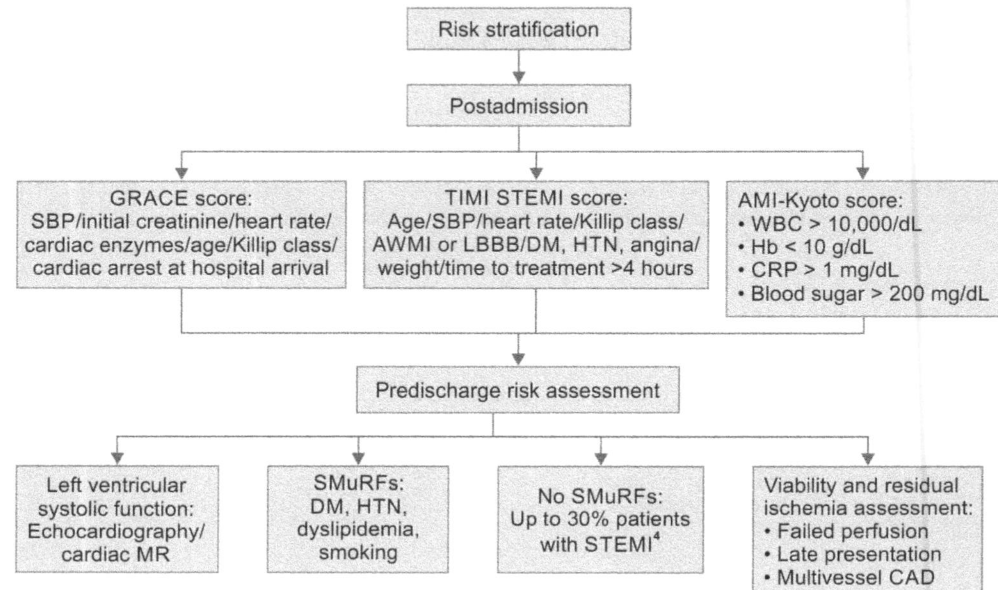

(AWMI: anterior wall myocardial infarction; CAD: coronary artery disease; CRP: C-reactive protein; DM: diabetes mellitus; GRACE: Global Registry of Acute Coronary Events; Hb: hemoglobin; HTN: hypertension; LBBB: left bundle branch block; MR: magnetic resonance; SBP: systolic blood pressure; SMuRFs: standard modifiable cardiovascular risk factors; STEMI: ST-elevated myocardial infarction; TIMI: thrombolysis in myocardial infarction; WBC: white blood cell)

Role of echocardiogram in STEMI during hospital stay

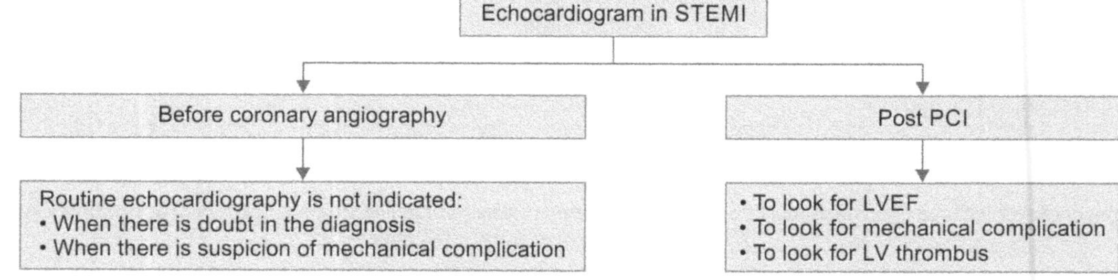

(LV: left ventricular; LVEF: left ventricular ejection fraction; PCI: percutaneous coronary intervention; STEMI: ST-elevated myocardial infarction)

Postdischarge strategy in STEMI patients: Lifestyle modification[3]

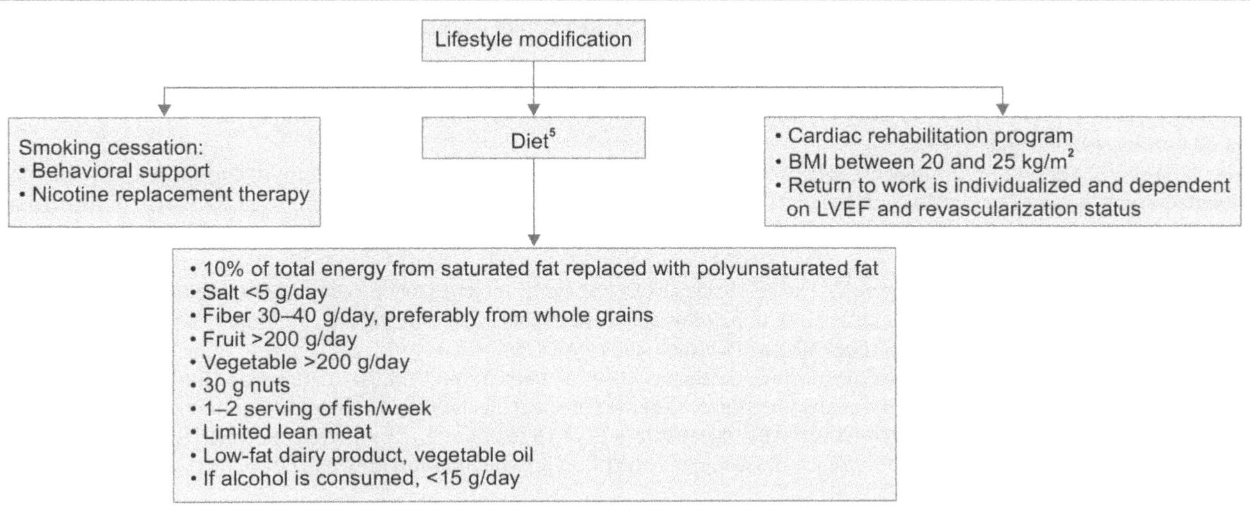

(BMI: body mass index; LVEF: left ventricular ejection fraction; STEMI: ST-elevated myocardial infarction)

Postdischarge strategy: Antiplatelet medication[3]

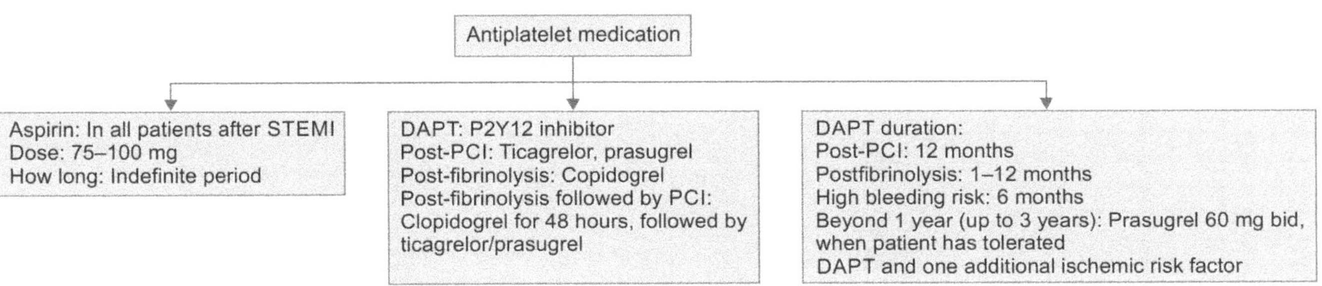

(DAPT: dual antiplatelet therapy; PCI: percutaneous coronary intervention)

Post-discharge strategy: Other medications[3]

Other medications (in absence of contraindication)

Lipid-lowering agent:
• High-intensity statin
• If the LDL target (LDL <70 mg/dL/>50% reduction) not achieved: To add ezetimibe
• If target not achieved, PCSK9 inhibitor
• If the current episode is a recurrence within 2 years and on high-intensity statin, LDL target should be <40 mg/dL

ACEi/ARB/ARNi:
• Patients with heart failure in initial phase/LVEF <40%/DM/HTN
• All patients with STEMI may be considered
• When to start: Within first 24 hours

MRA/SGLT-2 inhibitor[†]:
Patients with heart failure/LVEF <40%

Beta-blocker[3]:
• In all hemodynamically stable patient, those undergoing reperfusion should get IV.
• Beta-blocker followed by oral beta-blocker at presentation
• Oral beta-blocker should be continued in all patients with STEMI for an indefinite period

[†]SGLT-2 inhibitors: Still not included in guideline

(ACEi: angiotensin converting enzyme inhibitor; ARB: angiotensin receptor blocker; ARNi: angiotensin receptor-neprilysin inhibitor; DM: diabetes mellitus; HTN: hypertension; IV: intravenous; LDL: low-density lipoprotein; LVEF: left ventricular ejection fraction; MRA: mineralocorticoid receptor antagonist; PCSK9: proprotein convertase subtilisin/kexin type 9; SGLT-2: sodium-glucose cotransporter-2; STEMI: ST-elevation myocardial infarction)

REFERENCES

1. Berger AK, Duval S, Jacobs DR Jr, Barber C, Vazquez G, Lee S, et al. Relation of length of hospital stay in acute myocardial infarction to postdischarge mortality. Am J Cardiol. 2008;101(4):428-34.
2. Grines CL, Marsalese DL, Brodie B, Griffin J, Donohue B, Costantini CR, et al. Safety and cost- effectiveness of early discharge after primary angioplasty in low risk patients with acute myocardial infarction. PAMI-II investigators. Primary angioplasty in myocardial infarction. J Am Coll Cardiol. 1998;31(5):967-72.
3. Ibanez B, James S, Agewall S, Antunes MJ, Bucciarelli-Ducci C, Bueno H, et al; ESC Scientific Document Group. 2017 ESC Guidelines for the management of acute myocardial infarction in patients presenting with ST-segment elevation: The Task Force for the management of acute myocardial infarction in patients presenting with ST-segment elevation of the European Society of Cardiology (ESC). Eur Heart J. 2018;39(2):119-77.
4. Dziewierz A, Siudak Z, Rakowski T, Zasada W, Dubiel JS, Dudek D. Impact of multivessel coronary artery disease and noninfarct-related artery revascularization on outcome of patients with ST-elevation myocardial infarction transferred for primary percutaneous coronary intervention (from the EUROTRANSFER registry). Am J Cardiol. 2010;106(3):342-47.
5. Piepoli MF, Hoes AW, Agewall S, Albus C, Brotons C, Catapano AL, et al; Verschuren WM. 2016 European Guidelines on cardiovascular disease prevention in clinical practice: The sixth joint task force of the European Society of Cardiology and other societies on cardiovascular disease prevention in clinical practice (constituted by representatives of 10 societies and by invited experts). Developed with the special contribution of the European Association for Cardiovascular Prevention & Rehabilitation (EACPR). Eur Heart J. 2016;37(29):2315-81.

CHAPTER 22

Coronary Artery Disease: Chronic Coronary Syndrome

INTRODUCTION

The term chronic coronary syndrome (CCS) was proposed in 2019 ESC guideline.[1] Terms like stable coronary artery disease or chronic stable angina oversimplify a chronic progressive disease with its own morbidity and mortality. Angina is the pivotal point in the evaluation of CCS. Only 10–15% of patients with CCS present with typical angina, whereas rest of the patients present with atypical or nonanginal chest pain.[2]

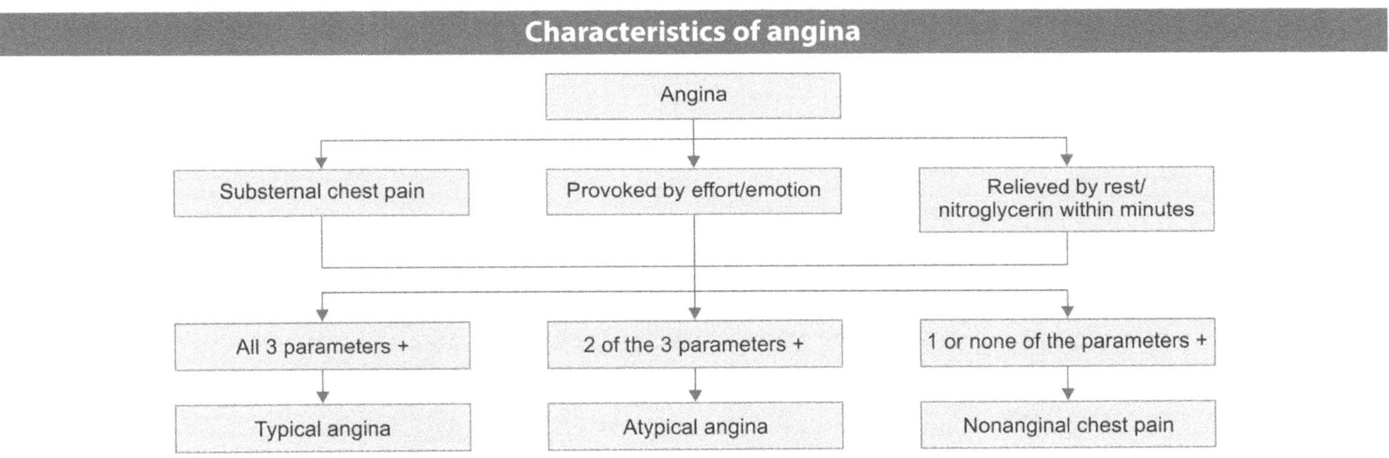

(ACS: acute coronary syndrome; CAD: coronary artery disease; CCS: chronic coronary syndrome; HF: heart failure)

Chronic coronary syndrome: Diagnostic strategy

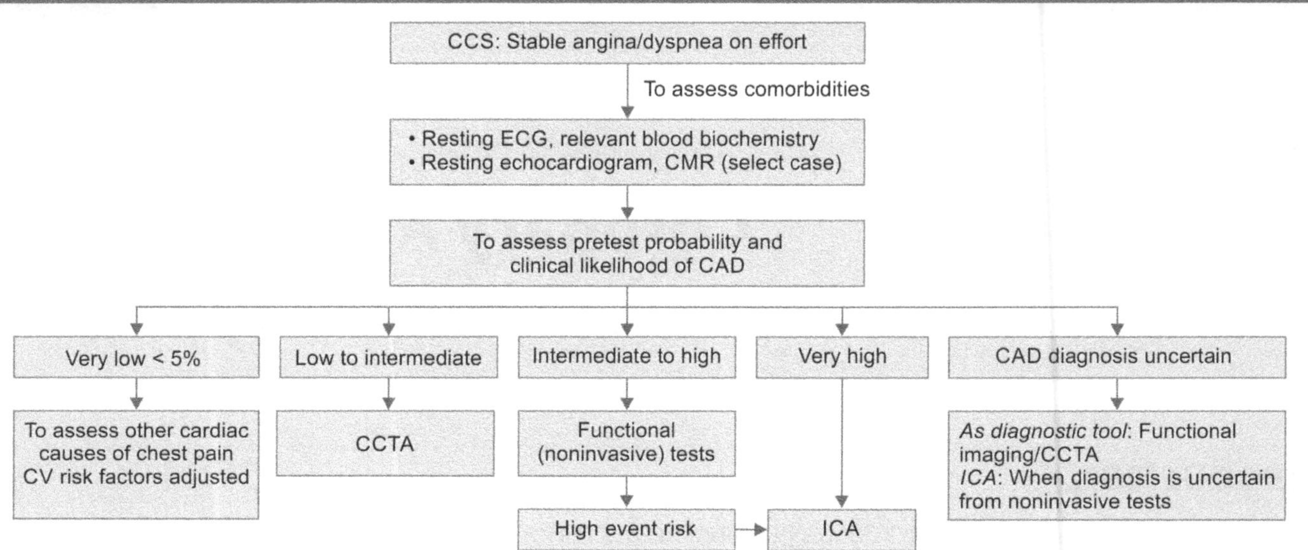

(CAD: coronary artery disease; CCS: chronic coronary syndrome; CCTA: coronary computed tomographic angiography; CMR: cardiovascular magnetic resonance; CV: cardiovascular; ECG: electrocardiogram; ICA: invasive coronary angiography)

Pretest probability of coronary artery disease according to type of chest pain[3]

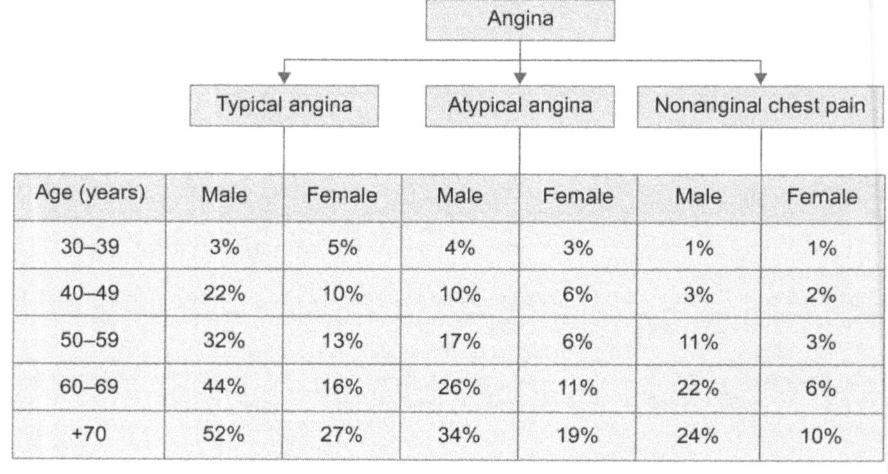

Age (years)	Typical angina		Atypical angina		Nonanginal chest pain	
	Male	Female	Male	Female	Male	Female
30–39	3%	5%	4%	3%	1%	1%
40–49	22%	10%	10%	6%	3%	2%
50–59	32%	13%	17%	6%	11%	3%
60–69	44%	16%	26%	11%	22%	6%
+70	52%	27%	34%	19%	24%	10%

Functional (noninvasive) test strategy in chronic coronary syndrome

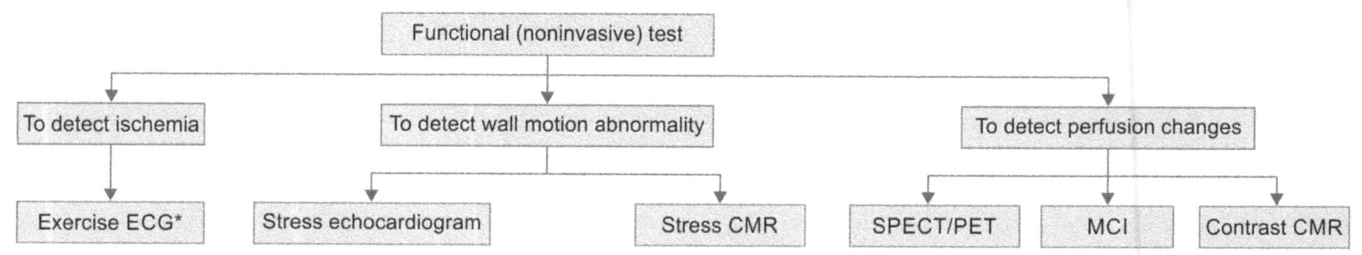

*Functional imaging test is preferred to exercise electrocardiogram[4]

(CMR: cardiac magnetic resonance; ECG: electrocardiogram; MCI: myocardial contrast imaging; PET: positron emission tomography; SPECT: single photon emission computed tomography)

Risk stratification algorithm

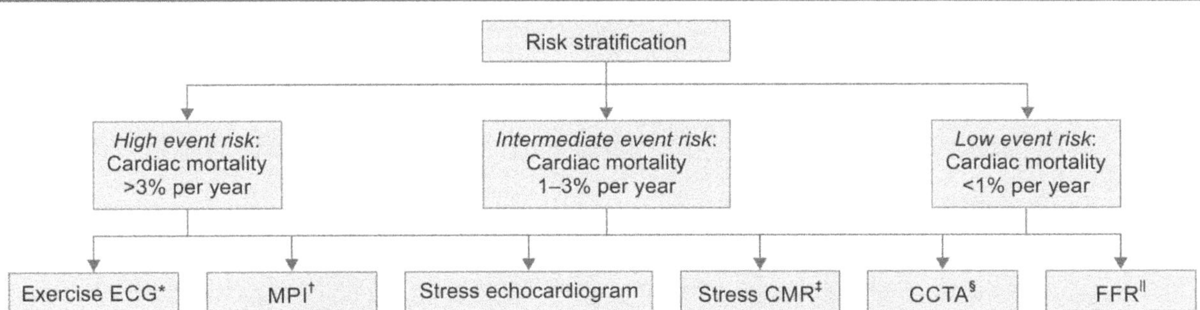

*Exercise ECG: The treadmill score[5] calculated as follows: Duration of exercise in minutes − (5 × the maximal ST-segment deviation during or after exercise, in millimeters) − (4 × the treadmill angina index). The numerical treadmill angina index was 0 for no angina, 1 for nonlimiting angina, and 2 for exercise-limiting angina. Treadmill scores ranged from −25 (indicating the highest risk) to +15 (indicating the lowest risk).

†Myocardial perfusion imaging (MPI): Ischemic area ≥10% of left ventricular myocardium; stress echocardiogram: ≥3 of the 16 segments show stress-induced hypokinesia or akinesia.

‡Cardiac magnetic resonance (CMR): ≥2 of the 16 segments show stress-induced perfusion defect.

§Coronary computed tomographic angiography (CCTA): Triple-vessel disease with proximal stenosis, left main disease, or proximal left anterior descending artery disease.

‖Functional flow reserve (FFR): ≥0.8

Chronic coronary syndrome: Lifestyle modification

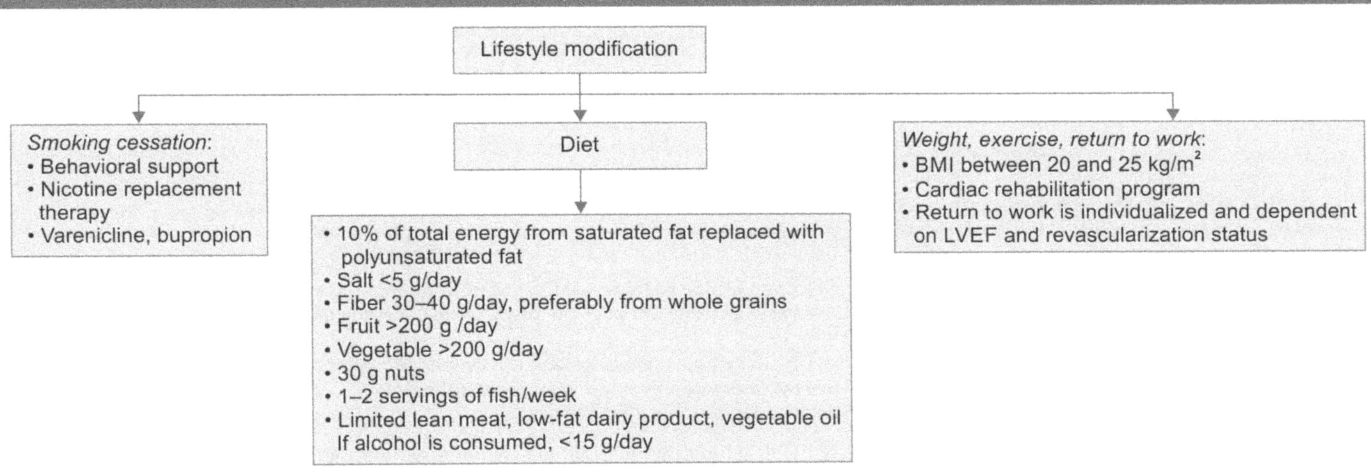

Chronic coronary syndrome: Medical management[1]

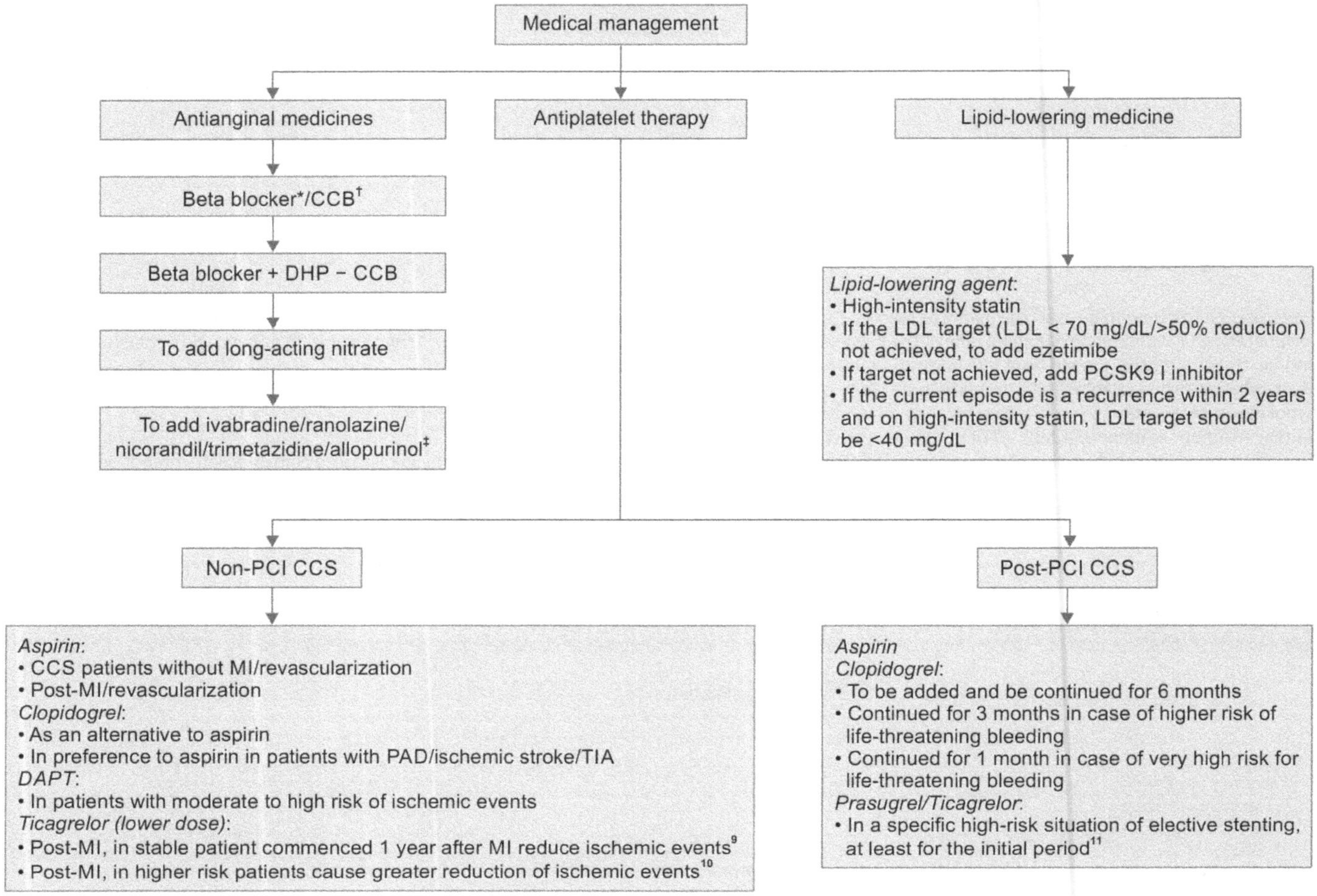
Medical management
Antianginal medicines
Beta blocker*/CCB†
Beta blocker + DHP - CCB
To add long-acting nitrate
To add ivabradine/ranolazine/nicorandil/trimetazidine/allopurinol‡
Antiplatelet therapy
Lipid-lowering medicine
Lipid-lowering agent:
• High-intensity statin
• If the LDL target (LDL < 70 mg/dL/>50% reduction) not achieved, to add ezetimibe
• If target not achieved, add PCSK9 I inhibitor
• If the current episode is a recurrence within 2 years and on high-intensity statin, LDL target should be <40 mg/dL
Non-PCI CCS
Aspirin:
• CCS patients without MI/revascularization
• Post-MI/revascularization
Clopidogrel:
• As an alternative to aspirin
• In preference to aspirin in patients with PAD/ischemic stroke/TIA
DAPT:
• In patients with moderate to high risk of ischemic events
Ticagrelor (lower dose):
• Post-MI, in stable patient commenced 1 year after MI reduce ischemic events9
• Post-MI, in higher risk patients cause greater reduction of ischemic events10
Post-PCI CCS
Aspirin
Clopidogrel:
• To be added and be continued for 6 months
• Continued for 3 months in case of higher risk of life-threatening bleeding
• Continued for 1 month in case of very high risk for life-threatening bleeding
Prasugrel/Ticagrelor:
• In a specific high-risk situation of elective stenting, at least for the initial period11

*Beta blocker: It is usually used as initial medicine. The resting heart rate is to be kept between 55 and 60 bpm, and the cardio-protective effect in CCS patients without MI or heart failure is less established.[6] However, in patients without MI or heart failure undergoing CABG, a beta blocker shows cardioprotective effect.

†CCB: Calcium-entry blocker can also be used as initial medicine. DHP (dihydropyridine) molecule can be used in combination with beta blocker. Amlodipine, as a single agent or in combination with beta blocker, is effective but underused, in reducing angina threshold.[7]

‡Allopurinol:[8] It was found to increase time to angina and ST-segment depression during exercise.

(CCS: chronic coronary syndrome; DAPT: dual antiplatelet therapy; DHP: dihydropyridine; LDL: low-density lipoprotein; MI: myocardial infarction; PAD: peripheral artery disease; PCI: percutaneous coronary intervention; PCSK9: proprotein convertase subtilisin/kexin type 9; TIA: transient ischemic attack)

Oral anticoagulant strategy in chronic coronary syndrome[9]

Oral anticoagulant
In sinus rhythm
Rivaroxaban 2.5 mg bid + aspirin: Greater reduction of ischemic events, more so in high-risk patients12
In AF, when OAC indicated
NOAC preferred over VKA
In long term, aspirin or clopidogrel may be added post-MI, with high risk for recurrent ischemic events (with low bleeding risk)
PCI and AF
VKA not interrupted prior to PCI. NOAC held 12–48 hours.
Before PCI pretreatment with aspirin and loading clopidogrel
Radial artery access preferred
Full-dose intraprocedural UFH and lower dose in them who are on VKA. OAC + aspirin + clopidogrel for ≥1 month, when thrombotic risk >> bleeding risk. OAC monotherapy 6–12 months. Dual therapy as OAC + aspirin/clopidogrel may be considered when ischemic risk is high

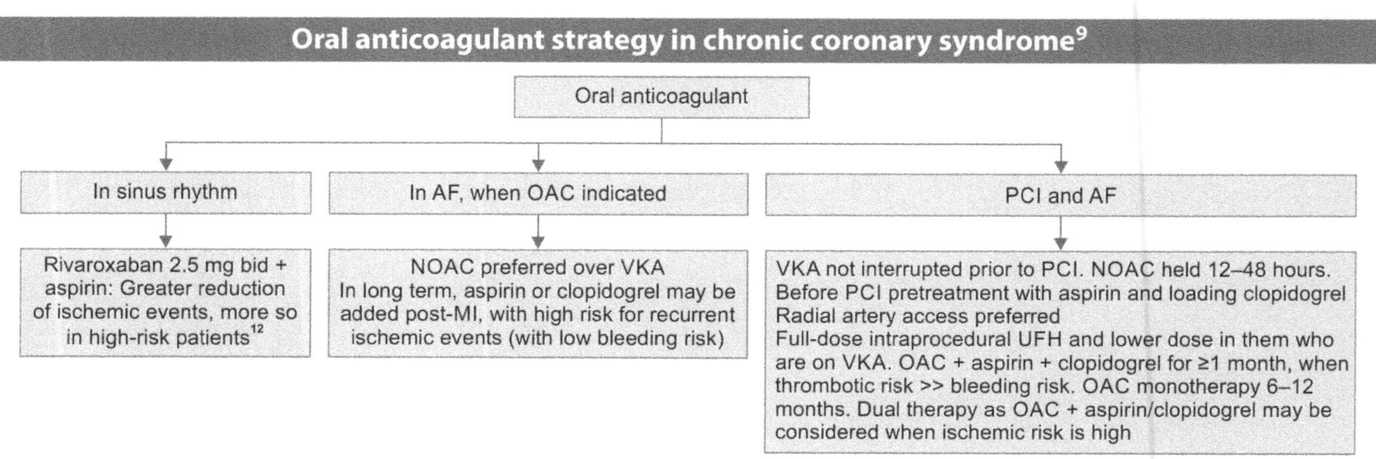

(AF: atrial fibrillation; MI: myocardial infarction; NAOC: novel oral anticoagulant drugs; PCI: percutaneous coronary intervention; VKA: vitamin K antagonists)

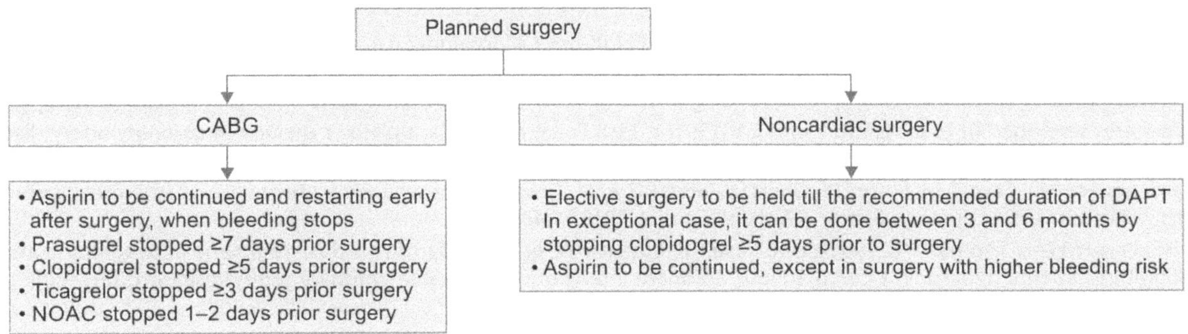

(CABG: coronary artery bypass graft; NAOC: novel oral anticoagulant drugs)

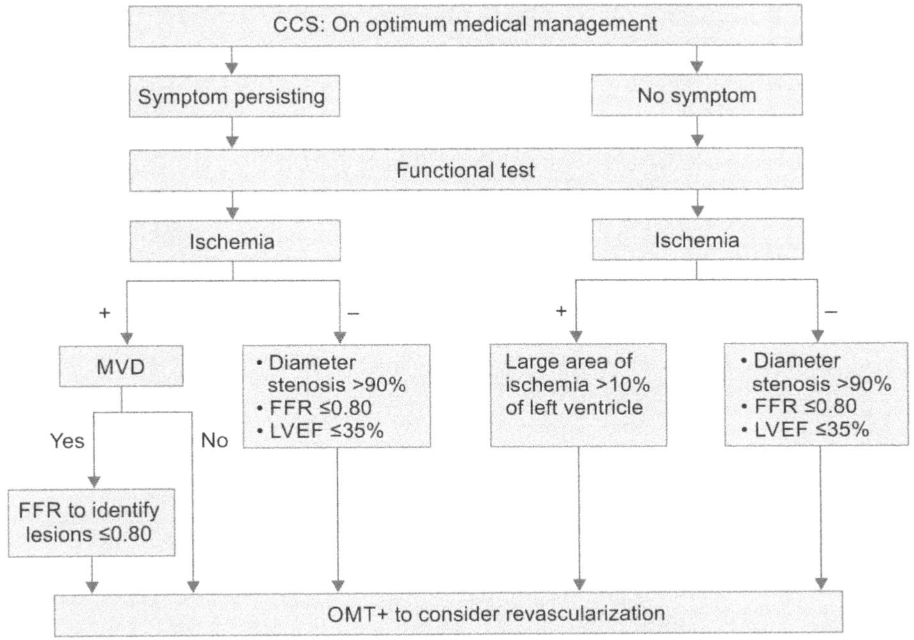

(CCS: chronic coronary syndrome; FFR: fractional flow reserve; LVEF: left ventricular ejection fraction; MVD: multi-vessel disease; OMT: optimal medical therapy)

REFERENCES

1. Knuuti J, Wijns W, Saraste A, Capodanno D, Barbato E, Funck-Brentano C, et al; ESC Scientific Document Group. 2019 ESC guidelines for the diagnosis and management of chronic coronary syndromes. Eur Heart J. 2020; 41(3):407-77.
2. Newby DE, Adamson PD, Berry C, Boon NA, Dweck MR, Flather M, et al; SCOT-HEART investigators. Coronary CT angiography and 5-year risk of myocardial infarction. N Engl J Med 2018;379:924-33.
3. Juarez-Orozco LE, Saraste A, Capodanno D, Prescott E, Ballo H, Bax JJ, et al. Impact of a decreasing pre-test probability on the performance of diagnostic tests for coronary artery disease. Eur Heart J Cardiovasc Imaging. 2019;20(11):1198-207.
4. Jorgensen ME, Andersson C, Norgaard BL, Abdulla J, Shreibati JB, Torp-Pedersen C, et al. Functional testing or coronary computed tomography angiography in patients with stable coronary artery disease. J Am Coll Cardiol. 2017;69:1761-70.
5. Mark DB, Shaw L, Harrell FE Jr, Hlatky MA, Lee KL, Bengtson JR, McCants CB, et al. Prognostic value of a treadmill exercise score in outpatients with suspected coronary artery disease. N Engl J Med. 1991;325:849-53.
6. Bangalore S, Steg G, Deedwania P, Crowley K, Eagle KA, Goto S, Ohman EM, et al; REACH Registry Investigators. β-Blocker use and clinical outcomes in stable outpatients with and without coronary artery disease. JAMA. 2012;308:1340-49.

7. Nissen SE, Tuzcu EM, Libby P, Thompson PD, Ghali M, Garza D, et al; CAMELOT Investigators. Effect of antihypertensive agents on cardiovascular events in patients with coronary disease and normal blood pressure: the CAMELOT study: a randomized controlled trial. JAMA. 2004;292:2217-25.

8. Noman A, Ang DS, Ogston S, Lang CC, Struthers AD. Effect of high-dose allopurinol on exercise in patients with chronic stable angina: a randomised, placebo controlled crossover trial. Lancet. 2010;375:2161-7.

9. Valgimigli M, Bueno H, Byrne RA, Collet JP, Costa F, Jeppsson A, et al. 2017 ESC focused update on dual anti-platelet therapy in coronary artery disease developed in collaboration with EACTS: The Task Force for dual antiplatelet therapy in coronary artery disease of the European Society of Cardiology (ESC) and of the European Association for Cardio-Thoracic Surgery (EACTS). Eur Heart J. 2018;39:213-60.

10. Bansilal S, Bonaca MP, Cornel JH, Storey RF, Bhatt DL, Steg PG, et al. Ticagrelor for secondary prevention of atherothrombotic events in patients with multivessel coronary disease. J Am Coll Cardiol. 2018;71:489-96.

11. Orme RC, Parker WAE, Thomas MR, Judge HM, Baster K, Sumaya W, et al. Study of two dose regimens of ticagrelor compared with clopidogrel in patients undergoing percutaneous coronary intervention for stable coronary artery disease (STEEL-PCI). Circulation. 2018;138:1290-300.

12. Eikelboom JW, Connolly SJ, Bosch J, Dagenais GR, Hart RG, Shestakovska O, et al; COMPASS Investigators. Rivaroxaban with or without aspirin in stable cardiovascular disease. N Engl J Med. 2017;377:1319-30.

13. Zhao Q, Zhu Y, Xu Z, Cheng Z, Mei J, Chen X, et al. Effect of ticagrelor plus aspirin, ticagrelor alone, or aspirin alone on saphenous vein graft patency 1 year after coronary artery bypass grafting: a randomized clinical trial. JAMA. 2018;319:1677-86.

CHAPTER 23

Coronary Artery Disease: Special Situations–Myocardial Infarction with Nonobstructive Coronary Artery

INTRODUCTION

Myocardial infarction with nonobstructive coronary artery (MINOCA) is not a very uncommon entity. Various registration studies indicate that in acute myocardial infarction (AMI) cases, coronary artery may not show any obstruction in 1–15% of cases.[1,2] In a recent NCDR (National Cardiovascular Data Registry) CathPCI registry, out of 286,780 patients admitted with AMI, 16,849 patients (5.9%) were categorized as MINOCA patients.[3]

Myocardial infarction with nonobstructive coronary artery patients are relatively younger, female. They are less likely dyslipidemic, diabetic, or hypertensive indicating atherosclerosis less likely as etiology. Insulin resistance and inflammation may precipitate the acute state. Their electrocardiogram (ECG) on presentation may show both ST-segment elevation and depression. In 2017, the European Society of Cardiology (ESC) in a position statement[4] defined MINOCA. They included MINOCA in the category of myocardial infarction. They included Takotsubo syndrome and myocarditis in the purview of MINOCA. However, in 2019 in the new definition of AMI,[5] MINOCA indicated only cases who presented with clinical ischemia. They excluded Takotsubo syndrome and myocarditis from the working diagnosis of MINOCA.

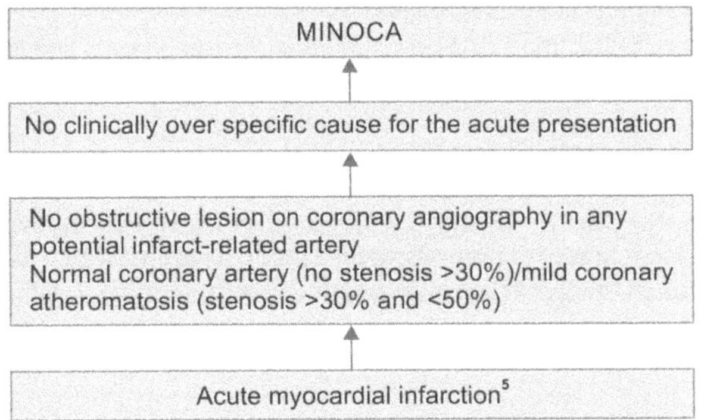

(MINOCA: myocardial infarction with nonobstructive coronary artery)

Myocardial infarction with nonobstructive coronary artery: Approach

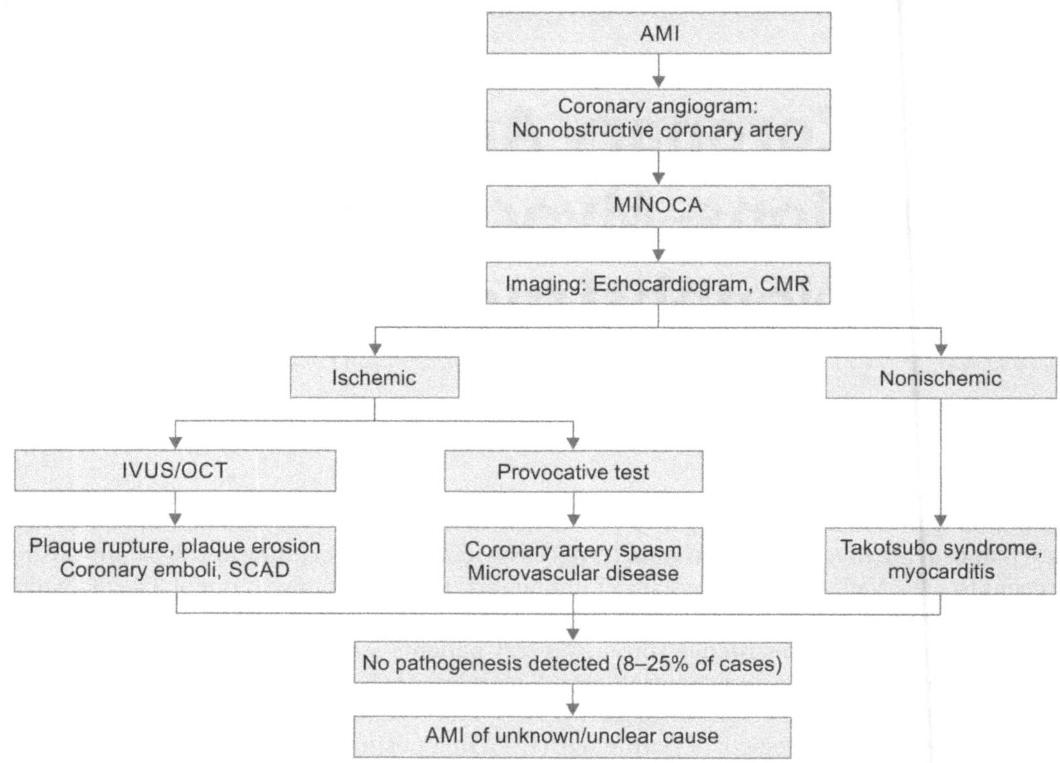

(AMI: acute myocardial infarction; CMR: cardiac magnetic resonance; IVUS: intravascular ultrasound; MINOCA: myocardial infarction with nonobstructive coronary artery; OCT: optical coherence tomography; SCAD: spontaneous coronary artery dissection)

REFERENCES

1. Pasupathy S, Air T, Dreyer RP, Tavella R, Beltrame JF. Systematic review of patients presenting with suspected myocardial infarction and nonobstructive coronary arteries. Circulation. 2015;131(10):861-70.
2. Safdar B, Spatz ES, Dreyer RP, Beltrame JF, Lichtman JH, Spertus JA, et al. Presentation, Clinical Profile, and Prognosis of Young Patients with Myocardial Infarction with Non-obstructive Coronary Arteries (MINOCA): Results from theVIRGO Study. J Am Heart Assoc. 2018;7(13):e009174.
3. Dreyer RP, Tavella R, Curtis JP, Wang Y, Pauspathy S, Messenger J, et al. Myocardial infarction with non-obstructive coronary arteries as compared with myocardial infarction and obstructive coronary disease: outcomes in a Medicare population. Eur Heart J. 2020;41(7):870-8.
4. Agewall S, Beltrame JF, Reynolds HR, Niessner A, Rosano G, Caforio AL, et al.; WG on Cardiovascular Pharmacotherapy. ESC working group position paper on myocardial infarction with non-obstructive coronary arteries. Eur Heart J. 2017;38(3):143-53.
5. Thygesen K, Alpert JS, Jaffe AS, Chaitman BR, Bax JJ, Morrow DA, et al. Fourth universal definition of myocardial infarction (2018). Eur Heart J. 2018;138:e618–e651.

CHAPTER 24

Coronary Artery Disease: Special Situations–Spontaneous Coronary Artery Dissection

INTRODUCTION

Spontaneous coronary artery dissection (SCAD) is an important cause of nonatherosclerotic acute coronary syndrome (ACS). This is a disease of younger females, presenting at the age between 48 and 52 years, with a 4:1 ratio of female to male.[1] SCAD is not very uncommon with an incidence of 38% of all ACS in female and 4% of all ACS in male.[2] Common associations are fibromuscular dysplasia, connective tissue disorder, peripartum period, and undue physical strain. Patients with SCAD on conservative management may deteriorate in 15–20% of cases within the following week. There are two mechanisms of SCAD. The first is inside-out theory in which the dissection or rupture of intima occurs followed by entry and accumulation of blood from the arterial lumen to the wall leading to a false lumen, compressing the main lumen. Another is outside-in theory in which there is formation of intramural hematoma leading to separation of intima media and tearing of intima in lumen.

Angiographically, there are three types of lesions. Type 1 (29%) lesion is a longitudinal filling defect indicating the radiolucent intimal flap and false lumen. The filling defect separates two structures, the arterial wall which is stained by contrast and the true actual lumen containing the contrast producing a double-lumen appearance.

In type 2 (67%) lesion, there is a diffuse smooth tubular lesion due to compression of the lumen by intramural hematoma, which can cause complete vessel occlusion. Intimal flap is not visible and there is abrupt change of vessel diameter between normal and diseased segment of the artery. Type 3 (4%) lesion consists of multiple focal tubular lesions due to intramural hematoma.

Regarding management, conservative strategy is recommended in most of the cases. PCI always has complication more in SCAD than in atherosclerotic coronary artery lesion. Guide wire, balloon, and stent all can increase dissection. Dissection can progress after stenting. Unusual long dissection length and malapposition pose risk for higher chance of restenosis and stent thrombosis. Coronary artery bypass graft (CABG) is an option when PCI is not feasible with a higher rate of graft failure as spontaneous healing of the dissection of the native vessel occurs frequently.

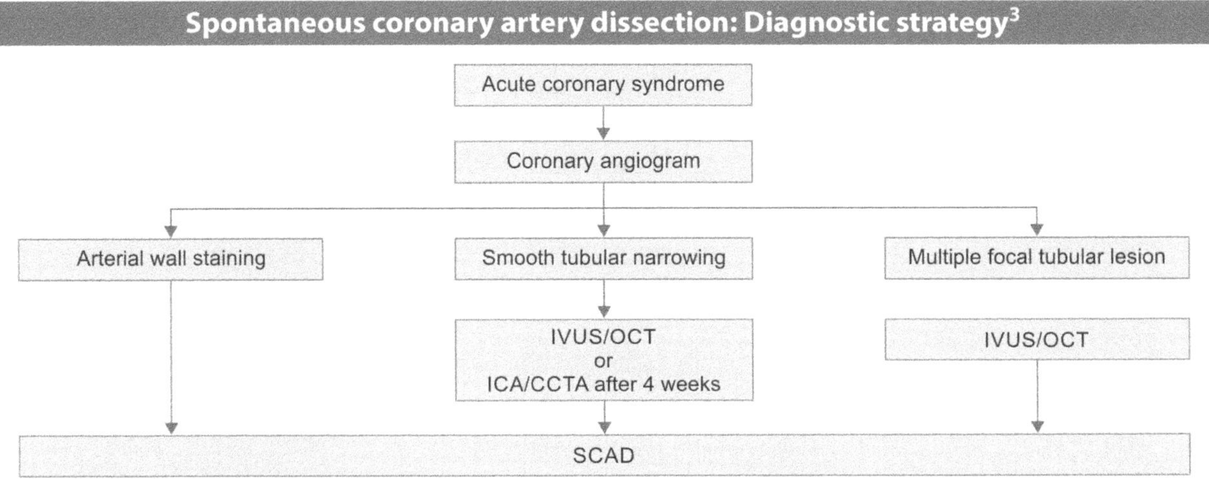

(CCTA: coronary computed tomography angiography; ICA: invasive coronary angiography; IVUS: intravascular ultrasound; OCT: optical coherence tomography; SCAD: spontaneous coronary artery dissection)

Spontaneous coronary artery dissection: Intervention strategy[4]

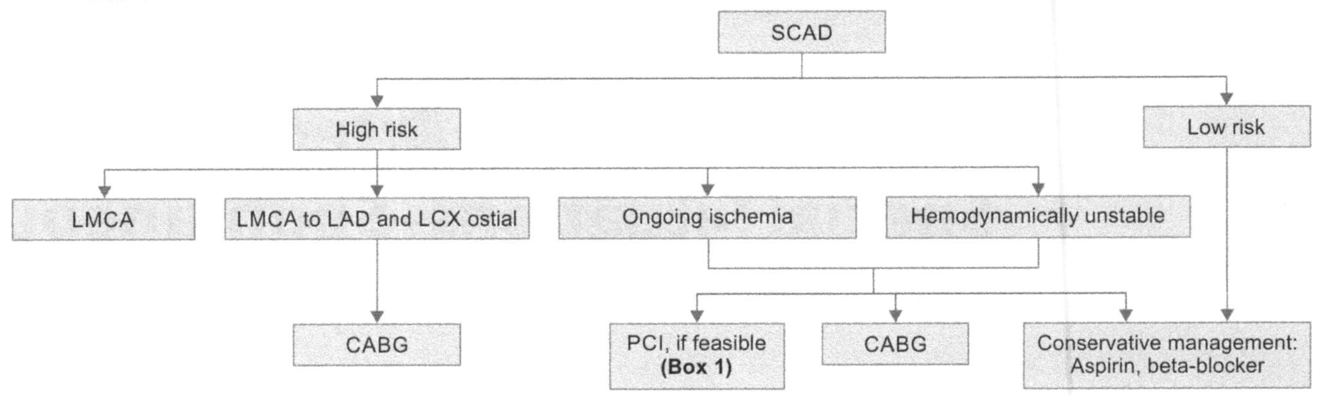

(CABG: coronary artery bypass graft; LAD: left anterior descending; LCX: left circumflex; LMCA: left main coronary artery; PCI: percutaneous coronary intervention)

BOX 1: Tips and tricks during PCI.

PCI: To prevent progression of intramural hematoma
- To seal the distal first and proximal at the end of the dissection before stenting the middle segment
- To use long stent to cover 5–10 mm on both proximal and distal end of dissection
- Minimum balloon inflation
- To use cutting balloon to fenestrate intramural hematoma to allow decompression of false lumen into the true lumen
- Liberal use of imaging

REFERENCES

1. Tweet MS Hayes SN, Pitta SR, Simari RD, Lerman A, Lennon RJ, et al. Clinical features, management, and prognosis of spontaneous coronary artery dissection. Circulation. 2012;126:579-88.
2. Nakashimia T Noguchi T, Haruta S, Yamamoto Y, Oshima S, Nakao K, et al. Prognostic impact of spontaneous coronary artery dissection in young female patients with acute myocardial infarction: a report from the Angina Pectoris-Myocardial Infarction Multicenter Investigators in Japan. Int J Cardiol. 2016;207:341-8.
3. Saw J. Coronary angiogram classification of spontaneous coronary artery dissection. Catheter Cardiovasc Interv. 2014;84(7):1115-22.
4. Saw J, Mancini GBJ, Humphries KH. Contemporary Review on Spontaneous Coronary Artery Dissection. J Am Coll Cardiol. 2016;68:297-312.

CHAPTER 25

Special Situations Chronic Kidney Disease and Coronary Artery Disease

INTRODUCTION

Chronic kidney disease (CKD) is a quite common and important risk factor for coronary artery disease. About 30–40% of patients undergoing percutaneous coronary intervention (PCI) have concomitant CKD. The chance of acute kidney injury (AKI) during PCI in a patient with CKD is high. There are various pathophysiological explanations, the most important of which is contrast-induced acute kidney injury (CI-AKI) or contrast-induced nephropathy (CIN). CI-AKI is defined as an increase in serum creatinine by ≥0.3 mg/dL within 48 hours of contrast media exposure or an increase to ≥50% within 1 week.[1] In advanced CKD, contrast volume/creatinine clearance ratio > 2 is an independent risk factor for CI-AKI.

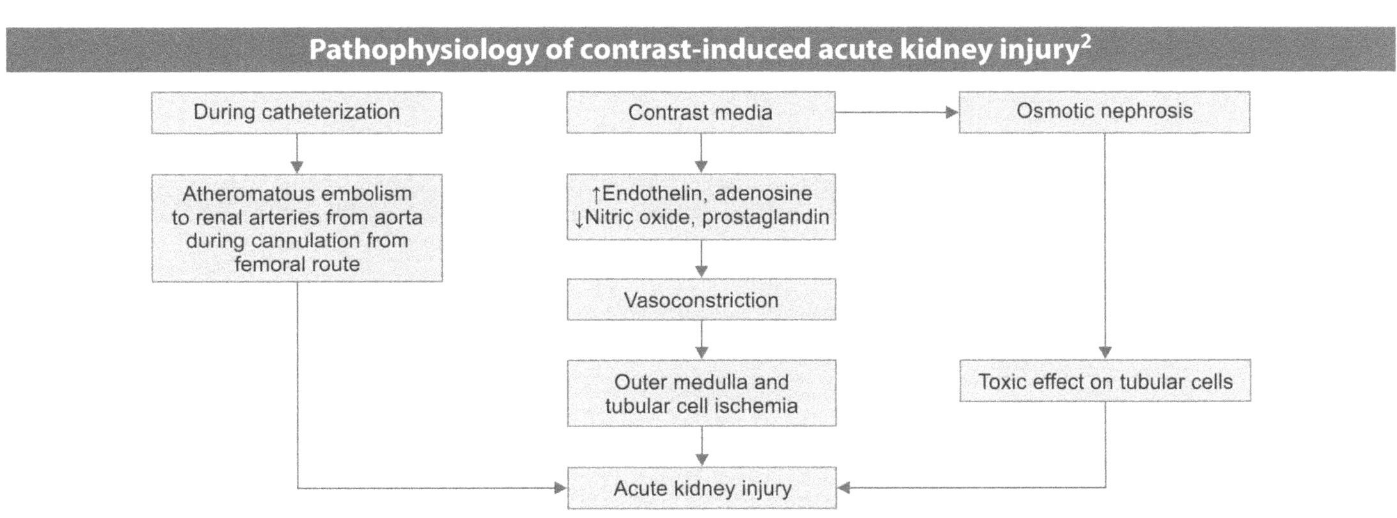

(ACS: acute coronary syndrome; AHF: acute heart failure; CI-AKI: contrast-induced acute kidney injury; CKD: chronic kidney disease; CS: cardiogenic shock; EF: ejection fraction; eGFR: estimated glomerular filtration rate; T2DM: type 2 diabetes mellitus)

Revascularization in patients with chronic kidney disease

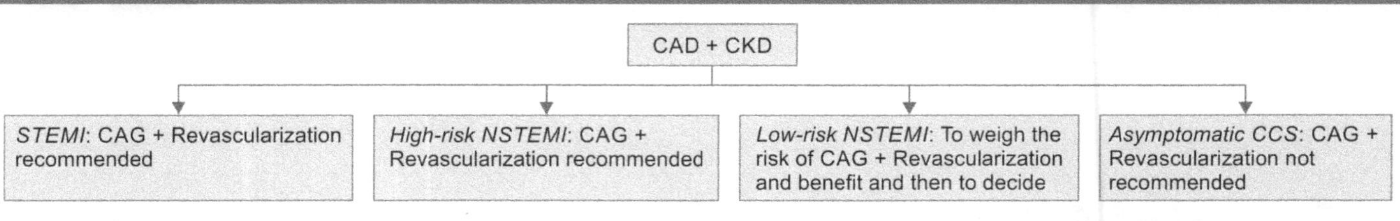

(CAD: coronary artery disease; CAG: coronary angiogram; CCS: chronic coronary syndrome; CKD: chronic kidney disease; NSTEMI: non-ST-elevation myocardial infarction; STEMI: ST-elevation myocardial infarction)

Periprocedural measures to prevent contrast-induced acute kidney injury

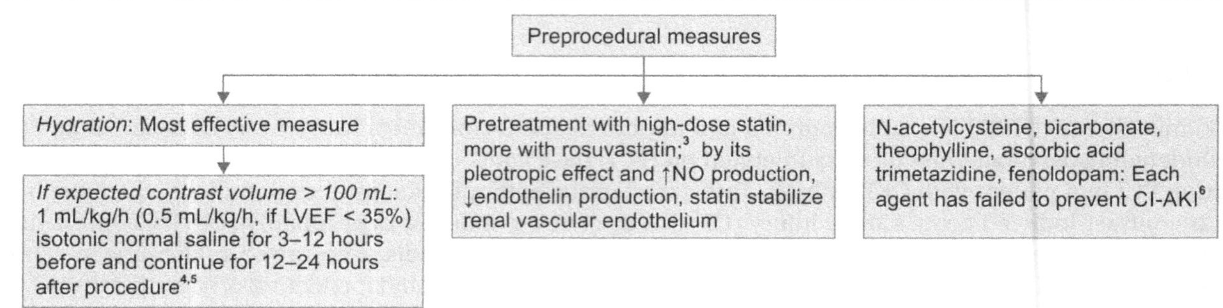

(CI-AKI: contrast-induced acute kidney injury; LVEF: left ventricular ejection fraction; NO: nitric oxide)

Contrast volume reduction to prevent contrast-induced acute kidney injury

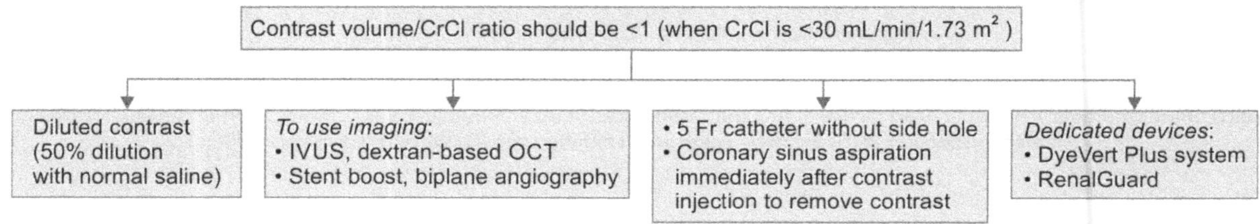

(CrCl: creatinine clearance; IVUS: intravascular ultrasound; OCT: optical coherence tomography)

Other measures to prevent contrast-induced acute kidney injury

REFERENCES

1. KDIGO Working Group. Section 4: contrast-induced AKI. Kidney Int Suppl (2011). 2012;2:69-88.

2. McCullough PA, Choi JP, Feghali GA, Schussler JM, Stoler RM, Vallabahn RC, et al. Contrast-induced acute kidney injury. J Am Coll Cardiol. 2016;68:1465-73.

3. Han Y, Zhu G, Han L, Hou F, Huang W, Liu H, et al. Short-term rosuvastatin therapy for prevention of contrast-induced acute kidney injury in patients with diabetes and chronic kidney disease. J Am Coll Cardiol. 2014;63:62-70.

4. Neumann FJ, Sousa-Uva M, Ahlsson A, Alfonso F, Banning AP, Benedetto U, et al. ESC Scientific Document Group. 2018 ESC/EACTS Guidelines on myocardial revascularization. Eur Heart J. 2019;40:87-165.

5. Stacul F, Adam A, Becker CR, Davidson C, Lameire N, McCullough PA, et al. Strategies to Reduce the Risk of Contrast-Induced Nephropathy. Am J Cardiol. 2006;98(6):59-77.

6. McCullough PA, Choi JP, Feghali GA, Schussler JM, Stoler RM, Vallabahn RC, et al. Contrast-induced acute kidney injury. J Am Coll Cardiol. 2016;68:1465-73.

7. Azzalini L, Vilca LM, Lombardo F, Poletti E, Laricchia A, Beneduce A, et al. Incidence of contrast-induced acute kidney injury in a large cohort of all-comers undergoing percutaneous coronary intervention: comparison of five contrast media. Int J Cardiol. 2018;273:69-73.

CHAPTER 26

Coronary Artery Bypass Graft Surgery: What the Cardiologist Should Know?

INTRODUCTION

"Is it still worth the pain to drain stenosed saphenous veins?" was the comment made by Puri and Bertrand in an editorial.[1] Coronary artery bypass graft (CABG) surgery is still a major therapeutic armamentarium in several situations of coronary artery disease.

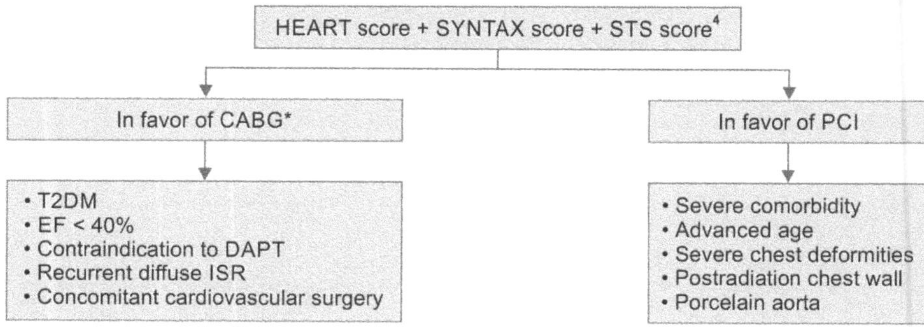

(CABG: coronary artery bypass graft; CS: cardiogenic shock; IRA: infarct-related artery; MI: myocardial infarction; PCI: percutaneous coronary intervention; STEMI: ST-elevation myocardial infarction)

*5–10% of NSTEMI patients require CABG.[5] Optimum time for surgery is individualized. The risk of ischemic events due to partially holding DAPT before surgery is <0.1%, whereas perioperative bleeding event due to antiplatelet is 10% at surgery.[6]

(CABG: coronary artery bypass graft; DAPT: dual antiplatelet therapy; HEART: history, ECG, age, risk factors, and troponin; ISR: in-stent restenosis; PCI: percutaneous coronary intervention; STS: society of thoracic surgeons; T2DM: type 2 diabetes mellitus)

CABG in chronic coronary syndrome[7]

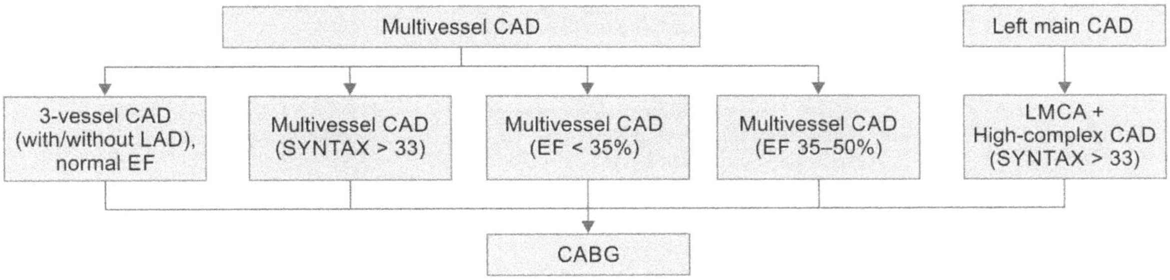

Multivessel CAD

Left main CAD

- 3-vessel CAD (with/without LAD), normal EF
- Multivessel CAD (SYNTAX > 33)
- Multivessel CAD (EF < 35%)
- Multivessel CAD (EF 35–50%)
- LMCA + High-complex CAD (SYNTAX > 33)

CABG

(CABG: coronary artery bypass graft; CAD: coronary artery disease; EF: ejection fraction; LAD: left anterior descending artery; LMCA: left main coronary artery)

CABG in chronic coronary syndrome[7]

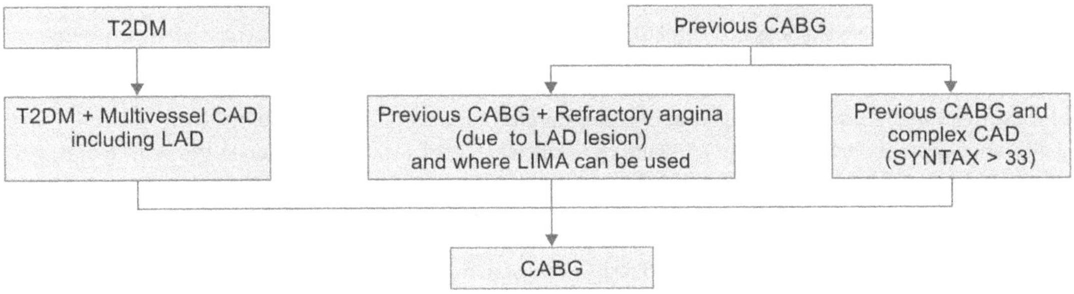

T2DM

Previous CABG

- T2DM + Multivessel CAD including LAD
- Previous CABG + Refractory angina (due to LAD lesion) and where LIMA can be used
- Previous CABG and complex CAD (SYNTAX > 33)

CABG

(CABG: coronary artery bypass graft; CAD: coronary artery disease; LAD: left anterior descending artery; LIMA: left internal mammary artery; T2DM: type 2 diabetes mellitus)

Antiplatelet strategy before CABG

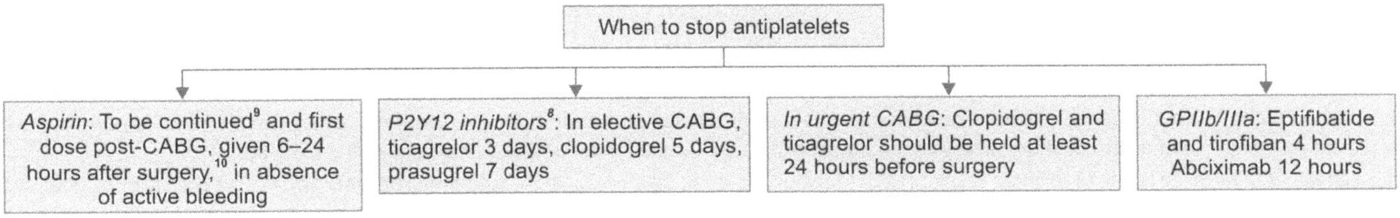

When to stop antiplatelets

- *Aspirin*: To be continued[9] and first dose post-CABG, given 6–24 hours after surgery,[10] in absence of active bleeding
- *P2Y12 inhibitors*[8]: In elective CABG, ticagrelor 3 days, clopidogrel 5 days, prasugrel 7 days
- *In urgent CABG*: Clopidogrel and ticagrelor should be held at least 24 hours before surgery
- *GPIIb/IIIa*: Eptifibatide and tirofiban 4 hours Abciximab 12 hours

(CABG: coronary artery bypass graft; GP: glycoprotein)

Other medicines, related to CABG to start before and after CABG

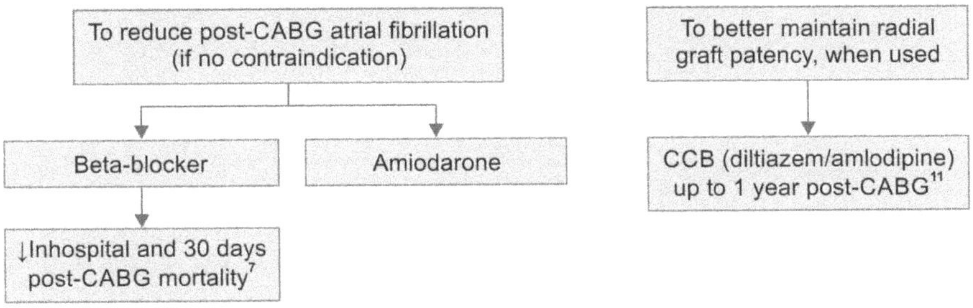

- To reduce post-CABG atrial fibrillation (if no contraindication)
  - Beta-blocker
    - ↓ Inhospital and 30 days post-CABG mortality[7]
  - Amiodarone
- To better maintain radial graft patency, when used
  - CCB (diltiazem/amlodipine) up to 1 year post-CABG[11]

(CABG: coronary artery bypass graft; CCB: calcium-channel blocker)

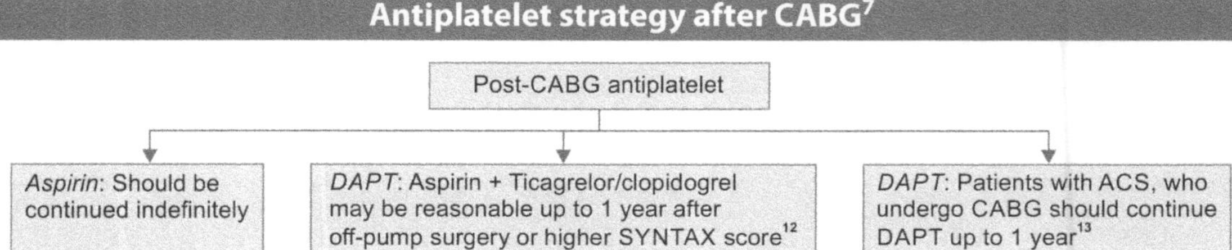

REFERENCES

1. Puri R, Bertrand OF. Is It Still Worth the Pain to "Drain" Stenosed Saphenous Veins?: Appraising Native Coronary Artery Versus Bypass Graft Percutaneous Coronary Interventions. JAAC Cardiovasc Interv. 2016;9:894-6.

2. Hochman JS, Sleeper LA, Webb JG, Sanborn TA, White HD, Talley JD, et al. Early revascularization in acute myocardial infarction complicated by cardiogenic shock. SHOCK Investigators. Should We Emergently Revascularize Occluded Coronaries for Cardiogenic Shock. N Engl J Med. 1999;341(9):625-4.

3. Weiss ES, Chang DD, Joyce DL, Nwakanma LU, Yuh DD. Optimal timing of coronary artery bypass after acute myocardial infarction: a review of California discharge data. J Thorac Cardiovasc Surg. 2008;135(3):503-11.

4. Osnabrugge RL, Speir AM, Head SJ, Fonner CE, Fonner E, Kappetein AP, Rich JB. Performance of EuroSCORE II in a large US database: implications for transcatheter aortic valve implantation. Eur J Cardiothorac Surg. 2014;46:400-8.

5. Ranasinghe I, Alprandi-Costa B, Chow V, Elliott JM, Waites J, Counsell JT, et al. Risk stratification in the setting of non-ST elevation acute coronary syndromes 1999-2007. Am J Cardiol. 2011;108(5):617-62.

6. Malm CJ, Hansson EC, Akesson J, Andersson M, Hesse C, Shams Hakimi C, et al. Preoperative platelet function predicts perioperative bleeding complications in ticagrelor-treated cardiac surgery patients: a prospective observational study. Br J Anaesth. 2016;117(3):309-15.

7. Lawton JS, Tamis-Holland JE, Bangalore S, Bates ER, Beckie TM, Bischoff JM, et al. 2021 ACC/AHA/SCAI Guideline for Coronary Artery Revascularization J Am Coll Cardiol. 2022;79:e21-e29.

8. Valgimigli M, Bueno H, Byrne RA, Collet JP, Costa F, Jeppsson A, et al. 2017 ESC Focused Update on Dual Antiplatelet Therapy in Coronary Artery Disease in collaboration with the European Association for Cardio-Thoracic Surgery (EACTS). The Task Force for the Management of Dual Antiplatelet Therapy in Coronary Artery Disease of the European Society of Cardiology (ESC). Eur Heart J. 2017;39(3):213-60.

9. Deja MA, Kargul T, Domaradzki W, Stacel T, Mazur W, Wojakowski W, et al. Effects preoperative aspirin in coronary artery bypass grafting: a double-blind, placebo-controlled, randomized trial. J Thorac Cardiovasc Surg. 2012;144(1):204-9.

10. Lim E, Ali Z, Ali A, Routledge T, Edmonds L, Altman DG, et al. Indirect comparison meta-analysis of aspirin therapy after coronary surgery. BMJ. 2003;327(7427):1309.

11. Gaudino M, Benedetto U, Fremes SE, Hare DL, Hayward P, Moat N, et al. Effect of calcium-channel blocker therapy on radial artery grafts after coronary bypass surgery. J Am Coll Cardiol. 2019;73:2299-306.

12. Zhao Q, Zhu Y, Xu Z, Cheng Z, Mei J, Chen X, et al. Effect of ticagrelor plus aspirin, ticagrelor alone, or aspirin alone on saphenous vein graft patency 1 year after coronary artery bypass grafting: a randomized clinical trial. JAMA. 2018;319:1677-86.

13. Levine GN, Bates ER, Bittl JA, Brindis RG, Fihn SD, Fleisher LA, et al. 2016 ACC/AHA guideline focused update on duration of dual anti-platelet therapy in patients with coronary artery dis- ease: a report of the American College of Cardiology/ American Heart Association Task Force on Clinical Practice Guidelines: an update of the 2011 ACCF/AHA/ SCAI guideline for percutaneous coronary intervention, 2011 ACCF/AHA guideline for coronary artery bypass graft surgery, 2012 ACC/AHA/ACP/AATS/PCNA/SCAI/ STS guideline for the diagnosis and management of patients with stable ischemic heart disease, 2013 ACCF/AHA guideline for the management of ST- elevation myocardial infarction, 2014 AHA/ACC guideline for the management of patients with non- ST-elevation acute coronary syndromes, and 2014 ACC/AHA guideline on perioperative cardiovascular evaluation and management of patients undergoing noncardiac surgery. J Am Coll Cardiol. 2016;68:1082-115.

Heart Failure

CHAPTER 27

Heart Failure: Definition and Types

INTRODUCTION

In 1988, Eugene Braunwald proposed a definition of heart failure (HF), which became the most quoted definition for heart failure over decades,—"A pathophysiological state in which an abnormality of cardiac function is responsible for the failure of the heart to pump blood at a rate commensurate with the requirements of the metabolizing tissues and/or to be able to do so only from an elevated filling pressure."[1] In 2016 European Society of Cardiology (ESC) guideline,[2] HF was defined as "HF is a clinical syndrome characterized by typical symptoms (e.g., breathlessness, ankle swelling and fatigue) that may be accompanied by signs (e.g., elevated jugular venous pressure, pulmonary crackles and peripheral edema) caused by a structural and/or functional cardiac abnormality, resulting in a reduced cardiac output and/or elevated intracardiac pressures at rest or during stress." In 2001, Coronel et al. expressed —"heart failure is the label for a cardiovascular syndrome that is lacking uniform criteria for definition."[3] Then, it takes 2 decades to get a universal definition of HF. In a recent landmark event in HF, the society for HF around the world proposed[4] a universal definition of HF,— "a clinical syndrome with symptoms and/or signs caused by a structural and/or functional cardiac abnormality and corroborated by elevated natriuretic peptide levels and/or objective evidence of pulmonary or systemic congestion."

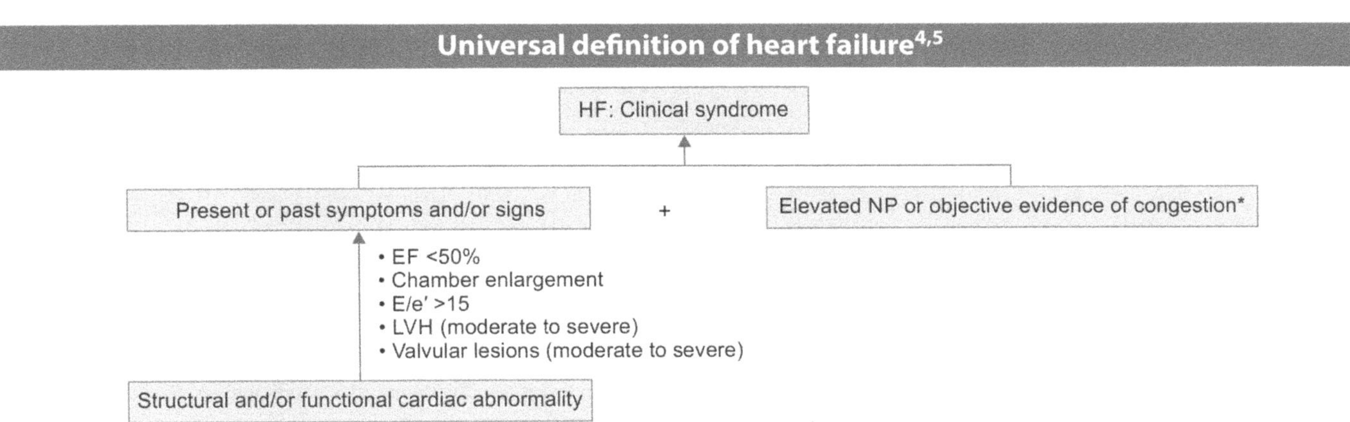

*Objective evidence of congestion: X-ray chest/elevated filling pressure by echocardiogram/or hemodynamic measurement at rest or with exercise.

(EF: ejection fraction; HF: heart failure; LVH: left ventricular hypertrophy; NP: natriuretic peptide)

Staging of heart failure[4,5]

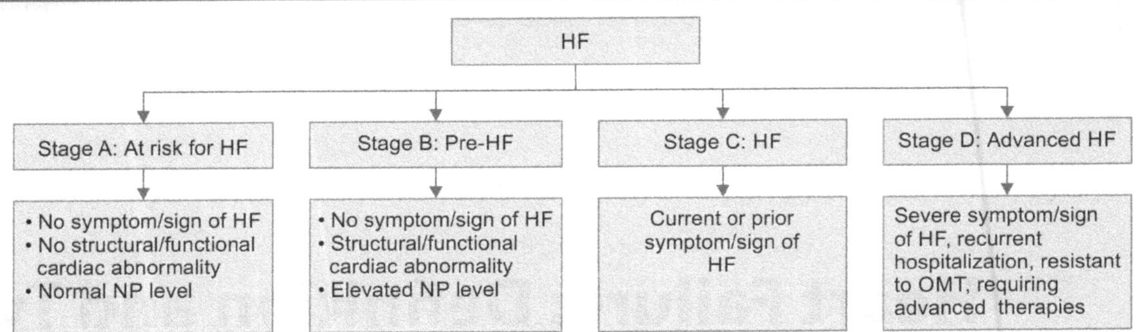

(HF: heart failure; NP: natriuretic peptide; OMT: osteopathic manipulation treatment)

Different heart failure types according to left ventricular ejection fraction: Universal heart failure definition[4,5]

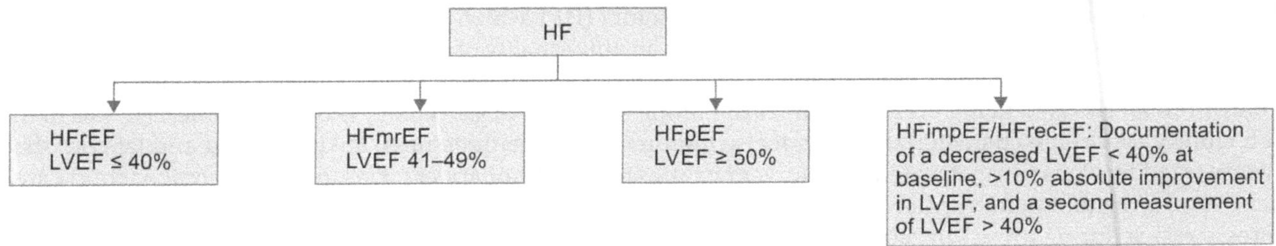

(HF: heart failure; HFrEF: heart failure with reduced ejection fraction; HFmrEF: heart failure with mildly reduced or midrange ejection fraction; HFpEF: heart failure with preserved ejection fraction; HFimpEF: heart failure with improved ejection fraction; HFrecEF: heart failure with recovered ejection fraction; LVEF: left ventricular ejection fraction)

Different heart failure types according to left ventricular ejection fraction: Lamp and Solomon[6]

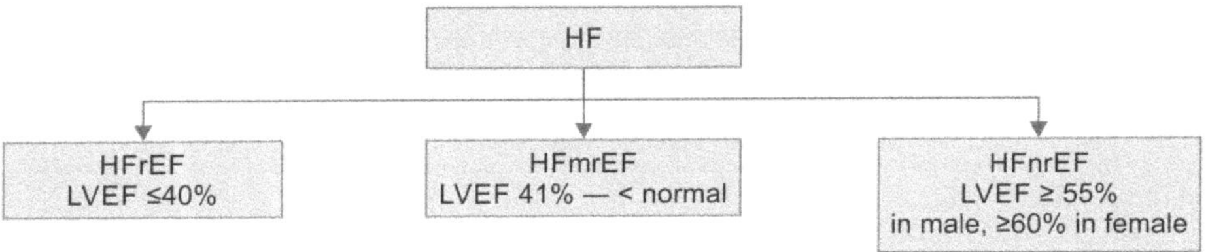

(HF: heart failure; HFrEF: heart failure with reduced ejection fraction; HFnrEF: heart failure with normal range ejection fraction; HFmrEF: heart failure with mildly reduced or midrange ejection fraction)

REFERENCES

1. Braunwald E. Clinical manifestations of heart failure. Heart Disease: A Textbook of Cardiovascular Medicine. In: Braunwald E (Ed). Pennsylvania: Saunders; 1988. pp. 471-84.
2. Ponikowski P, Voors AA, Anker SD, Bueno H, Cleland JGF, Coats AJS, et al. 2016 ESC Guidelines for the diagnosis and treatment of acute and chronic heart failure: the Task Force for the diagnosis and treatment of acute and chronic heart failure of the European Society of Cardiology (ESC) Developed with the special contribution of the Heart Failure Association (HFA) of the ESC. Eur Heart J. 2016;37:2129-200.
3. Coronel R, de Groot JR, van Lieshout JJ. Defining heart failure. Cardiovasc Res. 2001;50(3):419-22.
4. Bozkurt B, Coats A, Tsutsui H, Abdelhamid CM, Adamopoulos S, Albert N, et al. Universal definition and classification of heart failure: a report of the Heart Failure Society of America, Heart Failure Association of the European Society of Cardiology, Japanese Heart Failure Society and Writing Committee of the Universal Definition of Heart Failure: Endorsed by the Canadian Heart Failure Society, Heart Failure Association of India, Cardiac Society of Australia and New Zealand, and Chinese Heart Failure Association. Eur J Heart Fail. 2021;23:352-80.
5. 2022 AHA/ACC/HFSA Guideline for the Management of Heart Failure: A Report of the American College of Cardiology/American Heart Association Joint Committee on Clinical Practice Guidelines. J Am Coll Cardiol 2022;145:e895-e1032.
6. LAM CSP, Solomon SD. Classification of heart failure according to ejection fraction: JACC review topic of the week. J Am Coll Cardiol. 2021;77(25):3217-25.

CHAPTER 28

Heart Failure: Clinical Assessment

INTRODUCTION

As heart failure (HF) is a syndrome, clinical examination plays a contributory role in diagnostic workup. Both the components of HF, congestion and perfusion can be optimally assessed at bedside.

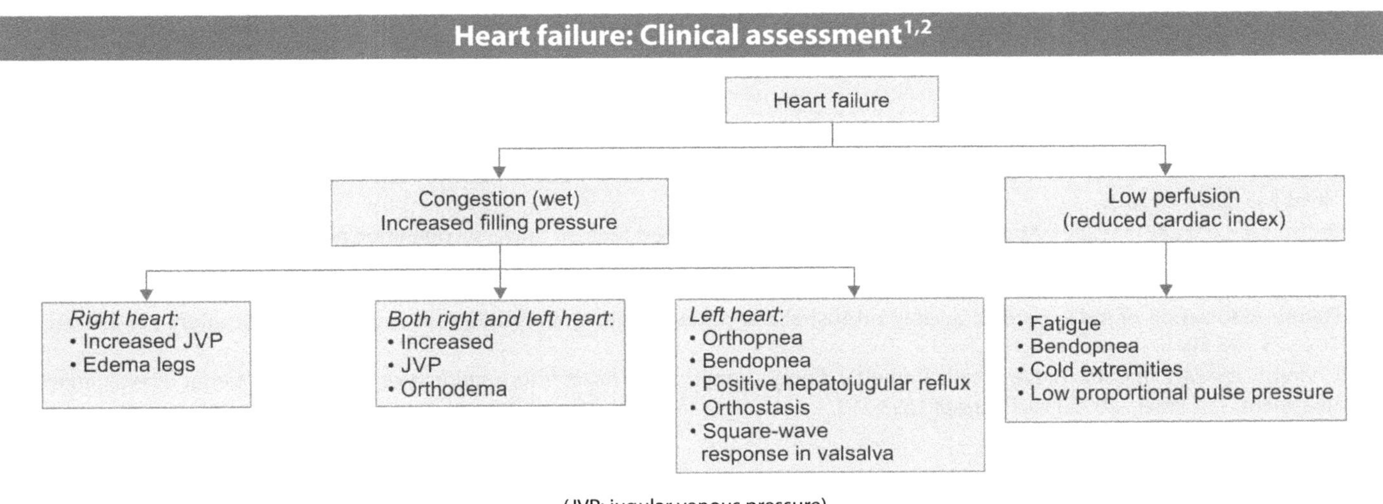

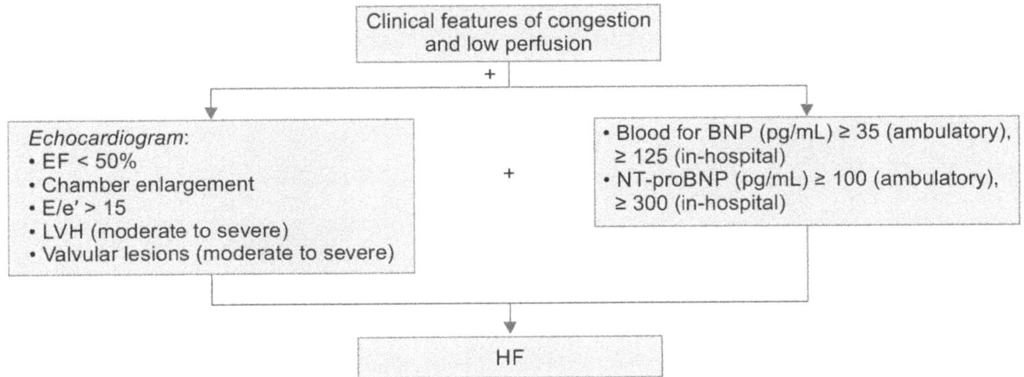

(BNP: brain natriuretic peptide; EF: ejection fraction; HF: heart failure; NT-proBNP: N-terminal pro-brain natriuretic peptide)

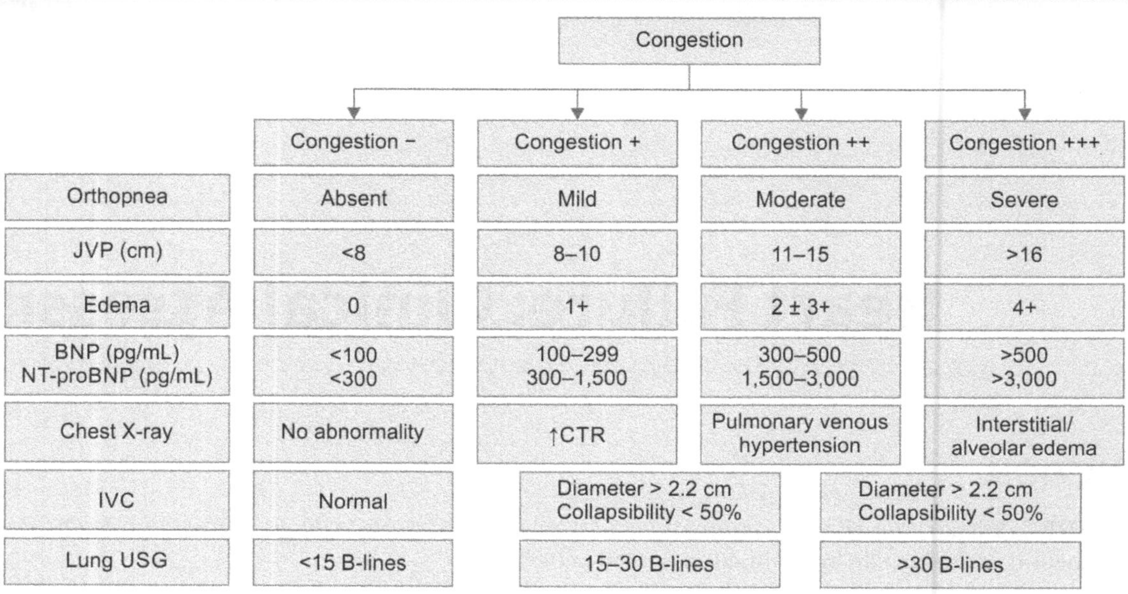

(BNP: brain natriuretic peptide; IVC: inferior vena cava; JVP: jugular venous pressure; NT-proBNP: N-terminal pro-brain natriuretic peptide; USG: ultrasonography)

REFERENCES

1. Sarkar A. Bedside cardiology, 2nd edition. New Delhi: Jaypee Brothers Medical Publishers; 2020.
2. Drazner MH, Hellkamp AS, Leier CV, et al. Value of clinician assessment of hemodynamics in advanced heart failure: the ESCAPE trial. Circ Heart Fail. 2008;1:170-7.
3. Bozkurt B, Coats A, Tsutsui H, Abdelhamid CM, Adamopoulos S, Albert N, et al. Universal definition and classification of heart failure: a report of the Heart Failure Society of America, Heart Failure Association of the European Society of Cardiology, Japanese Heart Failure Society and Writing Committee of the Universal Definition of Heart Failure: Endorsed by the Canadian Heart Failure Society, Heart Failure Association of India, Cardiac Society of Australia and New Zealand, and Chinese Heart Failure Association. Eur J Heart Fail. 2021;23:352-80.
4. Gheorghiade M, Filippatos G, De Luca L, Burnett J. Congestion in acute heart failure syndromes: an essential target of evaluation and treatment. Am J Med. 2006;119(12 Suppl 1):S3-S10.

CHAPTER 29

Management of Heart Failure with Reduced Ejection Fraction

INTRODUCTION

Either ARNI/ACEI/ARB (angiotensin receptor-neprilysin inhibitor/angiotensin-converting enzyme inhibitor/angiotensin receptor blocker) or beta-blocker can be started as a disease-modifying initial agent. Both can be started simultaneously. ARNI/ACEI/ARB is preferred to initiate in congested (wet) state, whereas beta-blocker is preferred in dry state.[1] ARN inhibitor is the drug of choice in ARNI/ACEI/ARB group. Initiation directly without pretreatment with ACEI/ARB is safe and effective.[2] Washout time is required only from switching from ACEI to ARNI and not required for ARB. When blood pressure is at the lower side (around 100 mm Hg), ARNI/ACEI/ARB should be uptitrated cautiously and doses of diuretic should be tried to lower down considering dry and wet status of the patient. Evidenced-based beta-blockers are Carvedilol, Metoprolol, and Bisoprolol. Sodium-glucose cotransporter-2 (SGLT-2) inhibitor induces natriuresis and osmotic diuresis, reduces arterial pressure, stiffness, and ventricular preload and afterload. It also shifts to ketone-based myocardial metabolism.[3] Regarding diuretics, any of the loop diuretics, Furosemide, Torsemide, or Bumetanide, can be initiated. Torsemide and Bumetanide have predictable and better bioavailability over Furosemide. Moreover, Torsemide may have a favorable effect in mitigating myocardial fibrosis as compared to Furosemide.[4] Soluble guanylate cyclase and myosin activator are the emerging molecules for heart failure **(Fig. 1)**.

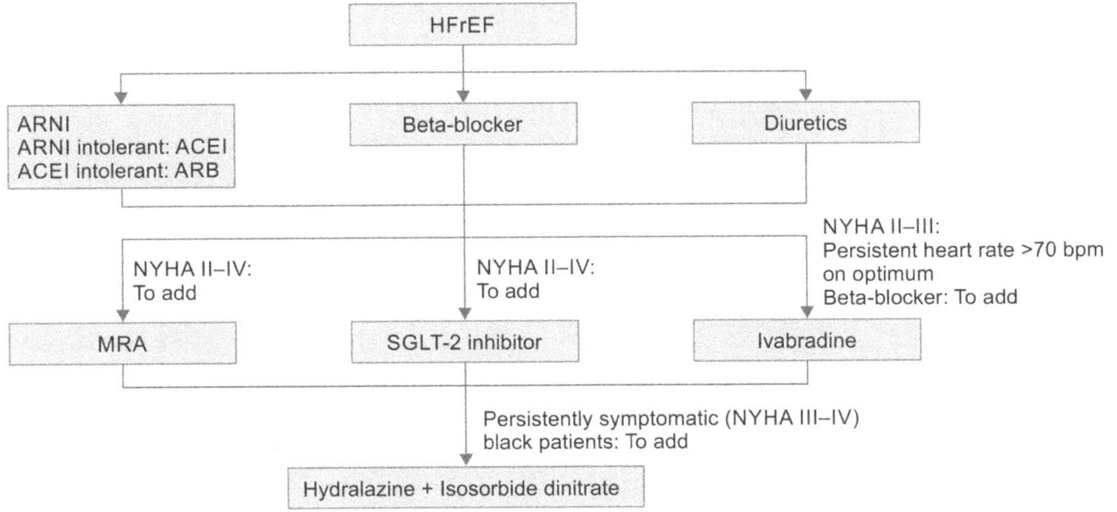

(ACEI: angiotensin-converting enzyme inhibitor; ARB: angiotensin receptor blocker; ARNI: angiotensin receptor-neprilysin inhibitor; HFrEF: heart failure with reduced ejection fraction; MRA: mineralocorticoid receptor antagonist; NYHA: New York Heart Association; SGLT-2: sodium-glucose cotransporter-2)

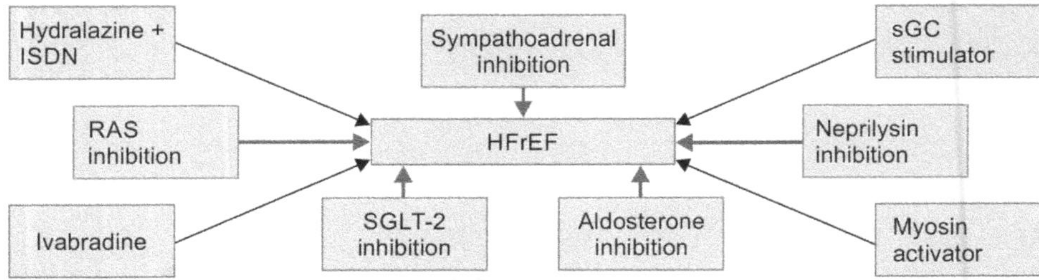

Fig. 1: Inner boxes showing disease-modifying agents used in all patients in HFrEF, outer boxes showing other agents used in selected patients. sGC and myosin activator are under investigation.[6]

(HFrEF: heart failure with reduced ejection fraction; ISDN: isosorbide dinitrate; RAS: renin–angiotensin system; sGC: soluble guanylate cyclase; SGLT-2: sodium-glucose cotransporter-2)

How to initiate angiotensin receptor-neprilysin inhibitor[5]

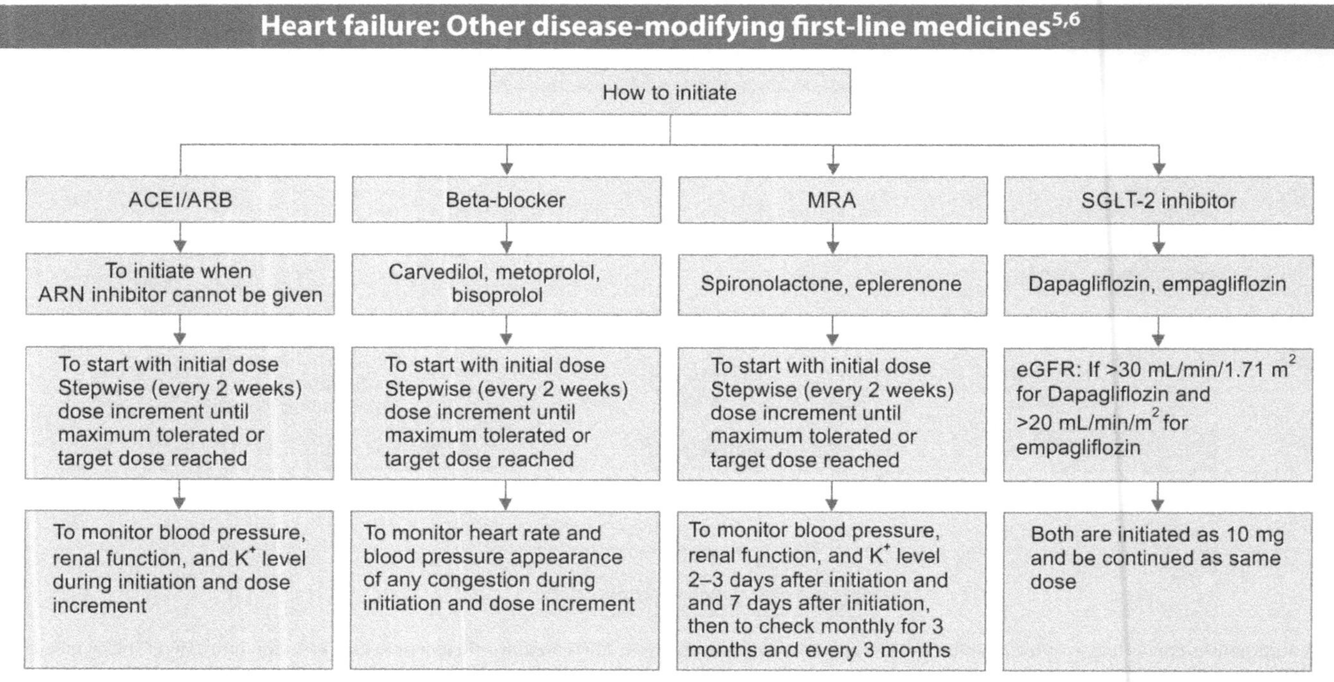

(ACEI: angiotensin-converting enzyme inhibitor; ARB: angiotensin receptor blocker; ARNI: angiotensin receptor-neprilysin inhibitor)

Heart failure: Other disease-modifying first-line medicines[5,6]

How to initiate			
ACEI/ARB	**Beta-blocker**	**MRA**	**SGLT-2 inhibitor**
To initiate when ARN inhibitor cannot be given	Carvedilol, metoprolol, bisoprolol	Spironolactone, eplerenone	Dapagliflozin, empagliflozin
To start with initial dose Stepwise (every 2 weeks) dose increment until maximum tolerated or target dose reached	To start with initial dose Stepwise (every 2 weeks) dose increment until maximum tolerated or target dose reached	To start with initial dose Stepwise (every 2 weeks) dose increment until maximum tolerated or target dose reached	eGFR: If >30 mL/min/1.71 m^2 for Dapagliflozin and >20 mL/min/m^2 for empagliflozin
To monitor blood pressure, renal function, and K$^+$ level during initiation and dose increment	To monitor heart rate and blood pressure appearance of any congestion during initiation and dose increment	To monitor blood pressure, renal function, and K$^+$ level 2–3 days after initiation and and 7 days after initiation, then to check monthly for 3 months and every 3 months	Both are initiated as 10 mg and be continued as same dose

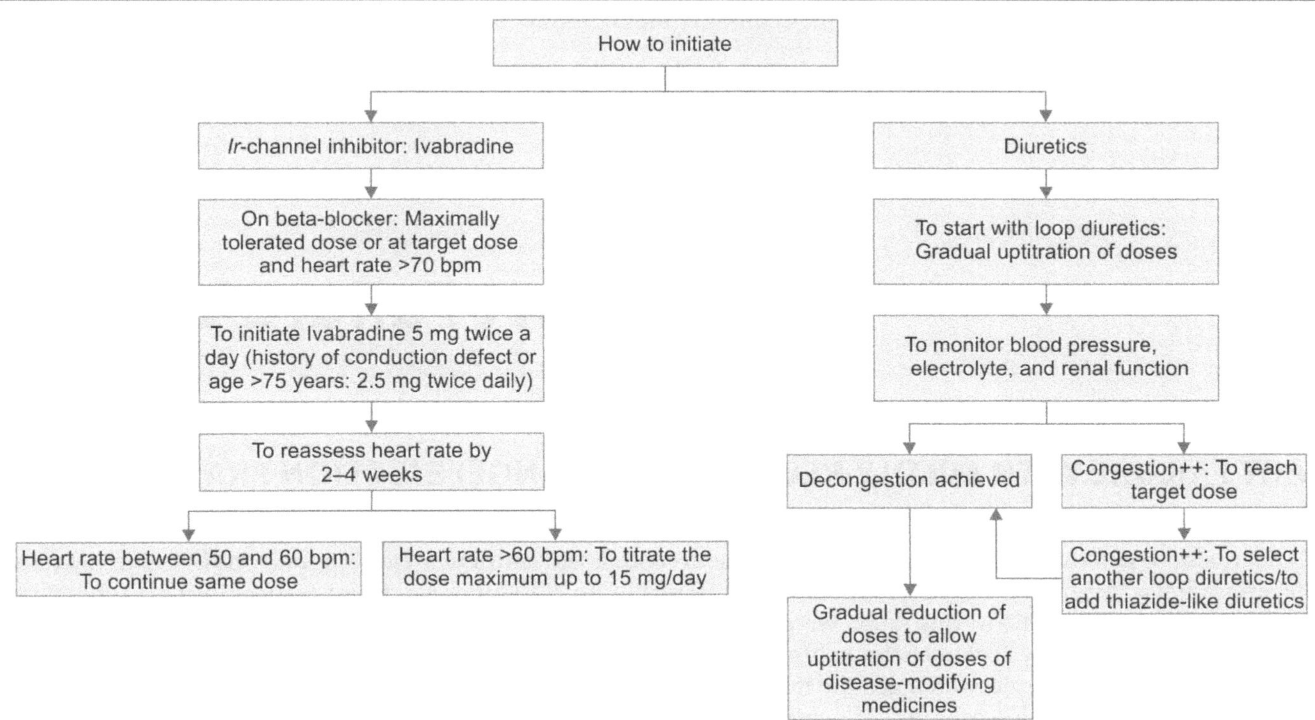

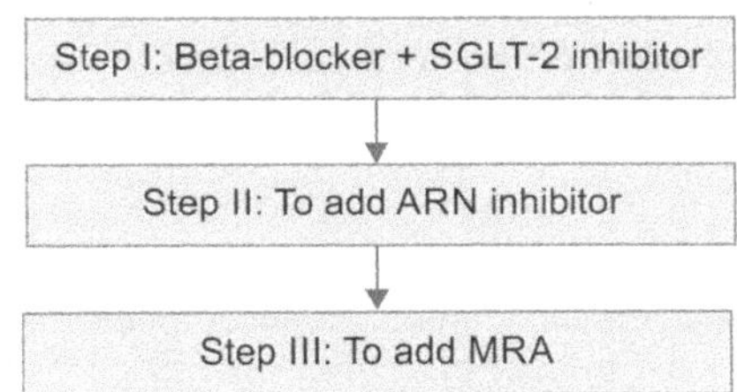

Note: All the steps, after initiation of therapy should be achieved within 4 weeks. Uptitration of individual agent should be started thereafter.

(ARN: angiotensin receptor-neprilysin; MRA: mineralocorticoid receptor antagonist; SGLT-2: sodium-glucose cotransporter-2)

REFERENCES

1. Maddox TM, Januzzi JL Jr, Allen LA, Breathett K, Butler J, Davis LL, et al. 2021 Update to the 2017 ACC Expert Consensus Decision Pathway for Optimization of Heart Failure Treatment: Answers to 10 Pivotal Issues About Heart Failure With Reduced Ejection Fraction. A Report of the American College of Cardiology Solution Set Oversight Committee. J Am Coll Cardiol. 2021;77:772-810.
2. Myhre PL, Vaduganathan M, Claggett B, Packer M, Desai AS, Rouleau JL, et al. B-type natriuretic peptide during treatment with sacubitril/valsartan: the PARADIGM-HF trial. J Am Coll Cardiol. 2019;73:1264-72.
3. Zelniker TA, Braunwald E. Mechanisms of cardiorenal effects of sodium-glucose cotransporter 2 inhibitors: JACC state-of-the-art review. J Am Coll Cardiol. 2020;75:422-34.
4. Lopez B, Querejeta R, Gonzalez A, Sanchez E, Larman M, Diez J. Effects of loop diuretics on myocardial fibrosis and collagen type I turnover in chronic heart failure. J Am Coll Cardiol 2004;43:2028-35.
5. Bozkurt B, Coats A, Tsutsui H. Universal definition and classification of heart failure: a report of the Heart Failure Society of America, Heart Failure Association of the European Society of Cardiology, Japanese Heart Failure Society and Writing Committee of the Universal Definition of Heart Failure: Endorsed by the Canadian Heart Failure Society, Heart Failure Association of India, Cardiac Society of Australia and New Zealand, and Chinese Heart Failure Association. Eur J Heart Fail. 2021;23:352-80.
6. Bhatt AS, Abraham WT, Lindenfeld J, Bristow M, Carson PE, Felker GM, et al. Treatment of HF in the ere of multiple therapies. J Am Coll Cardiol. HF 2021;9:1-12.
7. McMurray JJV, Packer M. How Should We Sequence the Treatments for Heart Failure and a Reduced Ejection Fraction? A Redefinition of Evidence-Based Medicine. Circulation 2021;143:875-7.

CHAPTER 30

Heart Failure Variants

HEART FAILURE WITH MILDLY REDUCED (MIDRANGE) EJECTION FRACTION

Heart failure with midrange ejection fraction (HFmrEF) was first introduced in 2016 European Society of Cardiology (ESC) heart failure guideline.[1] They described that "Patients with a left ventricular ejection fraction (LVEF) in the range of 40–49% represent a "grey area," which we now define as HFmrEF." In 2013 American Heart Association (AHA) heart failure guideline,[2] patients with LVEF in this range were described as borderline HFpEF (heart failure with preserved ejection fraction). Australian and New Zealand heart failure guidelines did not recognize HFmrEF as a clearly defined syndrome.[3] In 2021, several heart failure societies changed the terminology from "midrange" to "mildly reduced."[4]

HFmrEF is a heterogeneous condition in which only 33–35% of patients remain in this range of ejection fraction (EF) over a long-term follow-up. 25–37% of patients from this category are reclassified as heart failure with reduced ejection fraction (HFrEF) and 25–33% of patients are reclassified as HFpEF. The prevalence of HFmrEF in the heart failure population is 14–24%[5] with female dominance along with a common history of hypertension and atrial fibrillation. HFmrEF is also associated with an increased titer of biomarkers of heart failure, including biomarker of myocardial stretch (natriuretic peptide) and biomarker of inflammation, endothelin-1 and galectin-3. The 1-year mortality rate of HFmrEF (7.6%) is intermediate as compared to HFrEF (8.8%) and HFpEF (6.4%).

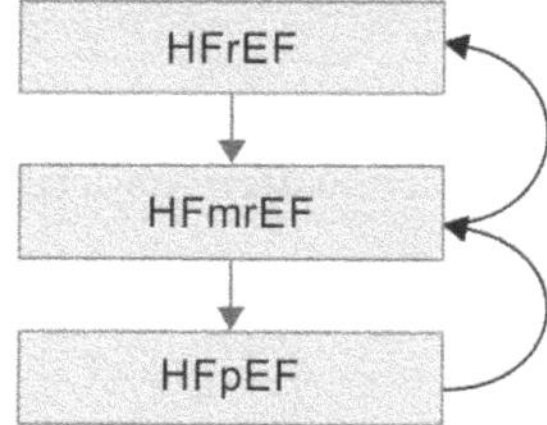

(HFpEF: heart failure with preserved ejection fraction; HFmrEF: heart failure with midrange ejection fraction; HFrEF: heart failure with reduced ejection fraction)

(ACEI: angiotensin converting enzyme inhibitor; ARB: angiotensin receptor blocker; ARNI: angiotensin receptor-neprilysin inhibitor; HFmrEF: heart failure with midrange ejection fraction; MRA: mineralocorticoid receptor antagonist; SGLT-2: sodium-glucose cotransporter-2)

HEART FAILURE WITH RECOVERED/IMPROVED EJECTION FRACTION

Heart failure with recovered ejection fraction (HFrecEF) has been defined in the Journal of Applied Analysis and Computation (JAAC) scientific expert panel[11] as "(1) documentation of a decreased LVEF <40% at baseline; (2) ≥10% absolute improvement in LVEF; and (3) a second measurement of LVEF >40%. These improvements in LVEF are typically accompanied by a reduction in LV volumes." Gulati et al.[12] preferred the word "improved" [heart failure with improved ejection fraction (HFimpEF)] in place of "recovered" because "it highlights two important features of this clinical entity: (1) despite having very improved or even normalized LVEF, these patients may continue to have clinical HF and abnormal biomarker signs of functional impairment and (2) the improvement experienced by these patients does not necessarily reflect recovery from their underlying structural cardiomyopathic process." In the consensus statement[4] of a universal definition of heart failure, the term HFimpEF has been used.

Improvement in LVEF is associated with reduction in left ventricular end-diastolic volume, indicating reverse remodeling, the extent of which is directly related to improvement in cardiac survival. The improvement or recovery may occur either spontaneously in selected cases or after guideline-directed medical therapy (GDMT) or device therapy. Only 9% of 4,500 patients in Val-heFT (Valsartan Heart Failure *Trial)*[13] experienced improvement in EF > 40% in the first 12 months. In MADIT-CRT (multicenter automatic defibrillator implantation trial with cardiac resynchronization therapy) trial,[14] 79% of patients had improvement of EF to 36–50%, but only 7% had improvement of EF above 50%. Clinical outcome is better in HFimpEF than in HFrEF with 5-year survival being 80–90% as compared to 65–75% in HFrEF.[15] Reverse remodeling alters the genetic expression of contractile protein in cardiac resynchronization therapy (CRT)-responder with decreased expression of beta-myosin heavy chain with increased expression of alpha-myosin heavy chain and phospholamban.[16] Natural history of HFiEF indicates that a significant proportion of patients will develop recurrent heart failure with deterioration of LVEF. This is because many of HFiEF patients retain the molecular features of failing heart and reverse remodeling state represents just a less pathological platform, from where patients may be drifted to the downhill platform.

In the open-label randomized pilot TRED-HF (withdrawal of pharmacological treatment for heart failure in patients with recovered dilated cardiomyopathy) trial, GDMT was withdrawn in patients with HFimpEF in whom 80% develop recurrence of heart failure, defined by a fall in LVEF > 10% to <50%, an increase in left ventricular end-diastolic volume > 10% to greater than the normal range, a doubling of the N-terminal pro-brain natriuretic peptide (NT-proBNP) to > 400 ng/L, or clinical evidence of HF.[17] Arrhythmic risk remains high in patients with recovered EF with a 3.3% per year rate of appropriate implantable cardioverter-defibrillator (ICD) therapy among patients with LVEF > 45%.[18]

Pathological states where reverse remodeling may happen

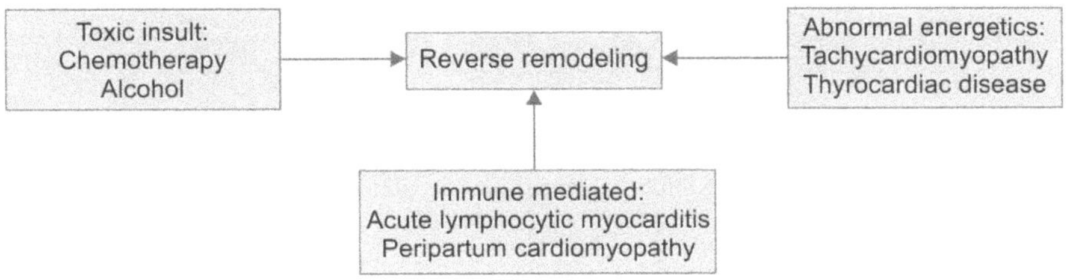

Factors favoring reverse remodeling

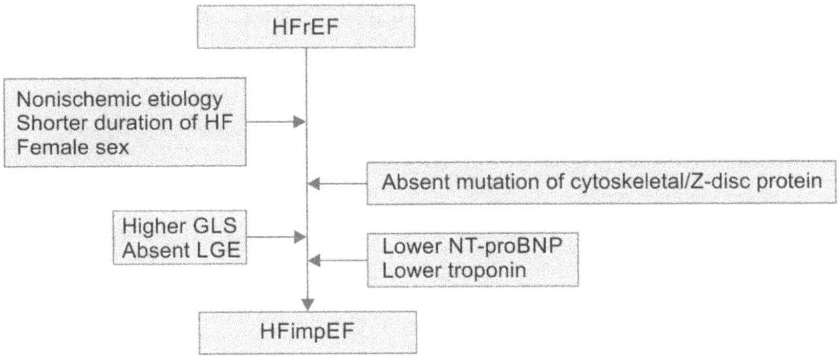

(HF: heart failure; HFimpEF: heart failure with improved ejection fraction; HFrEF: heart failure with reduced ejection fraction; GLS: global longitudinal strain; LGE: late gadolinium enhancement; NT-proBNP: N-terminal pro-brain natriuretic peptide)

What associations may convert heart failure with improved EF state again to reduced EF state

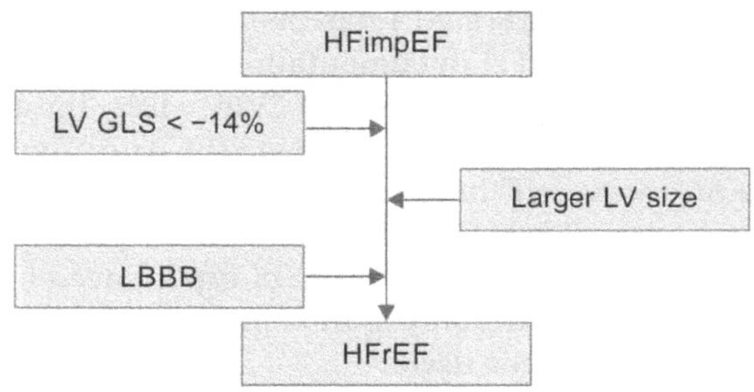

(HFimpEF: heart failure with improved ejection fraction; HFrEF: heart failure with reduced ejection fraction; LBBB: left bundle branch block; LV: left ventricular; LV GLS: left ventricular global longitudinal strain)

Follow-up in patients with HFimpEF

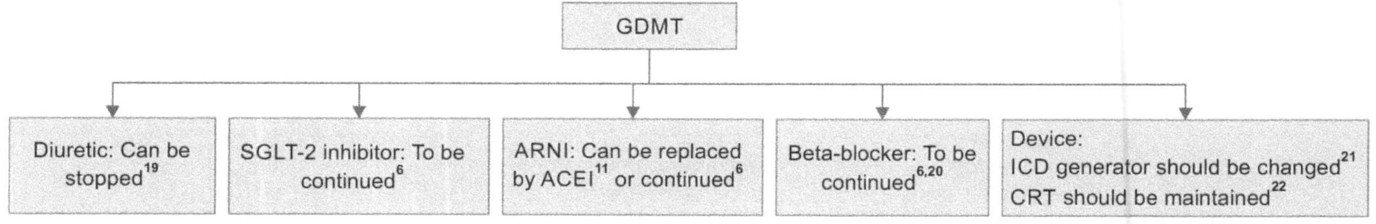

(CMR: cardiac magnetic resonance; ECG: electrocardiogram; LGE: late gadolinium enhancement; NT-proBNP: N-terminal pro-brain natriuretic peptide)

Should guideline-directed medical therapy and device to be continued in heart failure with improved EF?

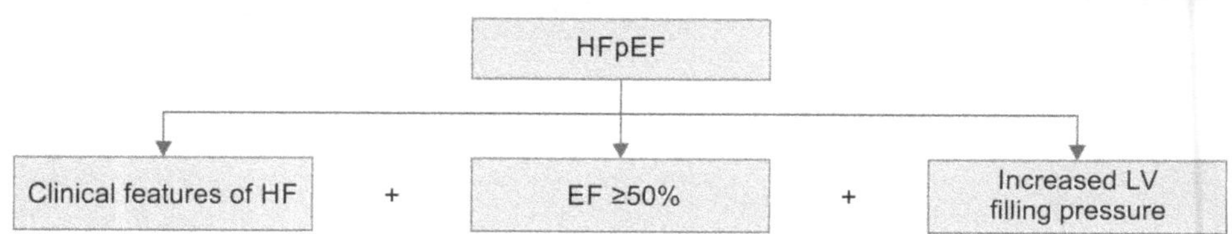

(ACEI: angiotensin-converting enzyme inhibitors; ARNI: angiotensin receptor-neprilysin inhibitors; CRT: cardiac resynchronization therapy; GDMT: guideline-directed medical therapy; ICD: implantable cardioverter defibrillator; SGLT-2: sodium-glucose cotransporter-2)

HEART FAILURE WITH PRESERVED EJECTION FRACTION

There is no consensus on what is preserved. In the last ESC guideline,[7] HFpEF has been defined as heart failure with EF[3] 50%. In the CHARM (candesartan in heart failure assessment of reduction in mortality and morbidity) study,[23] HFpEF was defined as EF >40%. An entity of heart failure with normal EF (male > 55% and female > 60%) has also been described[24] as heart failure with normal range ejection fraction (HFnrEF).

Heart failure with preserved EF: Definition[6]

(EF: ejection fraction; HF: heart failure; HFpEF: heart failure preserved ejection failure; LV: left ventricular)

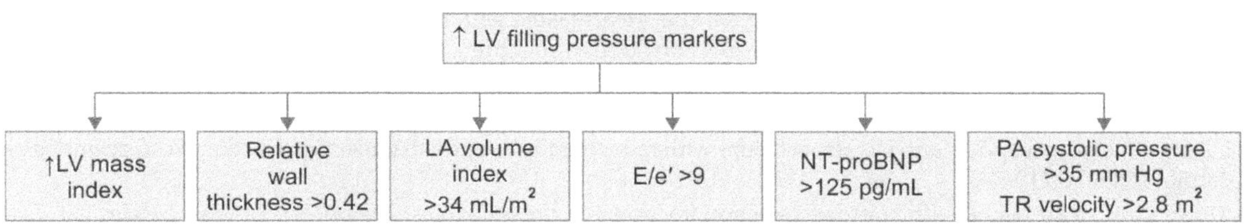

(LA: left atrial; LV: left ventricular; NT-proBNP: N-terminal pro-brain natriuretic peptide; TR: tricuspid regurgitation)

Management of heart failure with preserved EF[6,7]

HFpEF

Primary prevention:
Hypertension management
Statin in CVD and in high-risk CVD
SGLT-2 inhibitors in DM with high-risk CVD or CVD
Exercise, cessation of smoking
To avoid alcohol abuse, weight reduction

Management

Diuretics, preferably loop diuretics: Recommended

SGLT-2 inhibitor: Can be beneficial

MRA: May be considered in patients with LVEF on the lower end of spectrum

ARB: May be considered in patients with LVEF on the lower end of spectrum

ARNI: May be considered in patients with LVEF on the lower end of spectrum

(ARB: angiotensin-receptor blocker; ARNI: angiotensin receptor neprilysin inhibitor; CVD: cardiovascular disease; DM: diabetes mellitus; HFpEF: heart failure preserved ejection failure; LVEF: left ventricular ejection fraction; MRA: mineralocorticoid receptor antagonists; SGLT-2: sodium-glucose cotransporter-2)

REFERENCES

1. Ponikowski P, Voors AA, Anker SD, Bueno H, Cleland JGF, Coats AJS, et al. 2016 ESC Guidelines for the diagnosis and treatment of acute and chronic heart failure: the Task Force for the diagnosis and treatment of acute and chronic heart failure of the European Society of Cardiology (ESC) Developed with the special contribution of the Heart Failure Association (HFA) of the ESC. Eur Heart J. 2016;37:2129-200.

2. Yancy CW, Jessup M, Bozkurt B, Butler J, Casey DE Jr, Drazner MH, et al. 2013 ACCF/AHA guideline for the management of heart failure: a report of the American College of Car- diology Foundation/American Heart Association Task Force on Practice Guidelines. J Am Coll Cardiol. 2013;62:e147-239.

3. Atherton JJ, Sindone A, De Pasquale CG, , Driscoll A, MacDonald PS, Hopper I, et al.; NHFA CSANZ Heart Failure Guidelines Working Group. National Heart Foundation of Australia and Cardiac Society of Australia and New Zealand: guidelines for the prevention, detection, and management of heart failure in Australia 2018. Heart Lung Circ. 2018;27:1123-208.

4. Bozkurt B, Coats A, Tsutsui H, Abdelhamid CM, Adamopoulos S, Albert N, et al. Universal definition and classification of heart failure: a report of the Heart Failure Society of America, Heart Failure Association of the European Society of Cardiology, Japanese Heart Failure Society and Writing Committee of the Universal Definition of Heart Failure: Endorsed by the Canadian Heart Failure Society, Heart Failure Association of India, Cardiac Society of Australia and New Zealand, and Chinese Heart Failure Association. Eur J Heart Fail. 2021;23:352-80.

5. Koh AS, Tay WT, Teng THK, Vedin O, Benson L, Dahlstrom U, et al. A comprehensive population-based characterization of heart failure with mid-range ejection fraction. Eur J Heart Fail. 2017;19:1624–34.

6. Heidenreich PA, Bozkurt B, Aguilar D, Allen LA, Byun JJ, Colvin MM, et al. 2022 AHA/ACC/HFSA Guideline for the Management of Heart Failure: A Report of the American College of Cardiology/American Heart Association Joint Committee on Clinical Practice Guidelines. J Am Coll Cardiol. 2022;145:e895-e1032.

7. McDonagh TA, Metra M, Adamo M, Gardner RS, Baumbach A, Böhm M, et al; ESC Scientific Document Group. 2021 ESC Guidelines for the diagnosis and treatment of acute and chronic heart failure. Eur Heart J. 2021;42(36):3599-726.

8. Cleland JG. Beta-blockers for heart failure with reduced, mid-range, and preserved ejection fraction: an individual patient-level analysis of double-blind randomized trials. Eur Heart J. 2018;39:26-35.

9. Lund LH, Claggett B, Liu J, Lam CS, Jhund PS, Rosano GM, et al. Heart failure with mid-range ejection fraction in CHARM: characteristics, outcomes and effect of candesartan across the entire ejection fraction spectrum. Eur J Heart Fail. 2018;20:1230-9.

10. Solomon SD, Claggett B, Lewis EF, Desai A, Anand I, Sweitzer NK, et al; TOPCAT Investigators. Influence of ejection fraction on outcomes and efficacy of spironolactone in patients with heart failure with preserved ejection fraction. Eur Heart J. 2016;37:455-62.

11. Wilcox JE, Fang JC, Margulies KB, Mann DL. Heart failure with recovered left ventricular ejection fraction-JAAC scientific expert panel. J Am Coll Cardiol. 2020;76:719-34.

12. Gulati G, Udelson JE. Heart failure with improved ejection fraction: Is it possible to escape one's past? JAAC: Heart fail. 2018;6:725-33.

13. Florea VG, Rector TS, Anand IS, Cohn JN. Heart failure with improved ejection fraction: clinical characteristics, correlates of recovery, and survival: results from the Valsartan Heart Failure Trial. Circ Heart Fail. 2016;9:e003123.

14. Ruwald MH, Solomon SD, Foster E, Kutyifa V, Ruwald AC, Sherazi S, et al. Left ventricular ejection fraction normalization in cardiac resynchronization therapy and risk of ventricular arrhythmias and clinical outcomes: results from the Multicenter Automatic Defibrillator Implantation Trial with Cardiac Resynchronization Therapy (MADIT-CRT) trial. Circulation. 2014;130:2278-86.

15. Lupón J, Díez-López C, de Antonio M, Domingo M, Zamora E, Moliner P, et al. Recovered heart failure with reduced ejection fraction and outcomes: a prospective study. Eur J Heart Fail. 2017;19:1615-23.

16. Vanderheyden M, Mullens W, Delrue L, Goethals M, de Bruyne B, Wijns W, et al. Myocardial gene expression in heart failure patients treated with cardiac resynchronization therapy responders versus nonresponders. J Am Coll Cardiol. 2008;51:129-36.

17. Halliday BP, Wassall R, Lota AS, Khalique Z, Gregson J, Newsome S, et al. Withdrawal of pharmacological treatment for heart failure in patients with recovered dilated cardiomyopathy (TRED-HF): an open-label, pilot, randomised trial. Lancet. 2019;393:61-73.

18. Smer A, Saurav A, Azzouz MS, Salih M, Ayan M, Abuzaid A, et al. Meta-analysis of risk of ventricular arrhythmias after improvement in left ventricular ejection fraction during follow-up in patients with primary prevention implantable cardioverter defibrillators. Am J Cardiol. 2017;120:279-86.

19. Wilcox J, Yancy CW. Stopping medication for heart failure with improved ejection fraction. Lancet. 2019;393:8-10.

20. Waagstein F, Caidahl K, Wallentin I, Bergh CH, Hjalmarson A. Long-term beta-blockade in dilated cardiomyopathy. Effects of short- and long-term metoprolol treatment followed by withdrawal and readministration of metoprolol. Circulation. 1989;80:551-63.

21. Thomas IC, Wang Y, See VY, Minges KE, Curtis JP, Hsu JC. Outcomes following implantable cardioverter-defibrillator generator replacement in patients with recovered left ventricular systolic function: the National Cardiovascular Data Registry. Heart Rhythm. 2019;16:733-40.

22. Yu CM, Chau E, Sanderson JE, Fan K, Tang MO, Fung WH, et al. Tissue Doppler echocardiographic evidence of reverse remodeling and improved synchronicity by simultaneously delaying regional contraction after biventricular pacing therapy in heart failure. Circulation. 2002;105:438-45.

23. Pfeffer MA, Swedberg K, Granger CB, Held P, McMurray JJ, Michelson EL, et al.; CHARM Investigators and Committees. Effects of candesartan on mortality and morbidity in patients with chronic heart failure: the CHARM-Overall programme. Lancet. 2003;362:759-66.

24. LAM CSP, Solomon SD. Classification of Heart Failure According to Ejection Fraction. J Am Coll Cardiol. 2021;77:3217-25.

CHAPTER 31

Advanced Heart Failure

INTRODUCTION

Advanced heart failure is a clinical state, characterised by persistent and progressive severe symptoms and ventricular dysfunction despite guideline directed medical therapy. Advanced heart failure affects 0.5% of population with a prevalence of 5% among hospitalised patients.

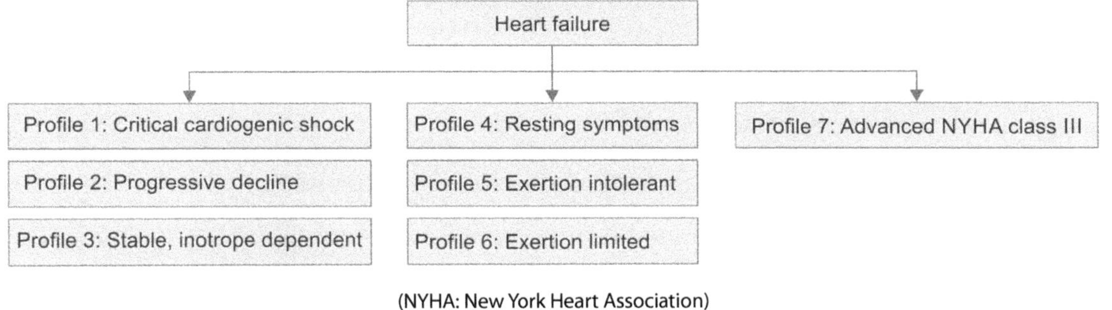

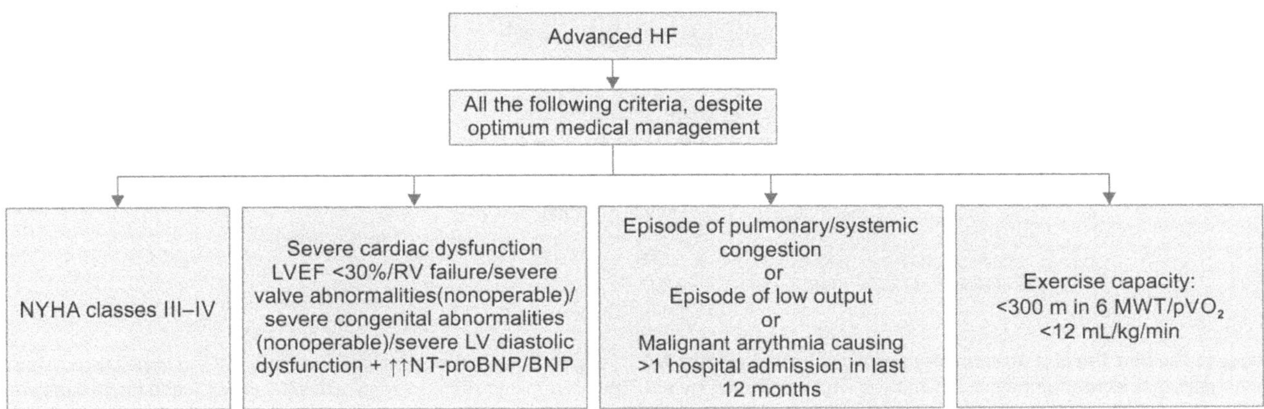

(BNP: brain natriuretic peptide; HF: heart failure; LVEF: left ventricular ejection fraction; MWT: minute walk test; N-proBNP: N-terminal pro-brain natriuretic peptide; NYHA: New York Heart Association; pVO₂: peak oxygen uptake; RV: right ventricular)

Management of advanced heart failure[2,3]

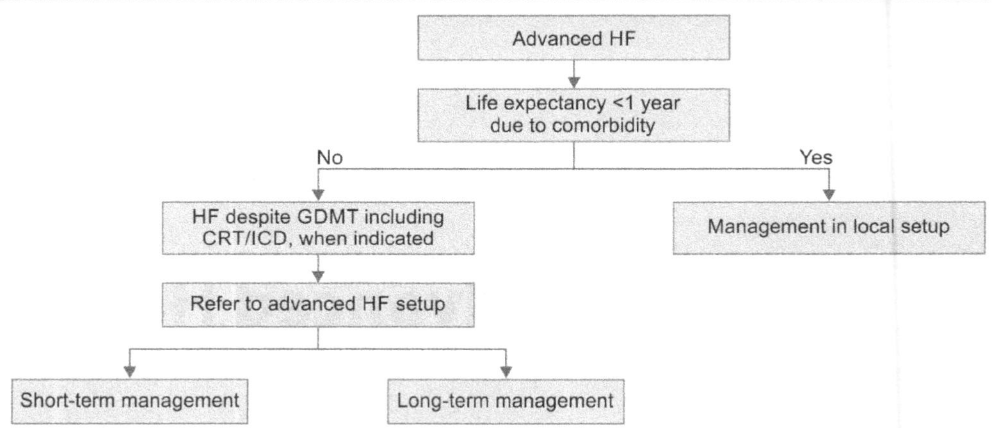

(CRT: cardiac resynchronization therapy; GDMT: guideline directed medical therapy; HF: heart failure; ICD: implantable cardioverter-defibrillator)

Management of advanced heart failure: Short-term management[2,3]

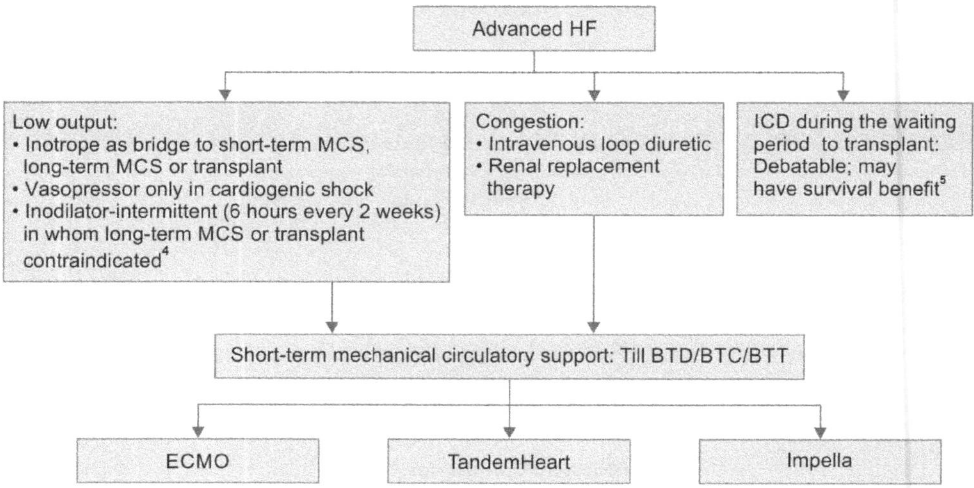

(BTC: bridge to candidacy; BTD: bridge to decision; BTT: bridge to transplant; ECMO: extracorporeal membrane oxygenation; HF: heart failure; ICD: implantable cardioverter-defibrillator; MCS: mechanical circulatory support)

Management of advanced heart failure: Long-term management[2,3]

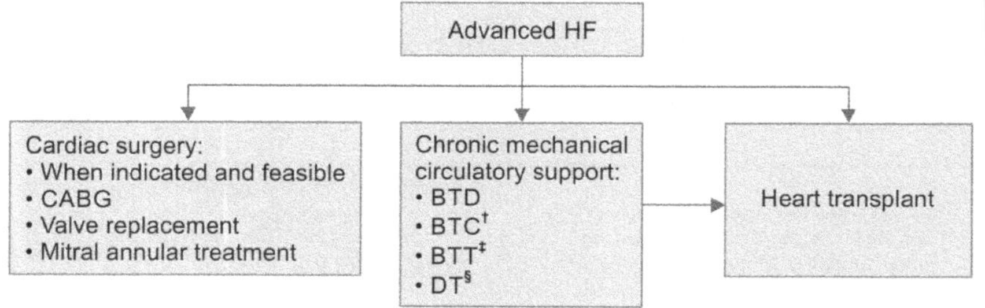

*BTD: bridge to decision: Use of short-term mechanical circulatory support (MCS) [extracorporeal membrane oxygenation (ECMO) or Impella] in patients with cardiogenic shock until hemodynamics and end-organ perfusion are stabilized, contraindications for long-term MCS are excluded (brain damage after resuscitation), and additional therapeutic options including long-term ventricular assist device (VAD) therapy or heart transplant can be evaluated.
†BTC: bridge to candidacy: Use of MCS to improve end-organ function and/or to make an ineligible patient eligible for heart transplantation.
‡BTT: bridge to transplant: Use of MCS to keep a patient alive who is otherwise at high risk of death before transplantation until a donor organ becomes available.
§DT: destination therapy: Long term use of MCS as an alternative to transplantation in patients with end-stage HF ineligible for transplantation.

(BTC: bridge to candidacy; BTD: bridge to decision; BTT: bridge to transplant; CABG: coronary artery bypass graft; DT: destination therapy; HF: heart failure)

REFERENCES

1. Kirklin JK, Naftel DC, Stevenson LW, Kormos RL, Pagani FD, Miller MA, et al. INTERMACS database for durable devices for circulatory support: First annual report. J Heart Lung Transplant. 2008;27:1065-72.
2. Crespo-Leiro MG, Metra M, Lund LH, Milicic D, Costanzo MR, Filippatos G, et al. Advanced heart failure: a position statement of the Heart Failure Association of the European Society of Cardiology. Eur J Heart Fail. 2018;20:1505-35.
3. McDonagh TA, Metra M, Adamo M, Gardner RS, Baumbach A, Böhm M, et al; ESC Scientific Document Group. 2021 ESC Guidelines for the diagnosis and treatment of acute and chronic heart failure. Eur Heart J. 2021;42(36):3599-726.
4. Comin-Colet J, Manito N, Segovia-Cubero J, Delgado J, Garcia Pinilla JM, Almenar L, et al; LION-HEART Study Investigators. Efficacy and safety of intermittent intravenous outpatient administration of levosimendan in patients with advanced heart failure: the LION-HEART multicentre randomised trial. Eur J Heart Fail. 2018;20:1128-36.

CHAPTER 32

Advanced Heart Failure: Cardiac Device Therapy

INTRODUCTION

Advanced heart failure is associated with high morbidity and mortality despite guideline directed medical therapy. During hospital admission with heart failure, in-patient mortality is 9.5% and 1-year mortality is 27%. Cardiac device therapy plays a very important role, beyond medical therapy in addressing the mortality.

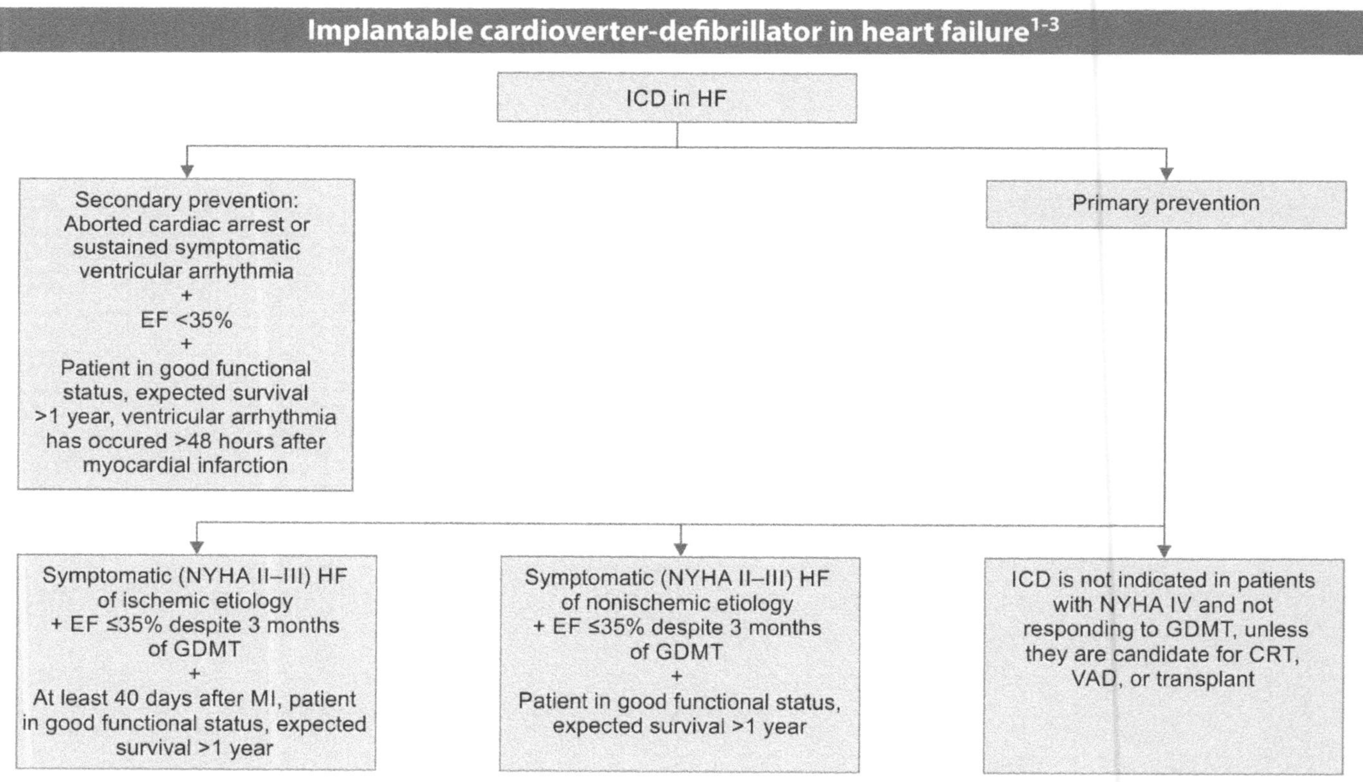

(CRT: cardiac resynchronization therapy; EF: ejection fraction; HF: heart failure; GDMT: guideline directed medical therapy; ICD: implantable cardioverter-defibrillator; MI: myocardial infarction; NYHA: New York Heart Association; VAD: ventricular assist device)

Cardiac synchronization therapy in heart failure[1-3]

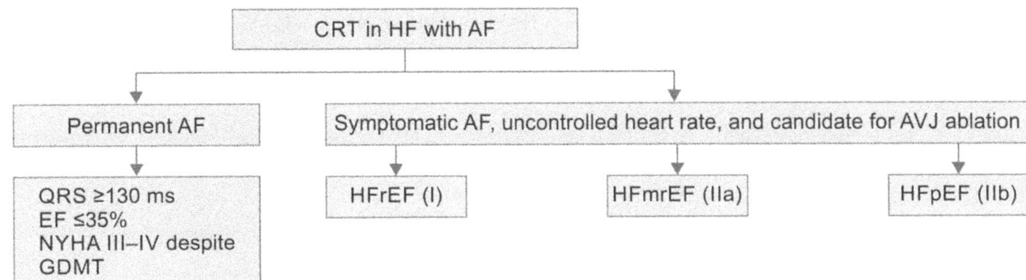

(AV: atrioventricular; CRT: cardiac synchronization therapy; GDMT: guideline directed medical therapy; HF: heart failure; LBBB: left bundle branch block; LVEF: left ventricular ejection fraction; RV: right ventricular; NYHA: New York Heart Association)

Cardiac synchronization therapy in heart failure with atrial fibrillation[1-3]

(AF: atrial fibrillation; AVJ: atrioventricular junction; CRT: cardiac synchronization therapy; EF: ejection fraction; GDMT: guideline directed medical therapy; HF: heart failure; HFmrEF: heart failure with midrange ejection fraction; HFpEF: heart failure with preserved ejection fraction; HFrEF: heart failure with reduced ejection fraction; NYHA: New York Heart Association)

NOVEL CARDIAC DEVICES

Device to treat secondary atrioventricular valve regurgitation[4]

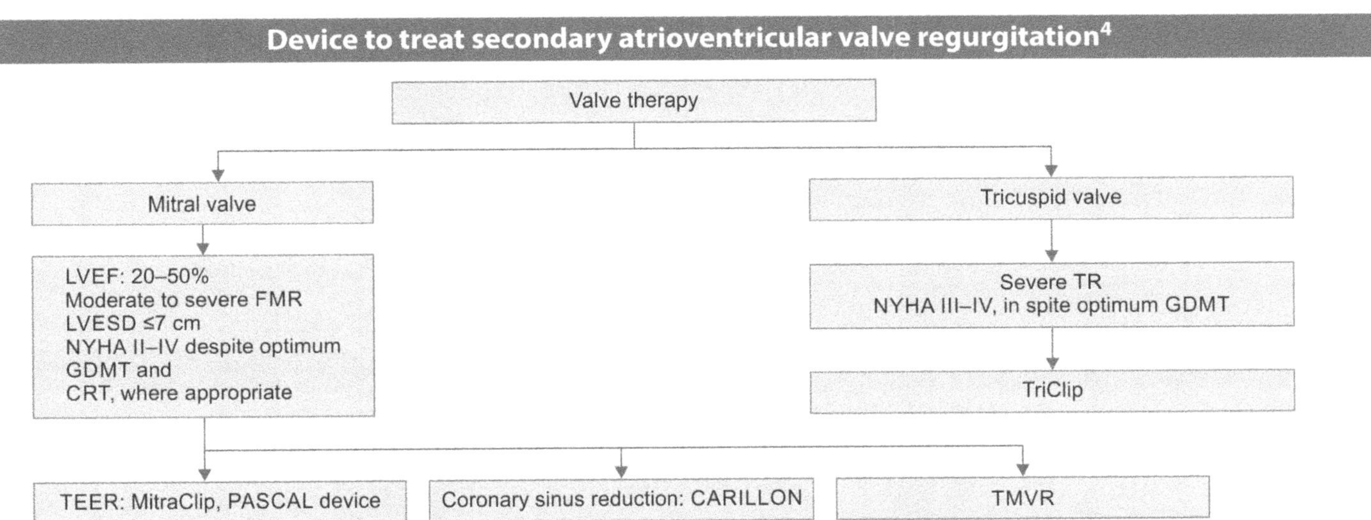

(CRT: cardiac resynchronization therapy; FMR: functional mitral regurgitation; GDMT: guideline directed medical therapy; LVEF: left ventricular ejection fraction; LVESD: left ventricular end-systolic dimension; NYHA: New York Heart Association; TEER: trans-catheter edge-to-edge repair; TMVR: trans-catheter mitral valve repair; TR: tricuspid regurgitation)

Device for autonomic modulation[4]

Autonomic modulation

LVEF ≤35%
NYHA II–III, despite optimum GDMT[5]

LVEF ≤35%
LVEDD ≤55 mm
QRS duration <130 ms
NYHA II–III despite optimum GDMT[6]

Splanchnic nerve stimulation

BAT

VNS

Implanted BAT pulse generator stimulates carotid baroreceptor leading to ↓in sympathetic activity and ↑in parasympathetic activity

(BAT: baroreflex activation therapy; GDMT: guideline directed medical therapy; LVEDD: left ventricular end-diastolic diameter; LVEF: left ventricular ejection fraction; NYHA: New York Heart Association; VNS: Vagus nerve stimulation)

Device for electrophysiological modulation[4]

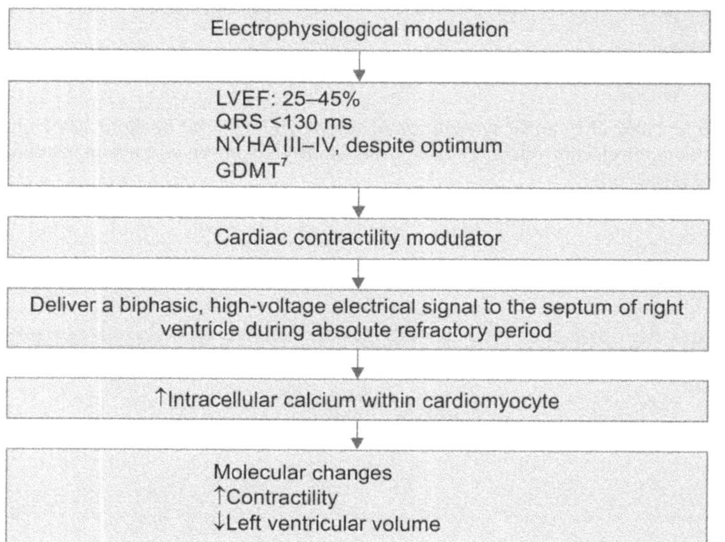

Electrophysiological modulation

LVEF: 25–45%
QRS <130 ms
NYHA III–IV, despite optimum GDMT[7]

Cardiac contractility modulator

Deliver a biphasic, high-voltage electrical signal to the septum of right ventricle during absolute refractory period

↑Intracellular calcium within cardiomyocyte

Molecular changes
↑Contractility
↓Left ventricular volume

(GDMT: guideline directed medical therapy; LVEF: left ventricular ejection fraction; NYHA: New York Heart Association)

Device for structural intervention[4]

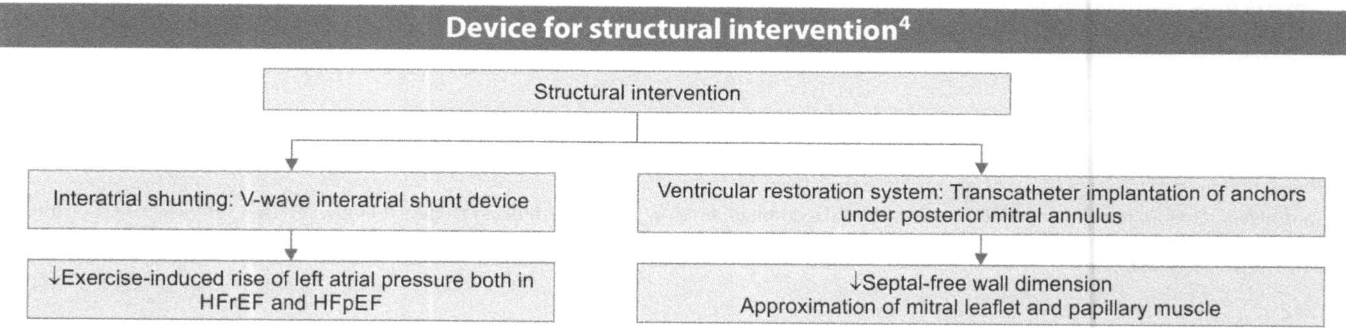

Structural intervention

Interatrial shunting: V-wave interatrial shunt device

Ventricular restoration system: Transcatheter implantation of anchors under posterior mitral annulus

↓Exercise-induced rise of left atrial pressure both in HFrEF and HFpEF

↓Septal-free wall dimension
Approximation of mitral leaflet and papillary muscle

(HFrEF: heart failure with reduced ejection fraction; HFpEF: heart failure with preserved ejection fraction)

REFERENCES

1. McDonagh TA, Metra M, Adamo M, Gardner RS, Baumbach A, Böhm M, et al; ESC Scientific Document Group. 2021 ESC Guidelines for the diagnosis and treatment of acute and chronic heart failure. Eur Heart J. 2021;42(36):3599-726.
2. Glikson M, Nielsen JC, Kronborg MB, Michowitz Y, Auricchio A, Barbash IM, et al. 2021 ESC guidelines on cardiac pacing and cardiac resynchronization therapy. Eur Heart J. 2021;42:3427-520.
3. Heidenreich PA, Bozkurt B, Aguilar D, Allen LA, Byun JJ, Colvin MM, et al. 2022 AHA/ACC/HFSA Guideline for the Management of Heart Failure: A Report of the American College of Cardiology/American Heart Association Joint Committee on Clinical Practice Guidelines. J Am Coll Cardiol. 2022;145:e895-e1032.
4. Fudim M, Abraham WT, Bardelben RS, Lindenfeld J, Ponikowski PP, Salah HM, et al. Device therapy in chronic heart failure. J Am Coll Cardiol. 2021;78:931-56.
5. Georgakopoulos D, Little WC, Abraham WT, Weaver FA, Zile MR. Chronic baroreflex activation: a potential therapeutic approach to heart failure with preserved ejection fraction. J Card Fail. 2011;17:167-78.
6. De Ferrari GM, Stolen C, Tuinenburg AE, Wright DJ, Brugada J, Butter C, et al. Long-term vagal stimulation for heart failure: eighteen month results from the neural cardiac therapy for heart Failure (NECTAR-HF) trial. Int J Cardiol. 2017;244:229-34.
7. Abraham WT, Kuck KH, Goldsmith RL, Lindenfeld J, Reddy VY, Carson PE, et al. A randomized controlled trial to evaluate the safety and efficacy of cardiac contractility modulation. J Am Coll Cardiol HF. 2018;6:874-83.

CHAPTER 33

Acute Heart Failure: Approach

INTRODUCTION

Acute heart failure (AHF) is defined as new or worsening symptoms and signs of heart failure.[1] There may be two types of acute presentation of heart failure (HF): de novo HF in which the patients present with newly developed symptoms without any prior history of heart failure and acutely decompensated HF (ADHF) in which the patients with a history of chronic HF present with increasing symptoms. The latter is far more common. More than 1 million patients are admitted every year with AHF in both Europe and USA. Up to 24% of them are readmitted. The most common risk factor is ischemic heart disease. Inhospital mortality of AHF is 4%, which postdischarge becomes 10% at 3 months and 30% at 1 year.[2] Congestion, both in pulmonary and systemic circulation, which is the final gateway through AHF manifests its ill effects. Both fluid retention and fluid redistribution are responsible for congestion.

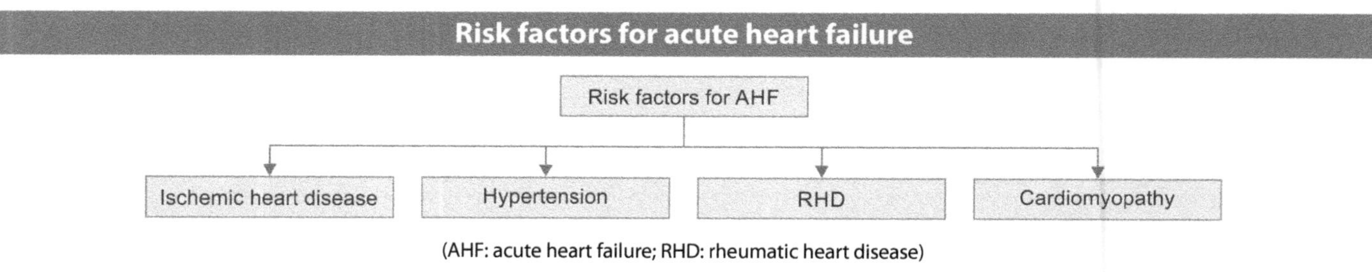

(AHF: acute heart failure; RHD: rheumatic heart disease)

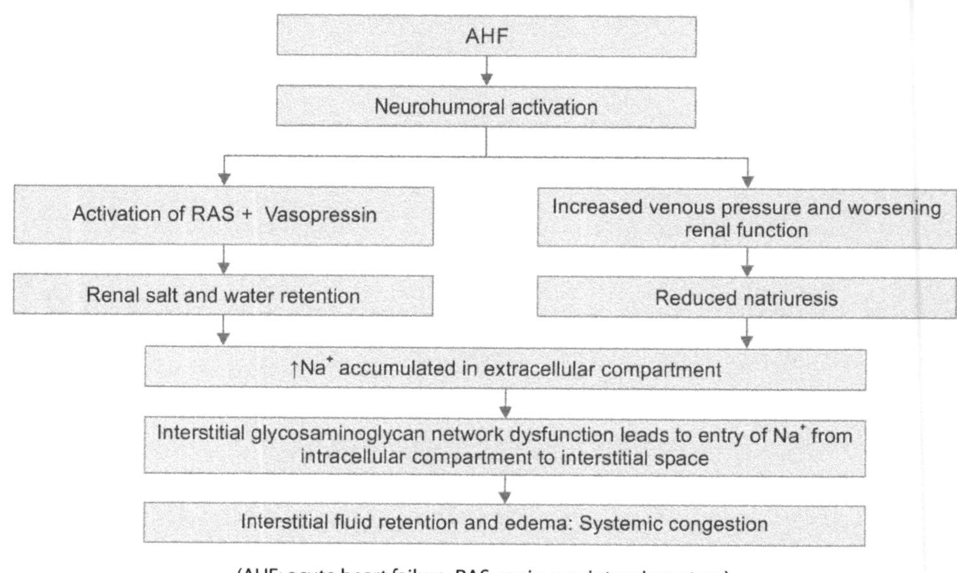

(AHF: acute heart failure; RAS: renin–angiotensin system)

Mechanism of congestion in acute heart failure: Fluid redistribution

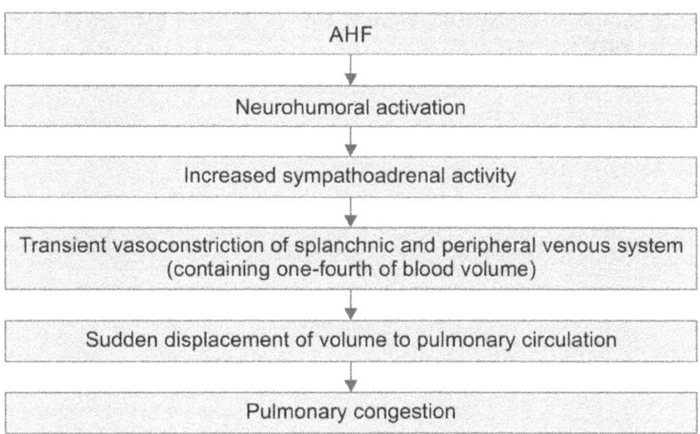

Congestion and renal function in acute heart failure

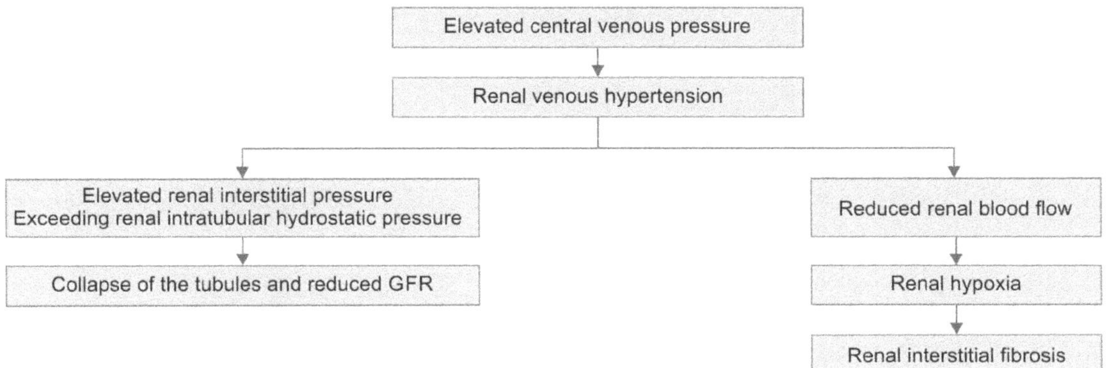

Acute heart failure: Diagnostic strategy[1,3]

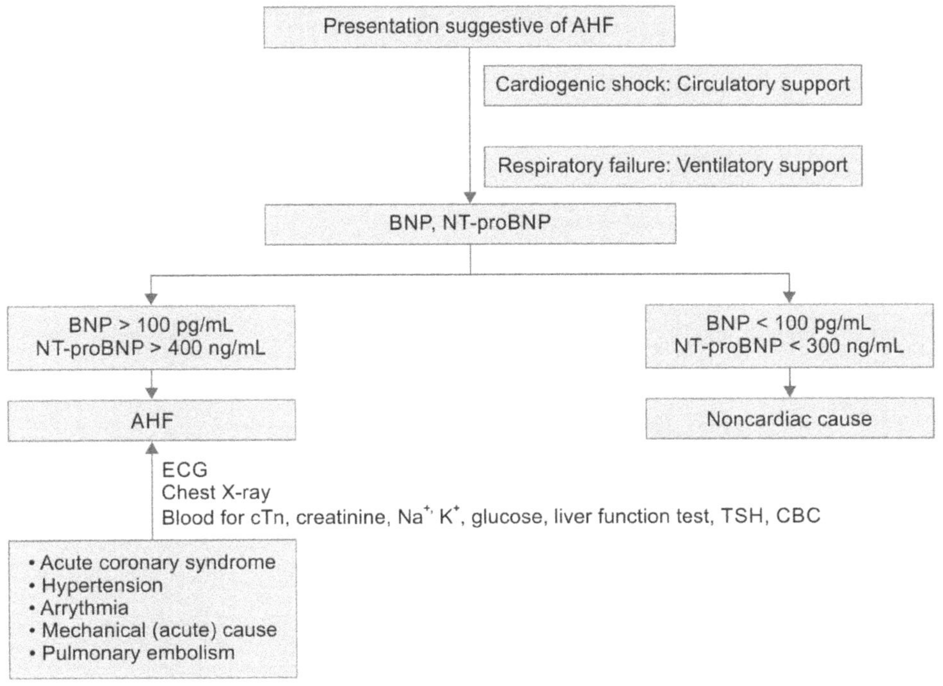

(AHF: acute heart failure; BNP: B-type natriuretic peptide; CBC: complete blood count; cTn: cardiac troponin; ECG: echocardiogram; GFR: glomerular filtration rate; NT-proBNP: N-terminal pro brain natriuretic peptide; TSH: thyroid stimulating hormone)

REFERENCES

1. Ponikowski P, Voors AA, Anker SD, Bueno H, Cleland JGF, Coats AJS, et al. 2016 ESC guidelines for the diagnosis and treatment of acute and chronic heart failure: The Task Force for the diagnosis and treatment of acute and chronic heart failure of the European Society of Cardiology (ESC) Developed with the special contribution of the Heart Failure Association (HFA) of the ESC. Eur. Heart J. 2016;37:2129-200.
2. Hamo CE, O'Connor C, Metra M, Udelson JE, Gheorghiade M, Butler J. A critical appraisal of short-term endpoints in acute heart failure clinical trials. J Card Fail. 2018;24:783-92.
3. McDonagh TA, Metra M, Adamo M, Gardner RS, Baumbach A, Böhm M, et al; ESC Scientific Document Group. 2021 ESC Guidelines for the diagnosis and treatment of acute and chronic heart failure. Eur Heart J. 2021;42(36):3599-726.

CHAPTER 34

Acute Heart Failure: Management

INTRODUCTION

Acute heart failure (AHF) management is challenging, because of the heterogeneity of patient population and incomplete understanding of the pathophysiology. Majority of the patients with AHF present with congestion. Hypoperfusion is present in a smaller portion of patients. Diuretics and vasoactive medicines are the mainstay of therapy. Though AHF responds dramatically to immediate treatment, post-discharge mortality and rehospitalization rate reach 10–20% and 20–30% respectively within 3–6 months.

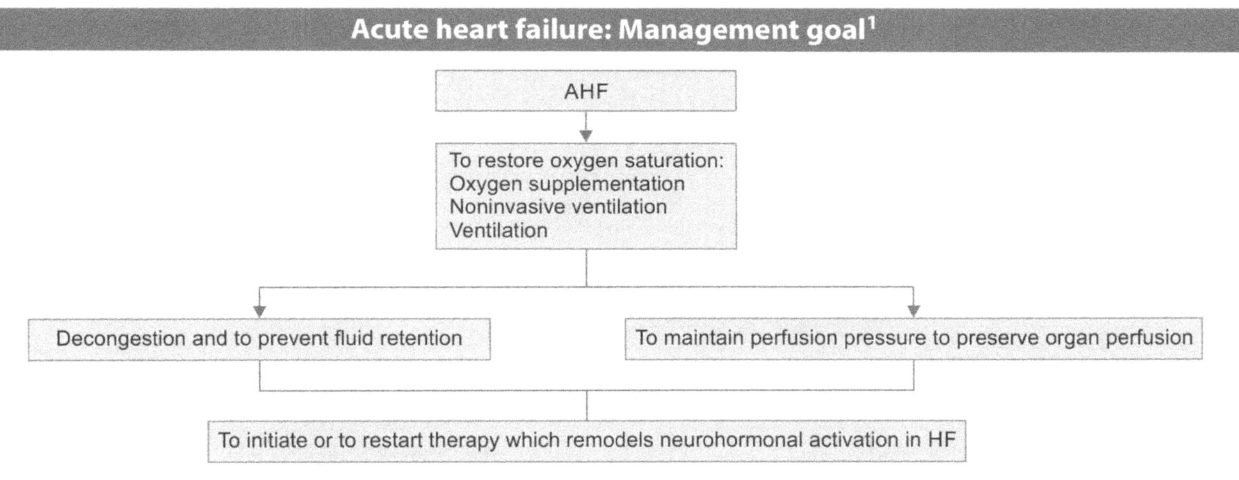

(AHF: acute heart failure; HF: heart failure)

Acute heart failure: Management strategy[1,2]

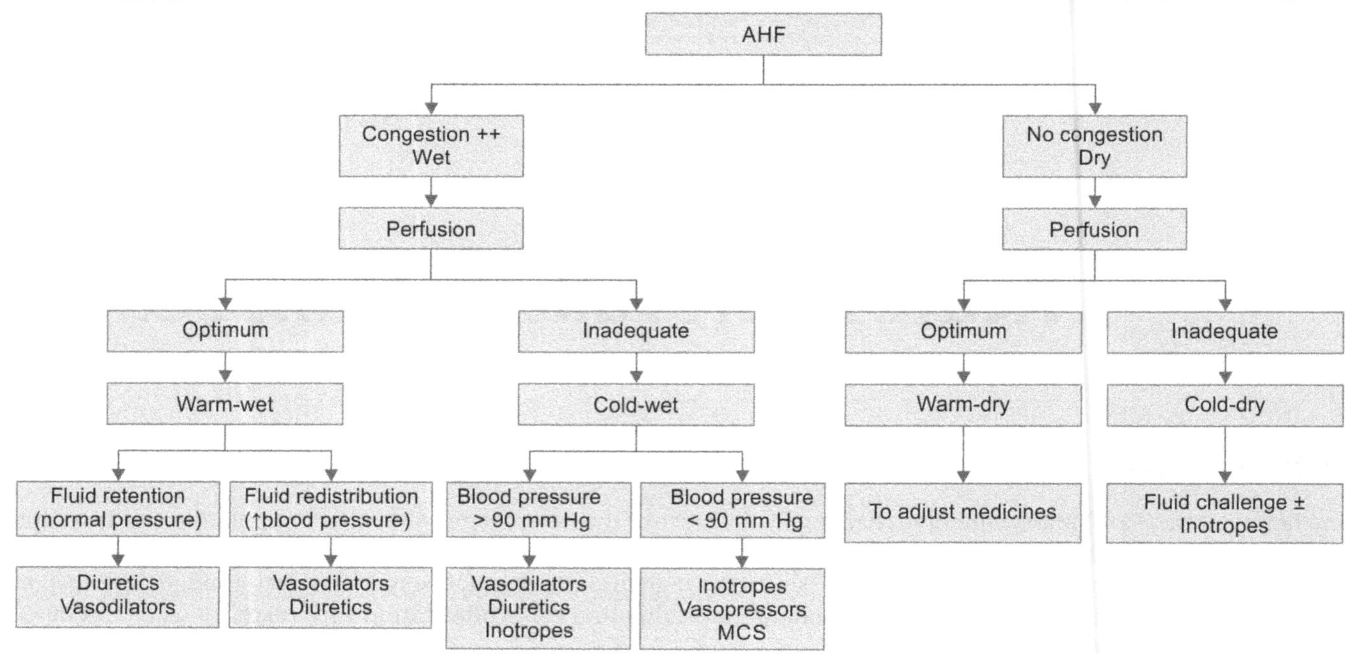

(AHF: acute heart failure; MCS: mechanical circulatory support)

Diuretics optimization strategy: First 24 hours[3]

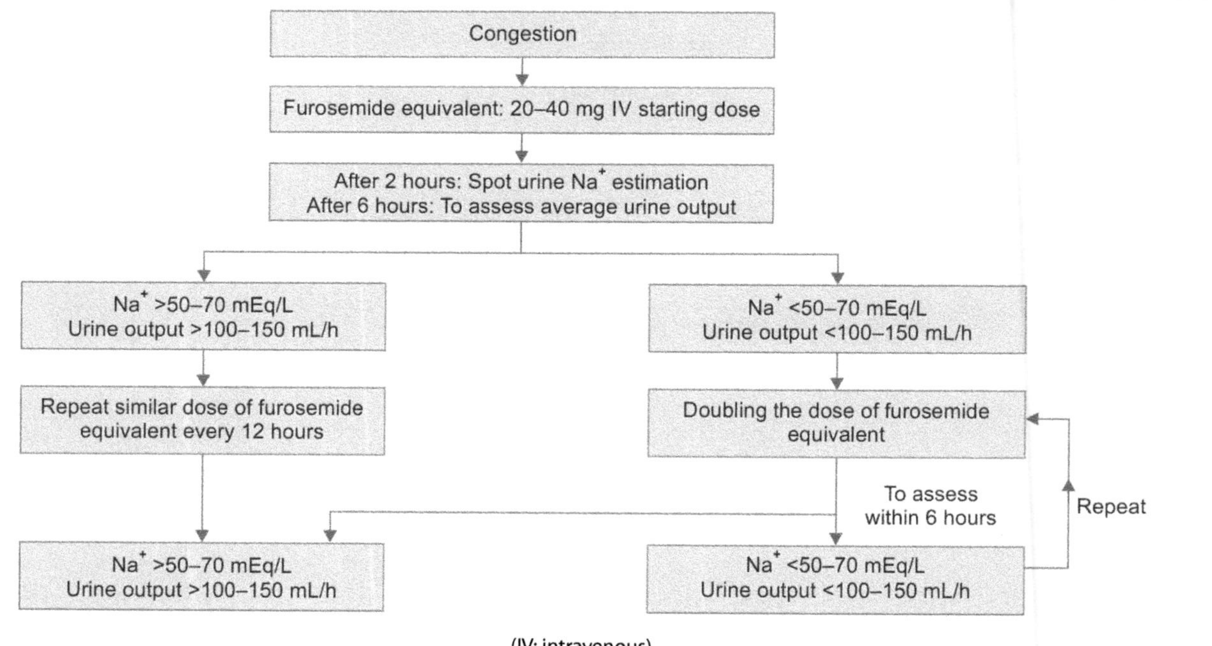

(IV: intravenous)

Diuretics optimization strategy: Second 24 hours[3]

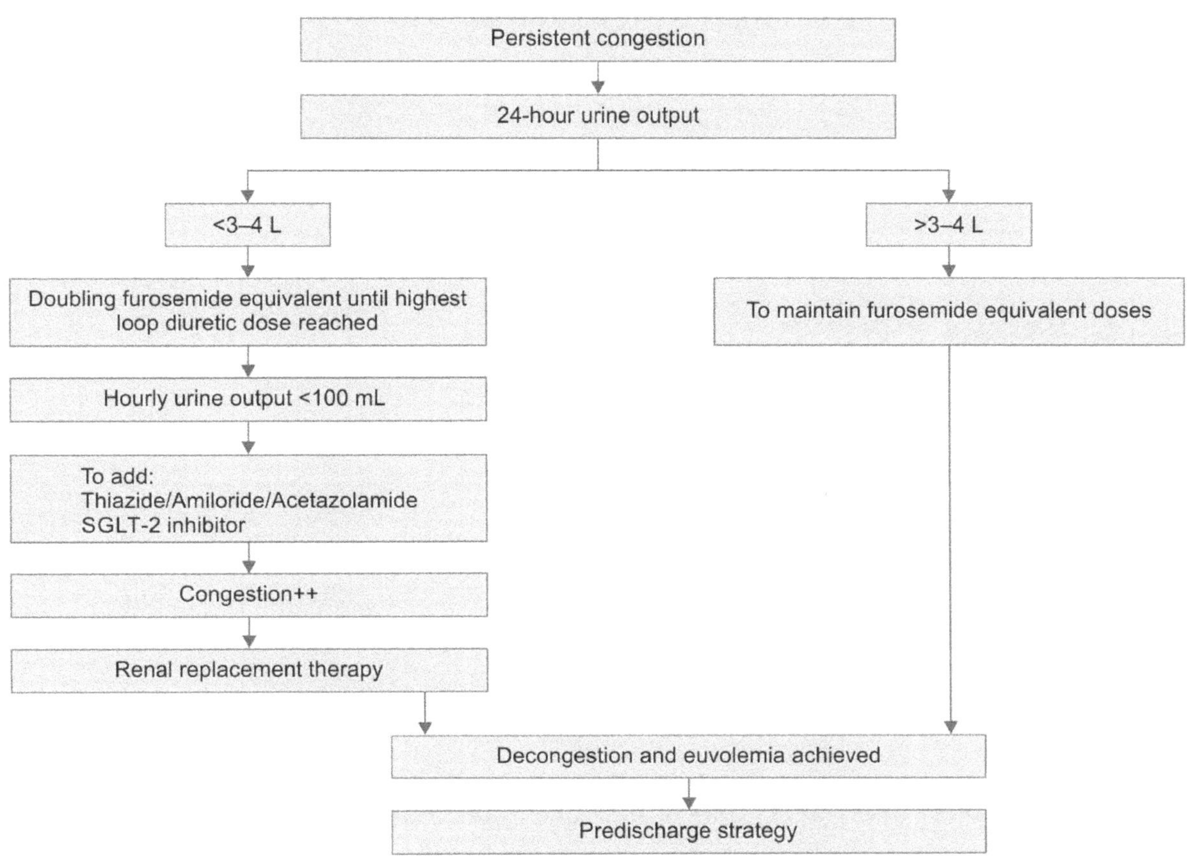

Clinical presentation of acute heart failure[4]

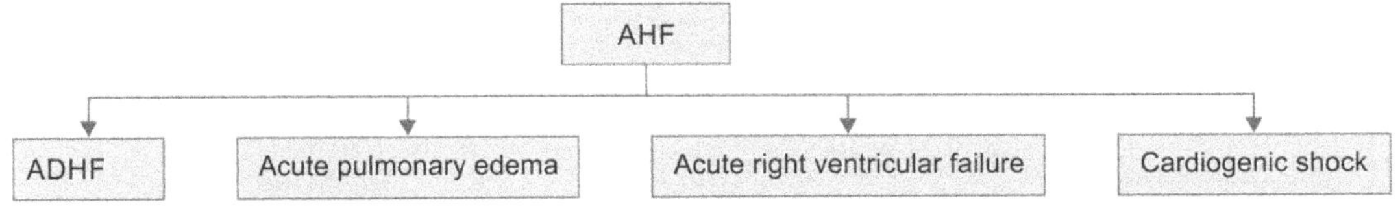

(ADHF: acute diastolic heart failure; AHF: acute heart failure)

Management of acute diastolic heart failure[4]

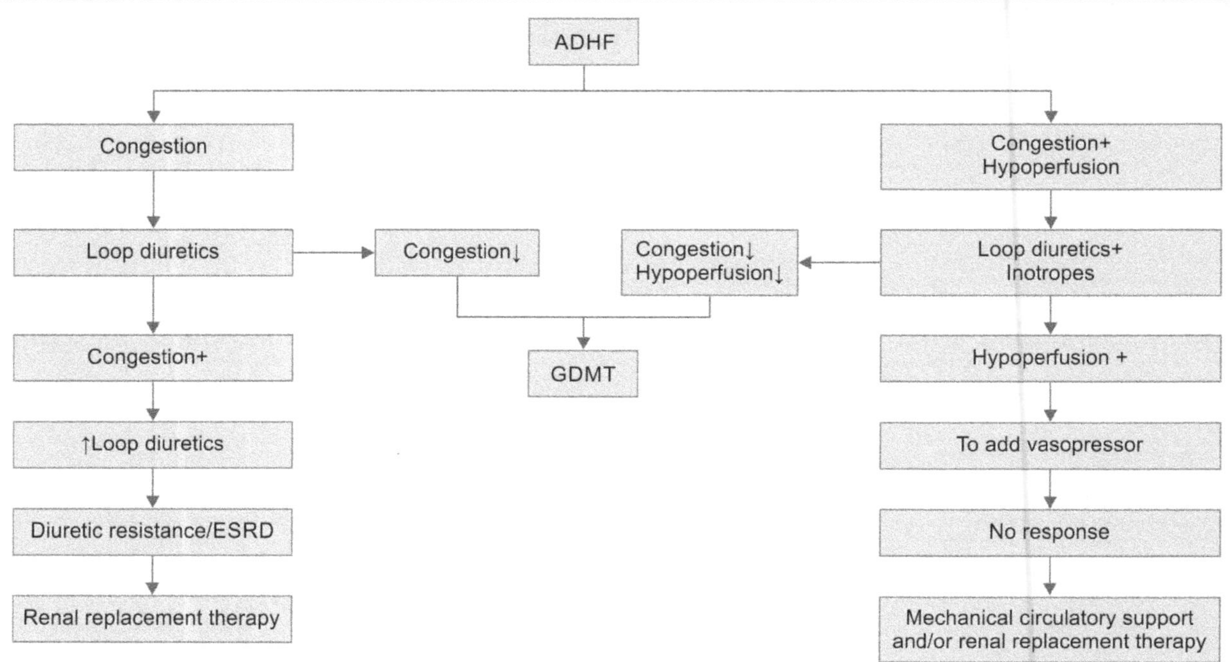

(ADHF: acute decompensated heart failure; ESRD: end-stage renal disease; GDMT: guideline-directed medical therapy)

Management of acute pulmonary edema[4]

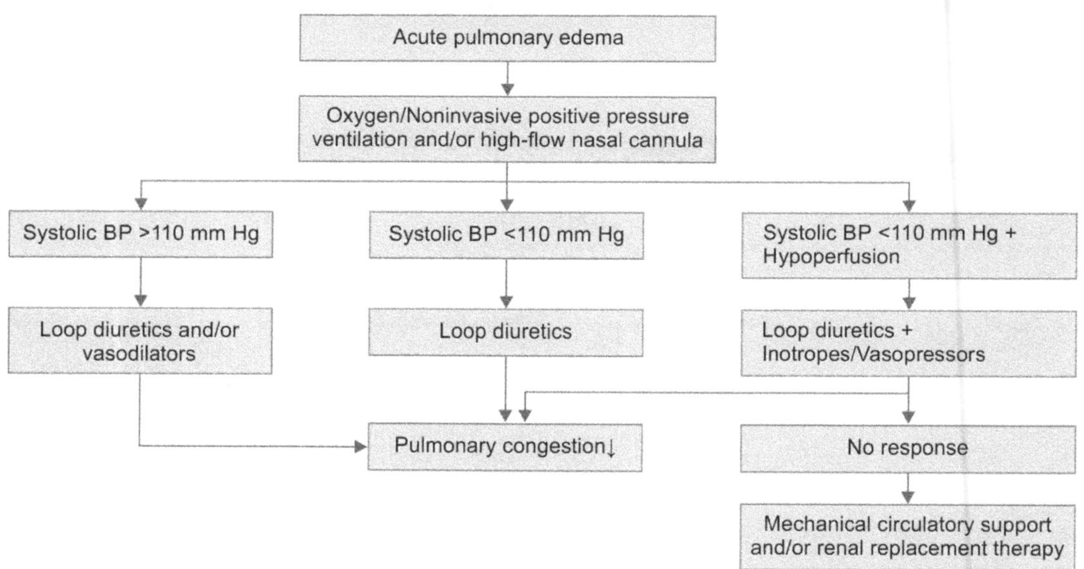

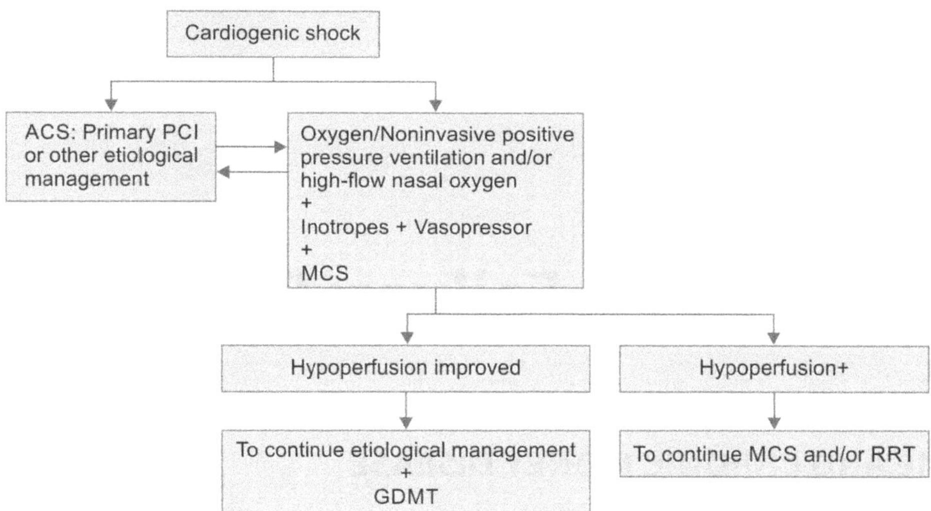

(ACS: acute coronary syndrome; PCI: percutaneous coronary intervention; GDMT: guideline directed medical therapy; MCS: mechanical circulatory support; RRT: renal replacement therapy)

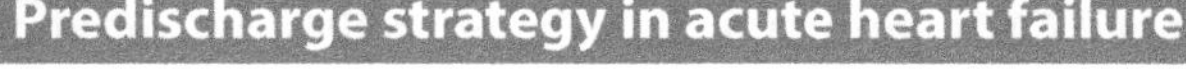

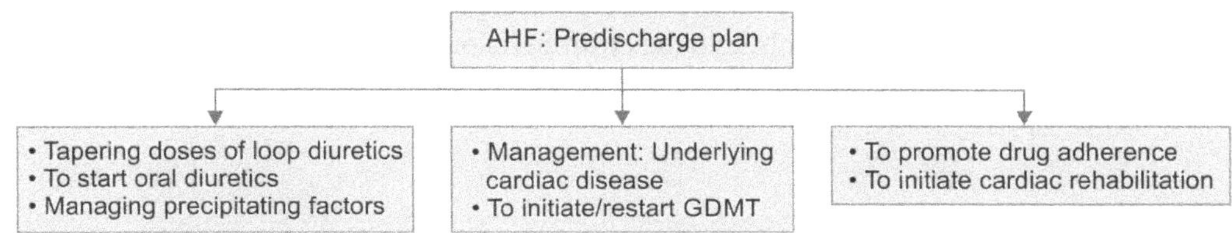

REFERENCES

1. Ponikowski P, Voors AA, Anker SD, Bueno H, Cleland JGF, Coats AJS, et al. 2016 ESC guidelines for the diagnosis and treatment of acute and chronic heart failure: The Task Force for the diagnosis and treatment of acute and chronic heart failure of the European Society of Cardiology (ESC) Developed with the special contribution of the Heart Failure Association (HFA) of the ESC. Eur Heart J. 2016;37:2129-200.
2. Hamo CE, O'Connor C, Metra M, Udelson JE, Gheorghiade M, Butler J, et al. A critical appraisal of short-term endpoints in acute heart failure clinical trials. J Card Fail. 2018;24:783-92.
3. Mullens W, Damman K, Harjola VP, Mebazaa A, Brunner-La Rocca HP, Martens P, et al. The use of diuretics in heart failure with congestion – a position statement from the Heart Failure Association of the European Society of Cardiology. Eur J Heart Fail. 2019;21:137-55.
4. McDonagh TA, Metra M, Adamo M, Gardner RS, Baumbach A, Böhm M, et al; ESC Scientific Document Group. 2021 ESC Guidelines for the diagnosis and treatment of acute and chronic heart failure. Eur Heart J. 2021;42(36):3599-726.

CHAPTER 35

Heart Failure: Special Situation

HEART FAILURE AND CHRONIC KIDNEY DISEASE

In heart failure with reduced ejection fraction (HFrEF), the prevalence of chronic kidney disease (CKD) is almost 10%.[1] Heart failure (HF) may predispose acute kidney injury and development of CKD due to affection of renal hemodynamic, whereas CKD by promoting sodium and fluid retention can precipitate HF. Most of the important clinical trials on HF have excluded patients with advanced CKD, because of which evidence in favor of contemporary guideline-directed medical treatment (GDMT) in HF with CKD is lacking. Despite the fact that HF with CKD has a poorer prognosis, patients get less aggressive GDMT. Patients with HF and advanced CKD, going for dialysis, not >40%, are on angiotensin-converting enzyme (ACE) inhibitor/angiotensin receptor blocker (ARB) and 60–75% on beta-blocker. There are several explanations, namely limited life span, comorbid conditions, limited clinical trials, and the apprehension of worsening renal function, for which clinicians are hesitant to use optimum GDMT. However, worsening renal function due to diuretics or ACE inhibitor or decompensated HF may not reflect true renal injury.[2]

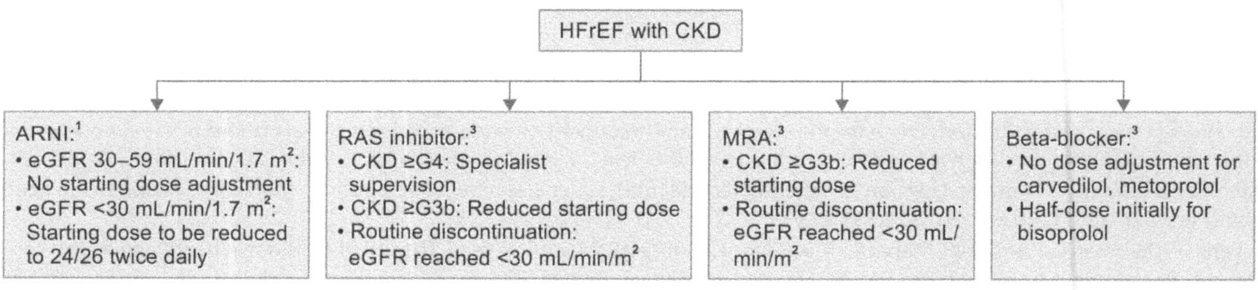

(ARNI: angiotensin receptor-neprilysin inhibitor; CKD: chronic kidney disease; eGFR: estimated glomerular filtration rate; HFrEF: heart failure with reduced ejection fraction; MRA: mineralocorticoid receptor antagonists)

HEART FAILURE WITH ATRIAL FIBRILLATION

Atrial fibrillation (AF) is an ominous complication of HF because AF is a marker of sicker patient, because it impairs cardiac function further and because it is associated with increased risk of thromboembolism. Rates of HF in a global AF registry were 33% in paroxysmal, 44% in persistent, and 56% in permanent AF.[4]

Many drugs belonging to GDMT, including ACE inhibitor/ARB, beta-blocker, and mineralocorticoid receptor antagonists (MRA), will reduce the incidence of AF. However, ivabradine may increase it, whereas cardiac resynchronization therapy (CRT) has no effect.[5] Amiodarone maintains sinus rhythm in more patients after cardioversion and itself can induce cardioversion and may be used in controlling symptoms in patients with paroxysmal AF.[6] Amiodarone should not better be used more than 6 months at a stretch. Dronedarone is contraindicated in AF with HF. Beta-blocker does not reduce mortality or recurrent hospitalization in HFrEF in presence of AF, shown by the metanalysis of 11 randomized controlled trials (RCTs).[7] Largest rate versus rhythm control study in AF, rhythm control did not show any advantage over rate control in relation to both primary and secondary endpoints.[8] That study did not include AF ablation as one of the modalities for rhythm control. However, recent large trials, which included pulmonary vein isolation as a modality for rhythm control. showed prognostic implication in rhythm control over rate control.[9]

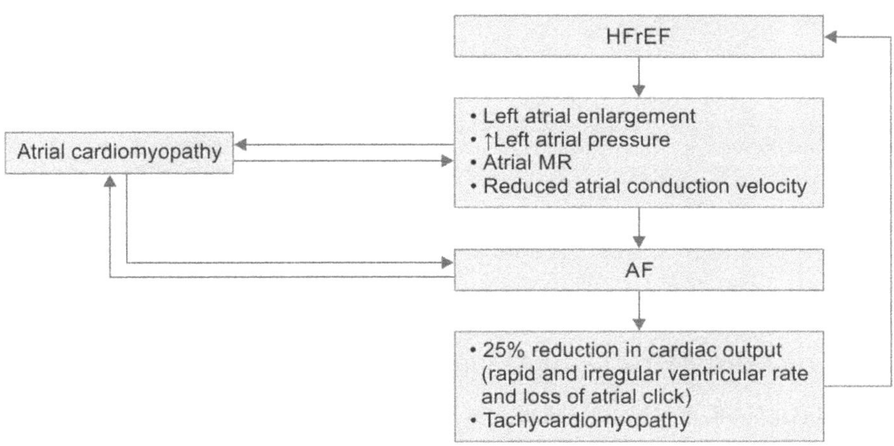

(AF: atrial fibrillation; HFrEF: heart failure with reduced ejection fraction; MR: mitral regurgitation)

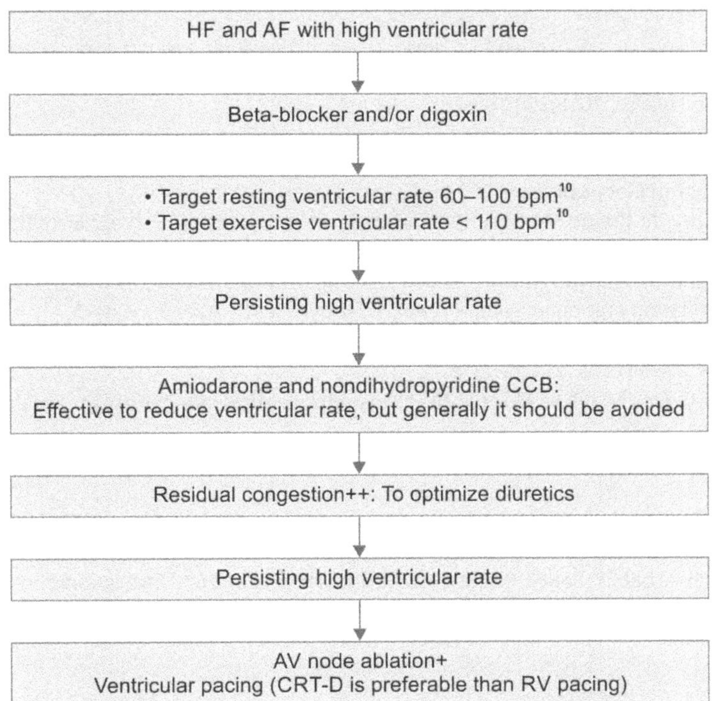

(AF: atrial fibrillation; AV: atrioventricular; CRT-D: cardiac resynchronization therapy with implantable cardioverter defibrillator; HF: heart failure; RV: right ventricular)

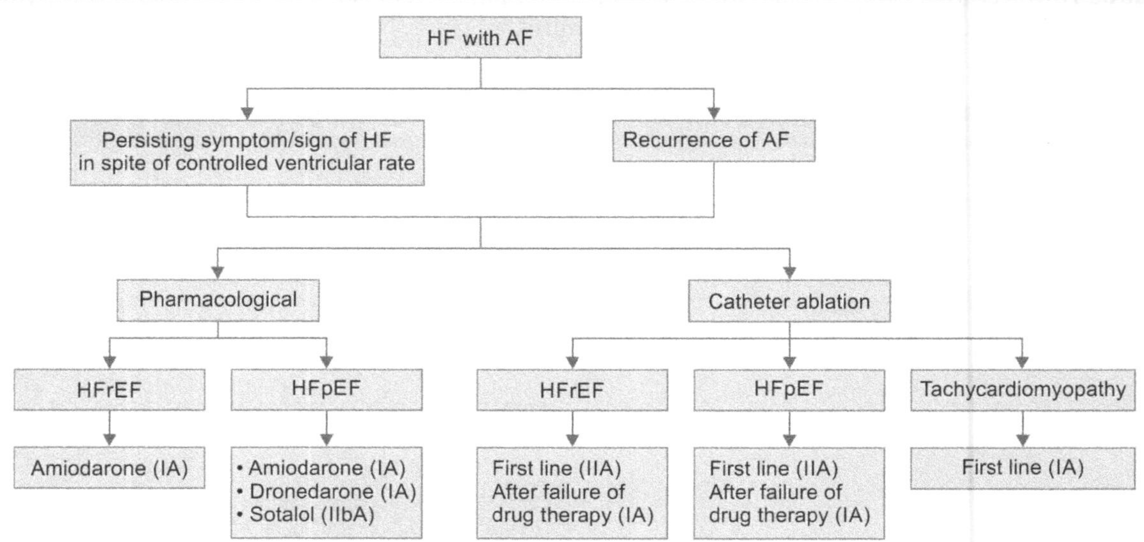

(AF: atrial fibrillation; HF: heart failure; HFpEF: heart failure with preserved ejection fraction; HFrEF: heart failure with reduced ejection fraction; OMT: osteopathic manipulative treatment)

REFERENCES

1. Levin A, Stevens PE, Bilous RW, Coresh J, De Francisco AL, De Jong PE, et al. Kidney disease: improving global outcomes (KDIGO) CKD work group. KDIGO 2012 clinical practice guideline for the evaluation and management of chronic kidney disease. Kidney Int. 2013;3(Suppl):1-150.

2. Fudim M, Loungani R, Doerfler SM, Coles A, Greene SJ, Cooper LB, et al. Worsening renal function during decongestion among patients hospitalized for heart failure: findings from the Evaluation Study of Congestive Heart Failure and Pulmonary Artery Catheterization Effectiveness (ESCAPE) trial. Am Heart J. 2018;204:163-73.

3. Chiang CE, Naditch-Brule L Murin J, Goethals M, Inoue H, O'Neill J, et al. Distribution and risk profile of paroxysmal, persistent, and permanent atrial fibrillation in routine clinical practice: insight from the real-life global survey evaluating patients with atrial fibrillation international registry Circ Arrhythm Electrophysiol. 2012;5:632-9.

4. Hess PL, Jackson KP, Hasselblad V, Al-Khatib SM. Is cardiac resynchronization therapy an antiarrhythmic therapy for atrial fibrillation? A systematic review and meta-analysis. Curr Cardiol Rep. 2013;15(2):330.

5. Shelton RJ, Clark AL, Goode K, Rigby AS, Houghton T, Kaye GC, et al. A randomised, controlled study of rate versus rhythm control in patients with chronic atrial fibrillation and heart failure: (CAFE-II Study). Heart. 2009;95:924-30.

6. Rienstra M, Damman K, Mulder BA, Van Gelder IC, McMurray JJ, Van Veldhuisen DJ. Beta-blockers and outcome in heart failure and atrial fibrillation: a meta-analysis. JACC Heart Fail. 2013;1:21-8.

7. Roy D, Talajic M, Nattel S, Wyse G, Dorian P, Lee KL, et al. Rhythm control versus rate control for atrial fibrillation and heart failure. N Engl J Med. 2008;358:2667-77.

8. Mulder BA, Rienstra M, Van Gelder IC, Blaauw Y. Update on management of atrial fibrillation in heart failure: a focus on ablation. Heart. 2022;108:422-8.

9. Van Gelder IC, Wyse DG, Chandler ML, Cooper HA, Olshansky B, Hagens VE, et al; RACE and AFFIRM Investigators. Does intensity of rate-control influence outcome in atrial fibrillation? An analysis of pooled data from the RACE and AFFIRM studies. Europace. 2006;8:935-42.

10. Hindricks G, Potpara T, Dagres N, Arbelo E, Bax JJ, Blomström-Lundqvist C, et al. 2020 ESC guidelines for the diagnosis and management of atrial fibrillation developed in collaboration with the European association for Cardio-Thoracic surgery (EACTS). Eur Heart J. 2021;42:373-498.

Pulmonary Hypertension

CHAPTER 36

Pulmonary Hypertension: Basic Approach

INTRODUCTION

Normal mean pulmonary arterial pressure is 14 ± 3.3 mm Hg, determined by right heart catheterization (RHC) studies.[1] Upper limit should be above the 97.5th percentile or 2 standard deviation or 20 mm Hg. Pulmonary hypertension (PH) has been defined as mean pulmonary artery pressure at rest >25 mm Hg determined by RHC study. The World Health Organization (WHO) in 1973 first offered this definition for PH.[2] There remains a gray zone between 20 and 25 mm Hg, which was defined as borderline PH. This definition continued till the 6th World Symposium on Pulmonary Hypertension held in 2018.[3] They redefined the level from 25 to 20 mm Hg, thus increasing the sensitivity of the diagnostic criteria. The reasoning was that a subset of patients with pulmonary artery pressure between 20 and 25 mm Hg may remain unnoticed and may develop significant PH with poorer outcome due to late diagnosis. General population with mean pulmonary artery pressure between 20 and 25 mm Hg shows higher mortality. At the same time, this population is also associated with some other confounders, such as increasing age, elevated body mass index, and coexistent left heart disease, all of which may contribute to the mortality. There always lies a probability of overdiagnosis and overtreatment of PH. "However, well-intentioned and provocative the recent hemodynamic threshold alterations might be, without further study there are currently insufficient data to support a PH diagnosis in this 'borderline' cohort. Moreover, there are no data to support treatment."[4]

Amongst the diagnosed cases of idiopathic pulmonary arterial hypertension (PAH), 25–30% of patients have an underlying genetic cause and they are classified as heritable PAH. *BMPR2* is the gene encoding bone morphogenetic protein receptor type II, the mutation of which is the genetic etiology associated with familial PAH in 70–80% of cases and with idiopathic PAH in 10–20% of cases.[5] The mutation has also been identified in PAH with anorexigenics, pulmonary veno-occlusive disease (PVOD), and congenital heart disease. Caveola, an invagination of the plasma membrane, is also important in the initiation of bone morphogenetic proteins (BMP) signaling. CAV1 is the major protein of caveola, the mutation of which reduces *BMPR2* membrane localization and signaling. *BMPR2* is highly expressive on pulmonary vascular endothelium, where it prevents endothelial cells apoptosis and excessive proliferation. Its deficiency promotes endothelial dysfunction, which is initiating even in pathobiology of PAH. *BMPR2* mutation is also responsible for uninhibited proliferation of smooth muscle cells of pulmonary artery and fibroblast in the interstitial tissue. The penetrance of disease phenotype of *BMPR2* mutation is 42% in female and only 12% in male. High penetrance in female may be related to estrogen metabolism. Patients with PAH associated with *BMPR2* mutation show four specific characteristics, namely presentation at earlier age, more deranged hemodynamic, poor response to vasodilatory challenge test, and less survival.[6]

The basic pathology in PH is the obstructive remodeling and loss of pulmonary vascular bed, the effects of which are increased pulmonary artery pressure and pulmonary vascular resistance. The events that occur at cellular as well as tissue level potentiate smooth muscle cells proliferation, endothelial cell dysfunction, and inflammation. All these lead to vasoconstriction, medial hypertrophy, intimal fibrosis, and initiation of plexiform lesions, which are mediated by three pathways, namely nitric oxide (NO), endothelin-1 (ET-1), and prostacyclin (PGI2). A fourth pathway, calcium channel, plays a minor role.

Clinical presentation suggestive of pulmonary hypertension

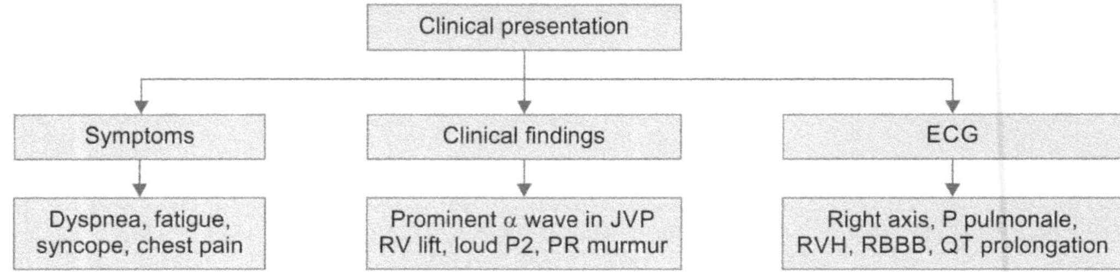

(ECG: electrocardiogram; JVP: jugular venous pressure; PR: pulmonic regurgitation; RBBB: right bundle branch block; RV: right ventricular; RVH: right ventricular hypertrophy)

Echocardiographic probabilities of pulmonary hypertension[7]

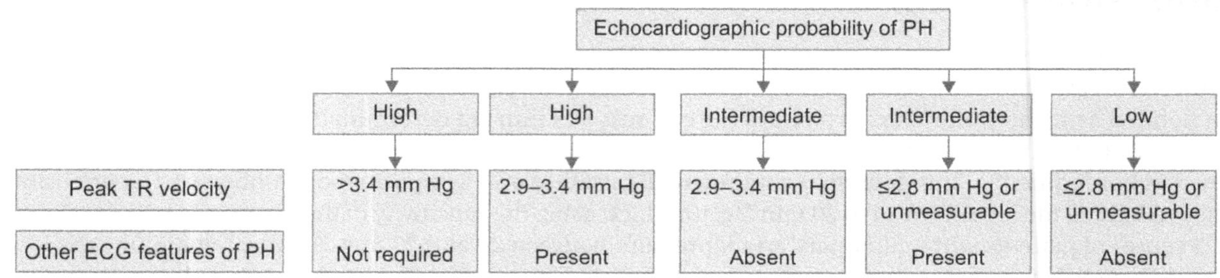

(ECG: electrocardiogram; PH: pulmonary hypertension; TR: tricuspid regurgitation)

Other echocardiographic features of pulmonary hypertension

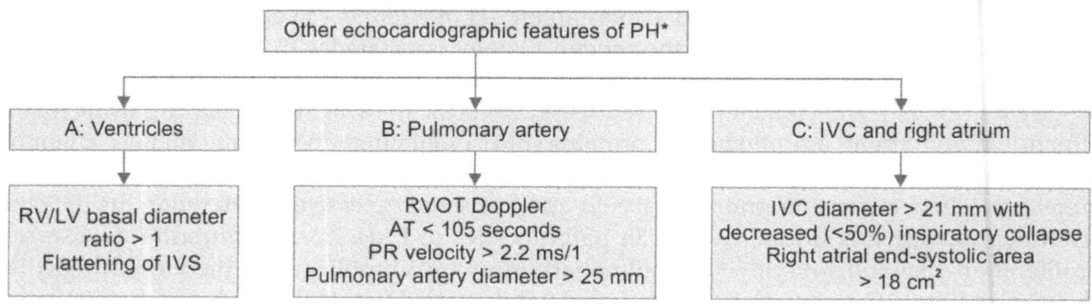

*At least two from different categories (A, B, or C) must be present to alter the probability of echocardiographic diagnosis of PH.

(AT: acceleration time; IVC: inferior vena cava; LV: left ventricle; PH: pulmonary hypertension; RV: right ventricle; RVOT: right ventricular outflow tract)

Diagnostic algorithm for pulmonary hypertension

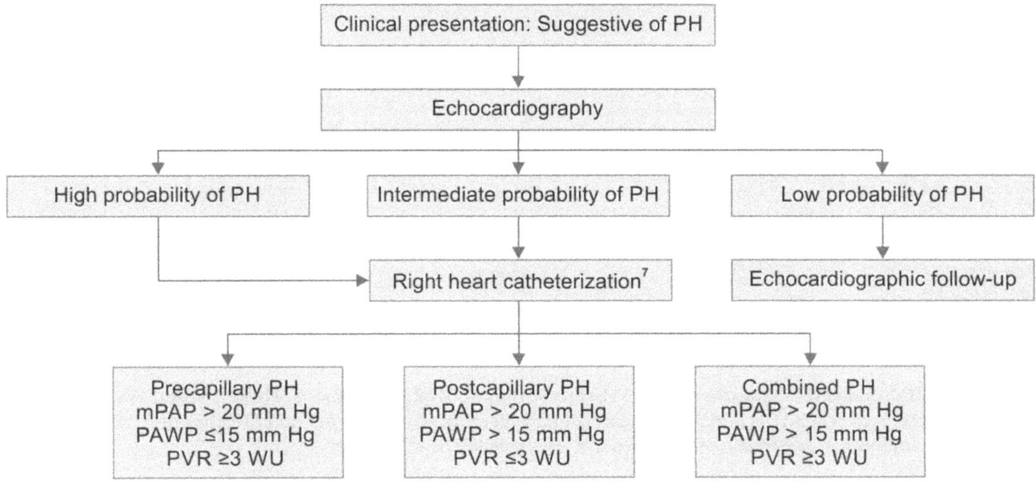

(PAWP: pulmonary artery wedge pressure; PH: pulmonary hypertension; PVR: pulmonary vascular resistance; mPAP: mean pulmonary artery pressure)

Classification of pulmonary hypertension[7]

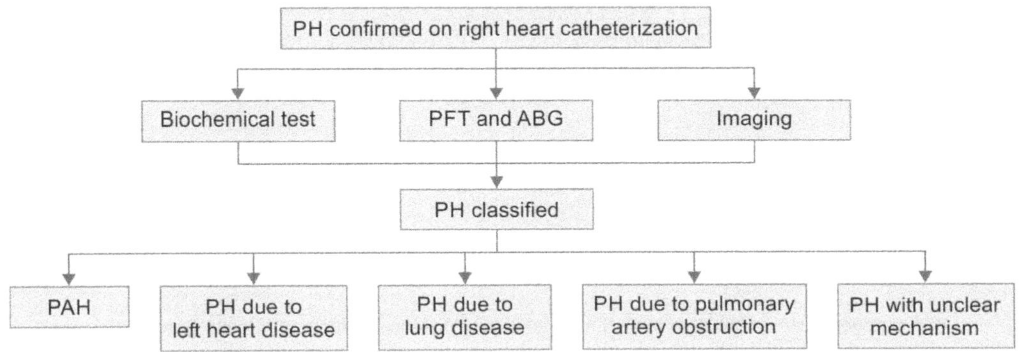

(ABG: arterial blood gas; PAH: pulmonary arterial hypertension; PFT: pulmonary function test; PH: pulmonary hypertension)

Basic investigations to classify pulmonary hypertension

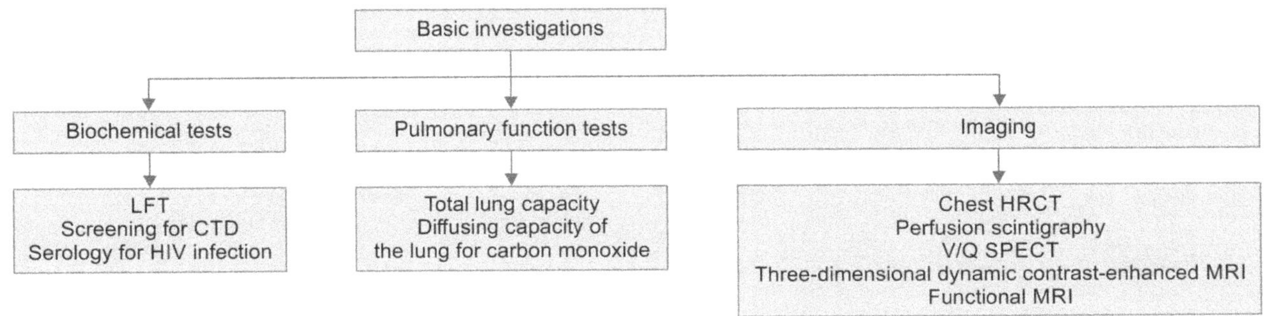

(CTD: connective tissue disease; HIV: human immunodeficiency virus; HRCT: high-resolution computed tomography; LFT: lung function test; MRI: magnetic resonance imaging; SPECT: single-photon emission computed tomography; V/Q: ventilation/perfusion)

Classification of pulmonary hypertension according to etiology[7]

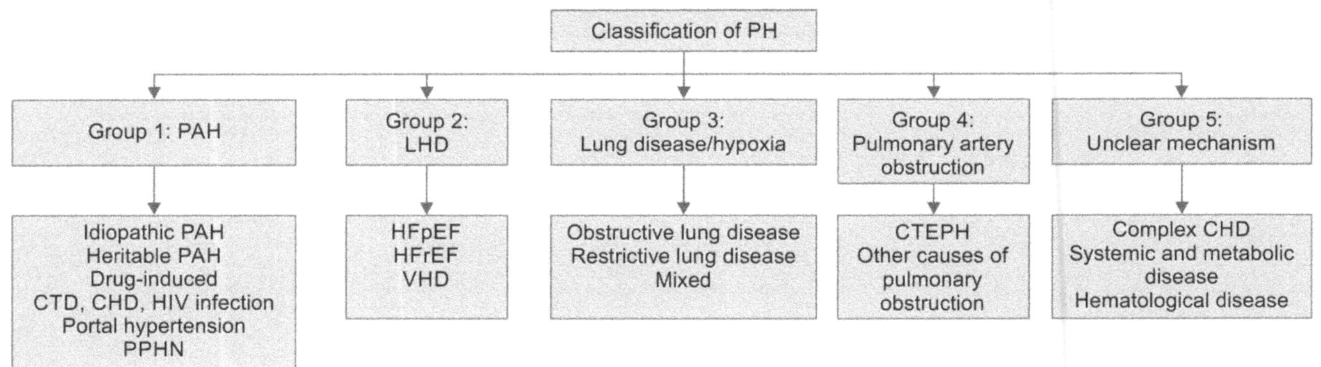

(CHD: congenital heart disease; CTD: connective tissue disease; CTEPH: chronic thromboembolic pulmonary hypertension; HIV: human immunodeficiency virus; HFpEF: heart failure with preserved ejection fraction; HFrEF: heart failure with reduced ejection fraction; LHD: left heart disease; PAH: pulmonary artery hypertension; PPHN: persistent pulmonary hypertension of the newborn; VHD: valvular heart disease)

Prognostic parameters in pulmonary arterial hypertension[7]

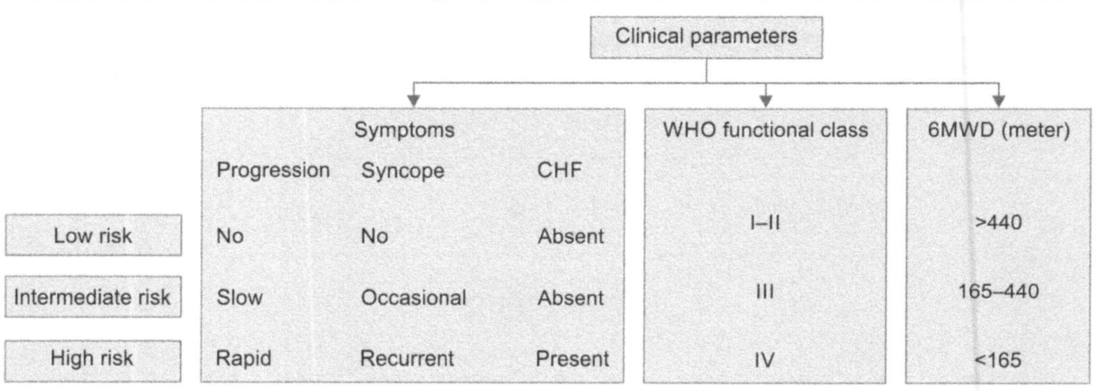

(CHF: congestive heart failure; 6MWD: 6-minute walking distance; WHO: World Health Organization)

Prognostic parameters in pulmonary arterial hypertension[7]

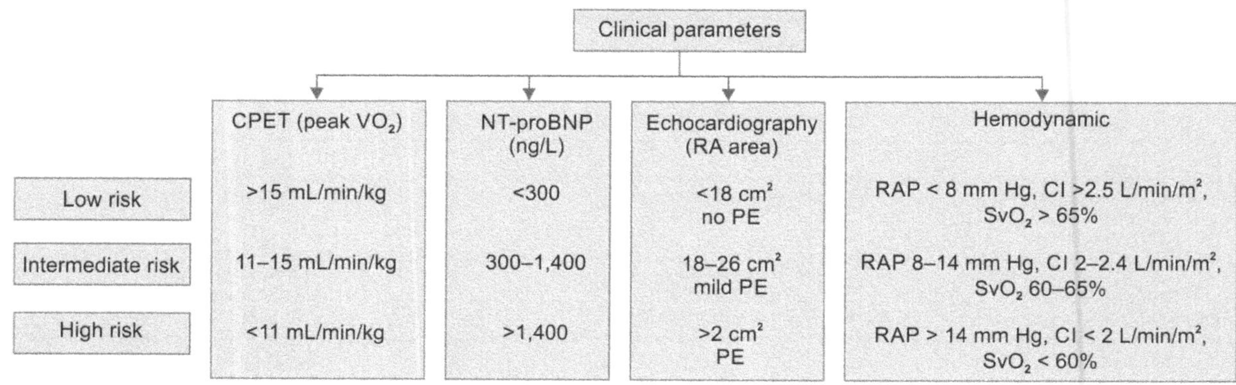

(CI: cardiac index; CPET: cardiopulmonary exercise test; NT-proBNP: N-terminal pro-brain natriuretic peptide; PE: pericardial effusion; RA: right atrial; RAP: right atrial pressure; SvO$_2$: mixed venous oxygen saturation)

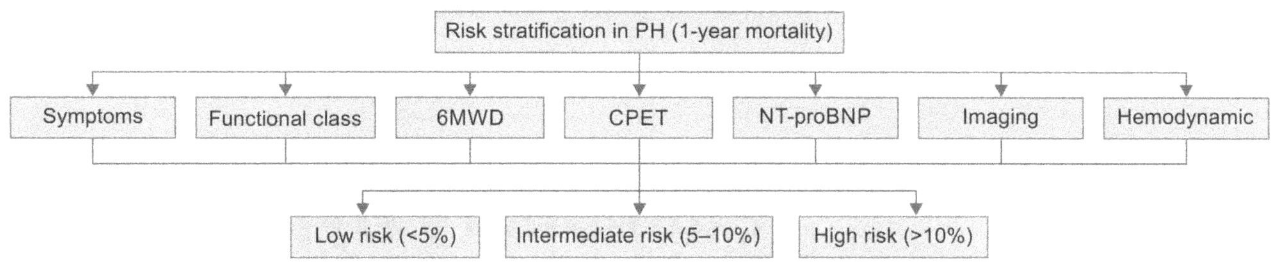

(6MWD: 6-minute walk distance; CPET: cardiopulmonary exercise test; NT-proBNP: N-terminal pro-brain natriuretic peptide)

REFERENCES

1. Kovacs G, Berghold A, Scheidl S, Olschewski H. Pulmonary arterial pressure during rest and exercise in healthy subjects: a systematic review. Eur Respir J. 2009;34:888-94.
2. Hatano S, Strasser T (Eds). Primary Pulmonary Hypertension. Report on a WHO Meeting. Geneva: World Health Organization; 1975.
3. Simonneau G, Montani D, Celermajer DS, Denton CP, Gatzoulis MA, Krowka M, et al. Haemodynamic definitions and updated clinical classification of pulmonary hypertension. Eur Respir J. 2019;53:1801913.
4. Ruopp NF, Farber HW. The new world symposium on pulmonary hypertension guideline. Circulation. 2019;140:1134-6.
5. Evans JD, Girerd B, Montani D, Wang XJ, Galie N, Austin ED. BMPR2 mutations and survival in pulmonary arterial hypertension: an individual participant data meta-analysis. Lancet Respir Med. 2016;4:129-37.
6. Sztrymf B, Coulet F, Girerd B, Yaici A, Jais X, Sitbon O, et al. Clinical outcomes of pulmonary arterial hypertension in carriers of BMPR2 mutation. Am J Respir Crit Care Med. 2008;177:1377-83.
7. Galiè N, Humbert M, Vachiery JL, Gibbs S, Lang I, Torbicki A, et al. 2015 ESC/ERS guidelines for the diagnosis and treatment of pulmonary hypertension: the joint Task force for the diagnosis and treatment of pulmonary hypertension of the European Society of cardiology (ESC) and the European respiratory Society (ERS): endorsed by: association for European paediatric and congenital cardiology (AEPC), International Society for heart and lung transplantation (ISHLT). Eur Respir J 2015;46:903-75.

CHAPTER 37

Pulmonary Hypertension: Management Algorithm

INTRODUCTION

Management algorithm is specifically targeted to patients with pulmonary hypertension (PH) belonging to group 1, i.e., pulmonary arterial hypertension (PAH). As mentioned earlier, three major pathways are target for therapy: nitric oxide (NO), endothelin (ET-1), and prostaglandin (PGI2). In a small number of patients, PAH is due to excessive vasoconstriction which is mediated by influx of calcium via calcium channels in vascular smooth muscle cells. Those calcium channels are the fourth target pathway for therapy. Any of the three calcium entry blockers (CEBs), namely nifedipine, diltiazem, or amlodipine, can be used. If the target is not reached by 3–6 months, other pulmonary vasodilators are added. The target is functional class I–II and remarkable hemodynamic response.[1]

There are two groups of drugs targeting NO pathway. First is the phosphodiesterase type-5 inhibitors (PDE5i), which include Sildenafil, Tadalafil, and Vardenafil. The other one is soluble guanylate cyclase (sGC) stimulators, which include Riociguat.

The ET pathway is targeted by endothelin receptor antagonists (ERA). Bosentan and Macitentan are dual ERA, because they bind to both endothelin A (ETA) and endothelin B (ETB) receptors, whereas Ambrisentan binds to ETA receptor only. The PGI2 pathway is targeted by prostacyclin analog and prostacyclin-receptor agonists. Parenteral prostanoids are Epoprostenol, synthetic analog, and Treprostinil, a tricyclic benzidine prostacyclin analog. The latter can be used in both intravenous (IV) and subcutaneous routes, including an implantable infusion pump. Inhalation prostanoids are Ileoprost and inhaled Treprostinil. Oral forms of protanoids are available as Treprostinil diolamine, Selexipag, and Ralinepag.

When monotherapy is decided, any of the pulmonary vasodilators can be chosen. For the high-risk group, IV prostacyclin is usually included in initial combination therapy. Alternative combination therapy may be used.

When the stage remains in intermediate to high after 3–6 months of follow-up, double combination therapy in case of having monotherapy or triple combination therapy in case of having double combination therapy is advised.

When the patient remains in intermediate or high risk, even after triple combination therapy, maximal medication therapy is advised. Maximal medication therapy means triple combination therapy including prostacyclin.

Four pathways, which lead to PH and the site of action of different pulmonary vasodilators

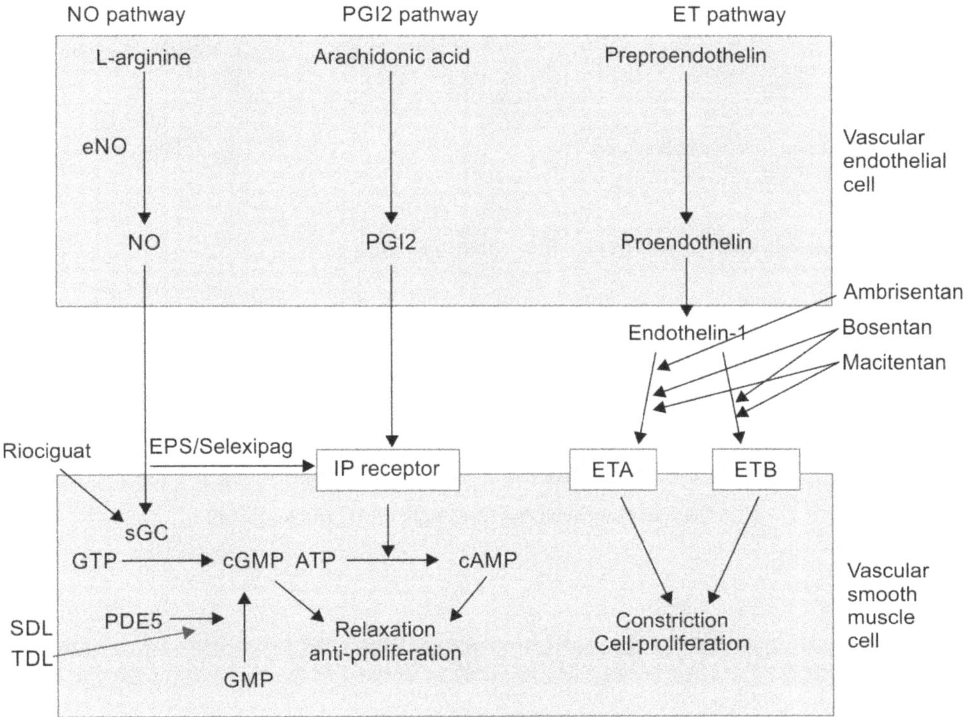

(ATP: adenosine triphosphate; cAMP : cyclic adenosine monophosphate; cGMP : cyclic guanosine monophosphate; eNOS : nitric oxide synthase; ETA: endothelin A; ETB: endothelin B; EPS: eprostenol; ET: endothelin; GTP : guanosine triphosphate;. IP: prostaglandin I2 receptor. NO : nitric oxide; PDE5 :phosphodiesterase type 5; sGC : soluble guanylate cyclase; SDL: sildenafil; TDL: tadalafil)

Different pulmonary vasodilators used in PAH

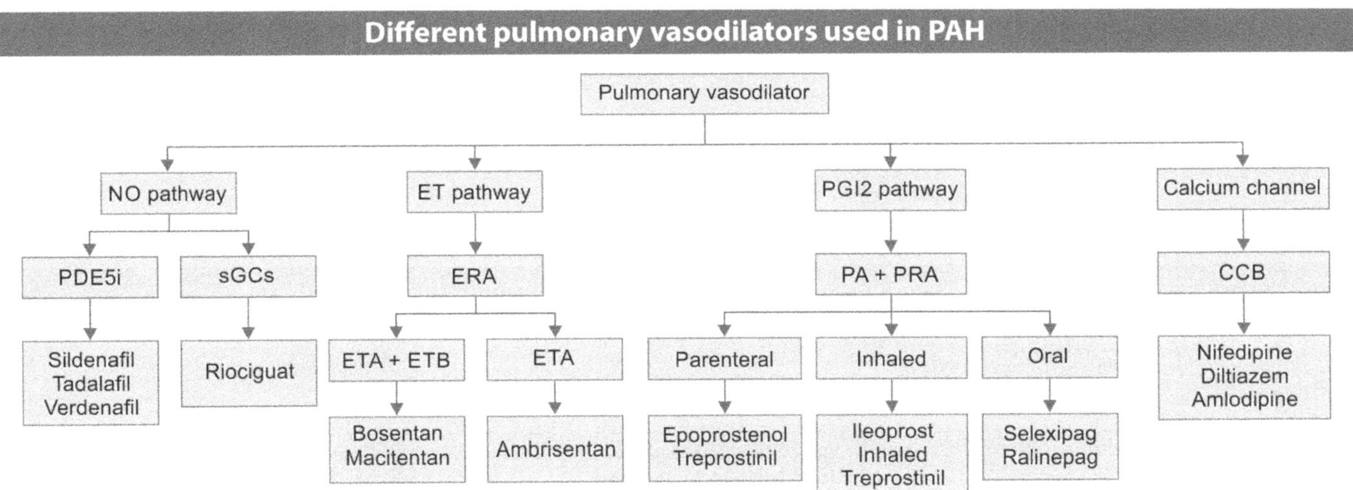

(CCB: calcium channel blocker; ERA: endothelin receptor antagonist; ETA: endothelin receptor A; ETB: endothelin receptor B; PA: prostacyclin analogue; PDE5i: phosphodiesterase 5-inhibitor; PRA: prostacyclin receptor agonist; sGCs: soluble guanylate cyclase stimulator)

Management outline of pulmonary arterial hypertension[2]

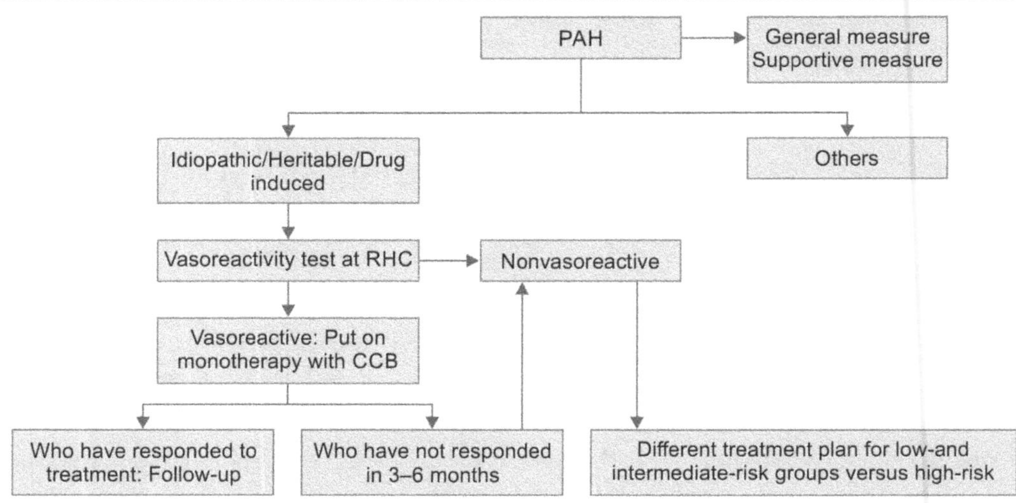

(CCB: calcium channel blocker; RHC: right heart catheterization)

General and supportive measures for pulmonary arterial hypertension

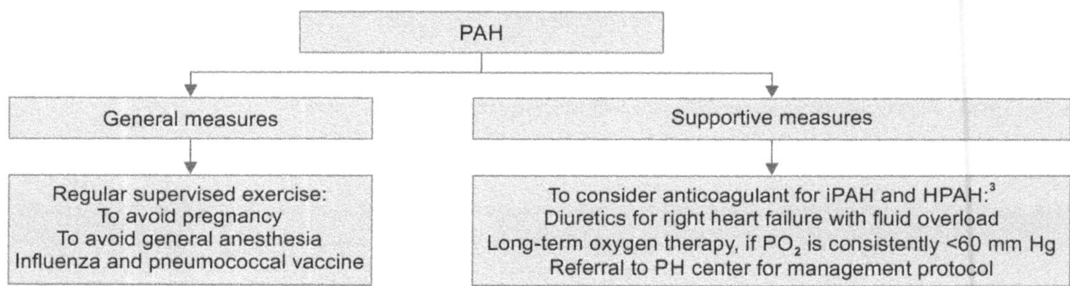

(HPAH: heritable pulmonary arterial hypertension; iPAH: idiopathic pulmonary arterial hypertension; PAH: pulmonary arterial hypertension; PH: pulmonary hypertension; PO_2: partial pressure of oxygen)

Criteria of responder to vasoreactive test in pulmonary arterial hypertension[1,2]

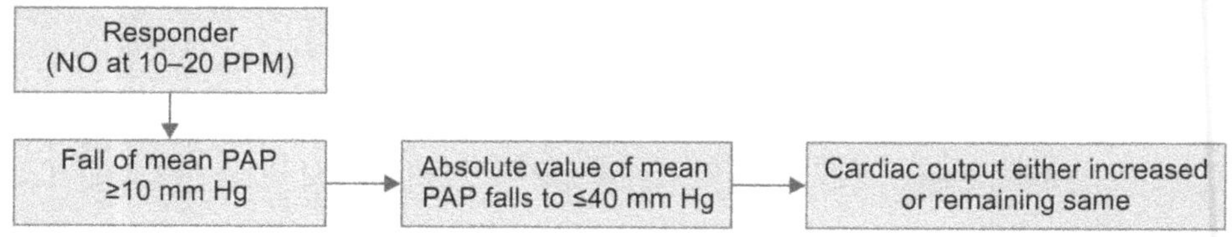

(NO: nitric oxide; PAP: pulmonary artery pressure; PPM: parts per million)

Treatment algorithm for low- or intermediate-risk group[2]

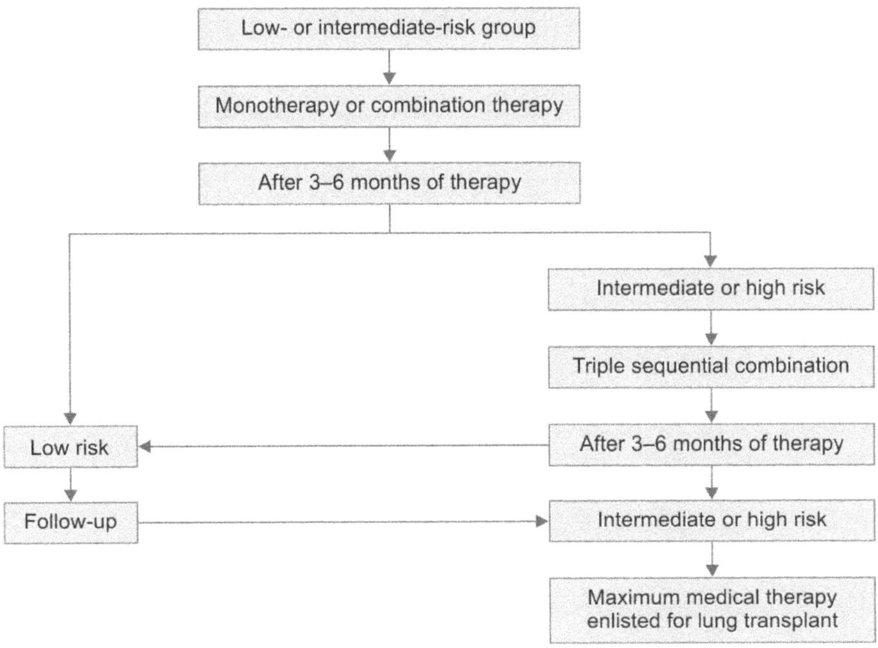

Treatment algorithm for high-risk group[2]

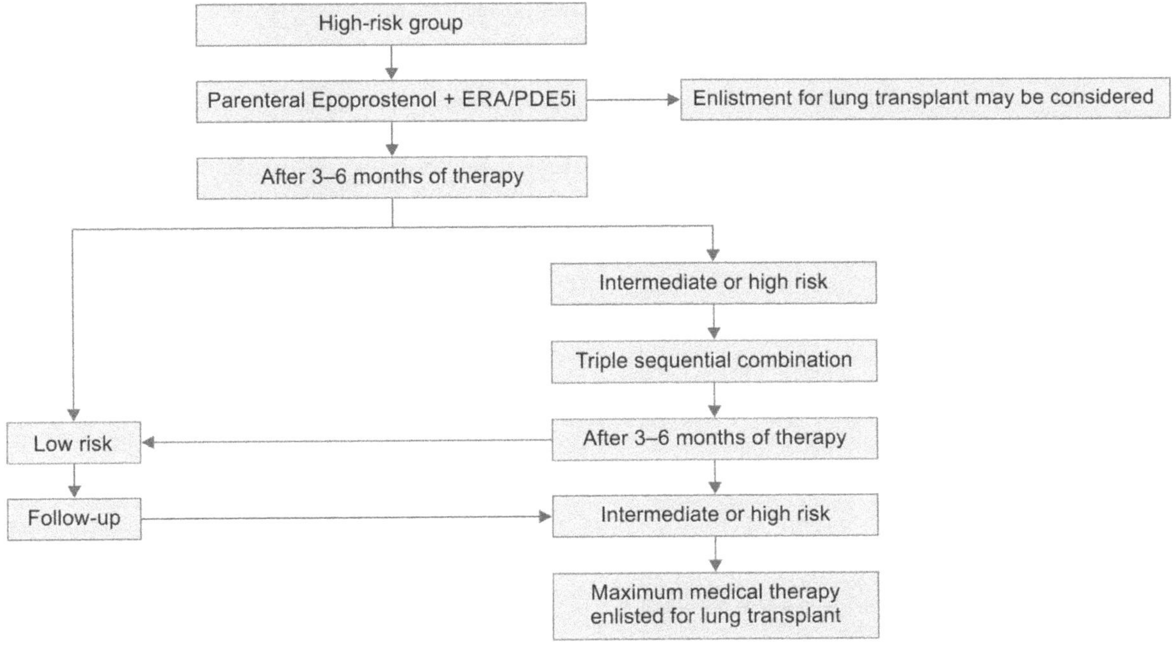

(ERA: endothelin receptor antagonists; PDE5i: phosphodiesterase 5-inhibitor)

Situation where monotherapy is preferred[4]

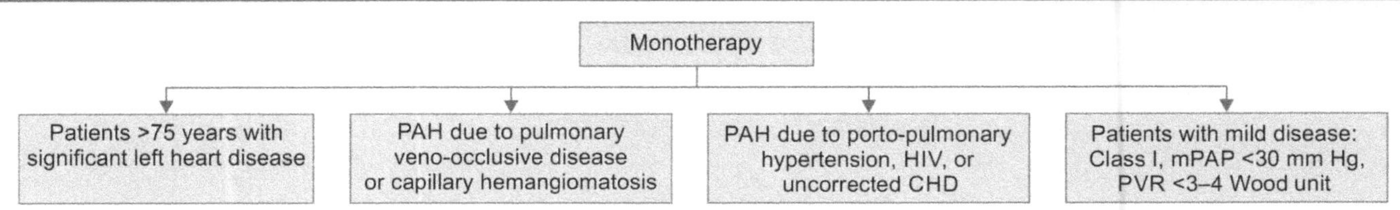

(CHD: coronary heart disease; HIV: human immunodeficiency virus; PAH: pulmonary arterial hypertension)

Different molecules used in combination therapy in different trials[5]

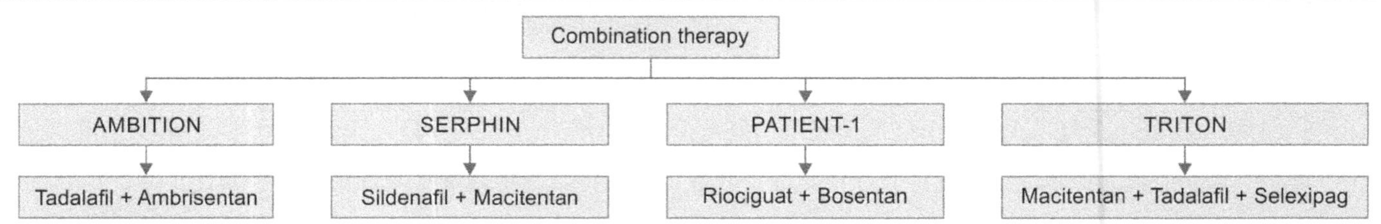

Drug choice in low- or intermediate-risk group[5]

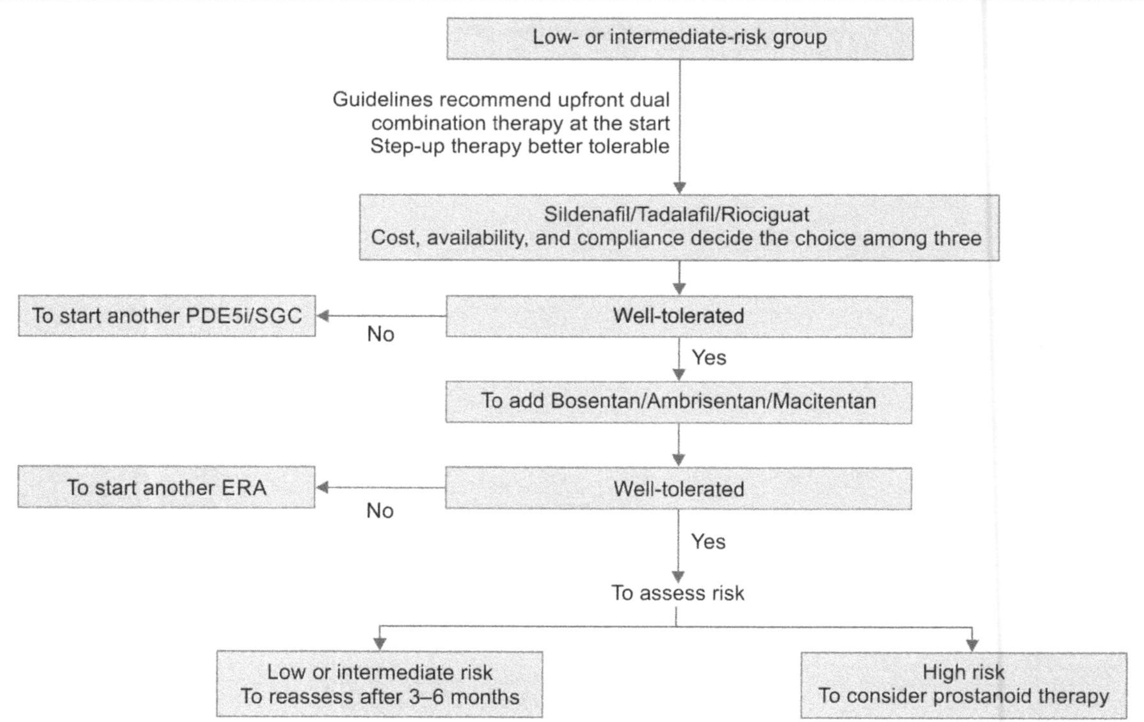

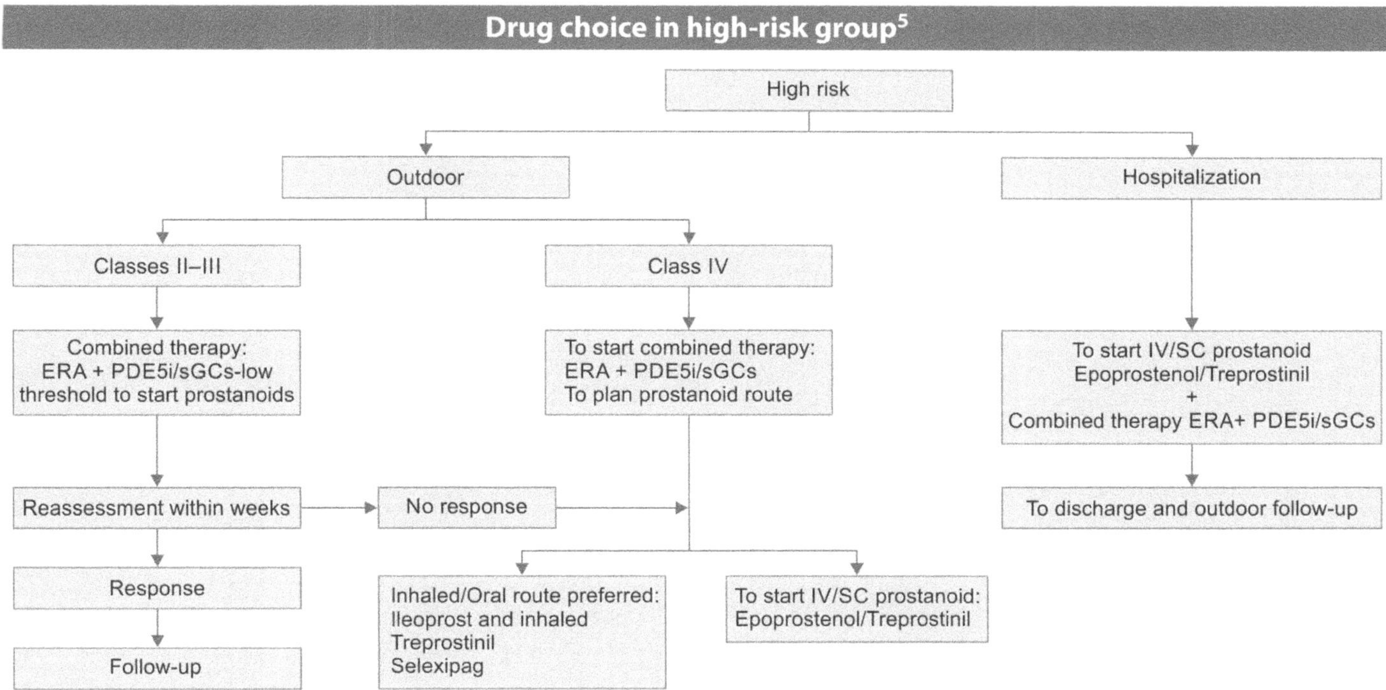

(ERA: endothelin receptor antagonist; IV: intravenous; PDE5i: phosphodiesterase 5-inhibitor; SC: subcutaneous; sGCs: soluble guanylate cyclase stimulator)

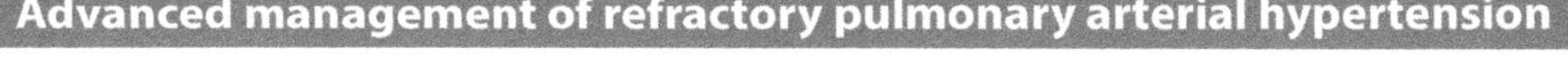

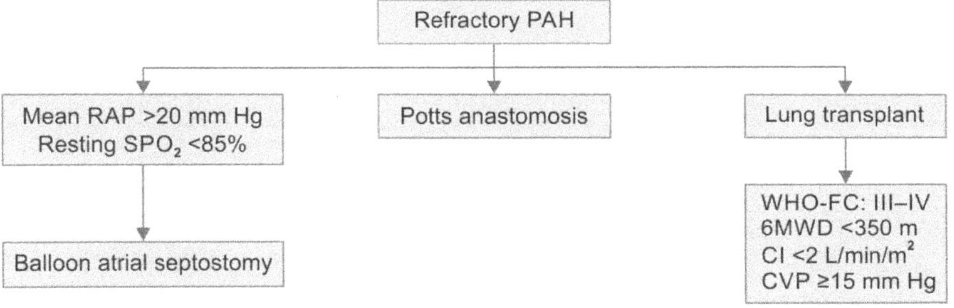

(CI: cardiac index; CVP: central venous pressure; RAP: right atrial pressure; 6MWD: 6-minute walk distance; PAH: pulmonary arterial hypertension; WHO: World Health Organization)

REFERENCES

1. Sitbon O, Humbert M, Jaïs X, Ioos V, Hamid AM, Provencher S, et al. Long-term response to calcium channel blockers in idiopathic pulmonary arterial hypertension. Circulation. 2005;111:3105-11.
2. Galiè N, Humbert M, Vachiery JL, Gibbs S, Lang I, Torbicki A, et al. 2015 ESC/ERS guidelines for the diagnosis and treatment of pulmonary hypertension: the joint Task force for the diagnosis and treatment of pulmonary hypertension of the European Society of cardiology (ESC) and the European respiratory Society (ERS): endorsed by: association for European paediatric and congenital cardiology (AEPC), International Society for heart and lung transplantation (ISHLT). Eur Respir J. 2015;46:903-75.
3. Preston IR, Roberts KE, Miller DP, Sen GP, Selej M, Benton WW, et al. Effect of warfarin treatment on survival of patients with pulmonary arterial hypertension (PAH) in the registry to evaluate early and long-term PAH disease management (reveal). Circulation 2015;132:2403-11.
4. Yaghi S, Novikov A, Trandafirescu T. Clinical update on pulmonary hypertension. J Investig Med. 2020;0:1-7.
5. Mayeux JD, Pan IZ, Dechand J. Management of pulmonary arterial hypertension. Curr Cardiovasc Risk Rep. 2021;15:2.

Myocarditis and Cardiomyopathy

CHAPTER 38

Myocarditis

INTRODUCTION

Myocarditis or more precisely acute myocarditis is defined by World Health Organization (WHO)/International Society and Federation of Cardiology (ISFC)[1] as an inflammatory disease of the myocardium diagnosed by established histological, immunological, and immunohistochemical criteria. There has been a shift in the time-old definition of myocarditis.

Inflammatory cardiomyopathy is defined as "myocarditis in association with cardiac dysfunction." A delayed diagnosis of acute myocarditis presents as inflammatory cardiomyopathy, which consists of mild elevation of troponin level disproportionate to the degree of left ventricular dysfunction and associated with dilated left ventricle.[2] Inflammatory cardiomyopathy and dilated cardiomyopathy are not mutually exclusive.

Fulminant myocarditis is defined as an acute and severe inflammation of the myocardium leading to myocyte necrosis, edema, and cardiogenic shock. Up to 30% cases of biopsy-proven myocarditis progress to inflammatory cardiomyopathy with fatal outcome.

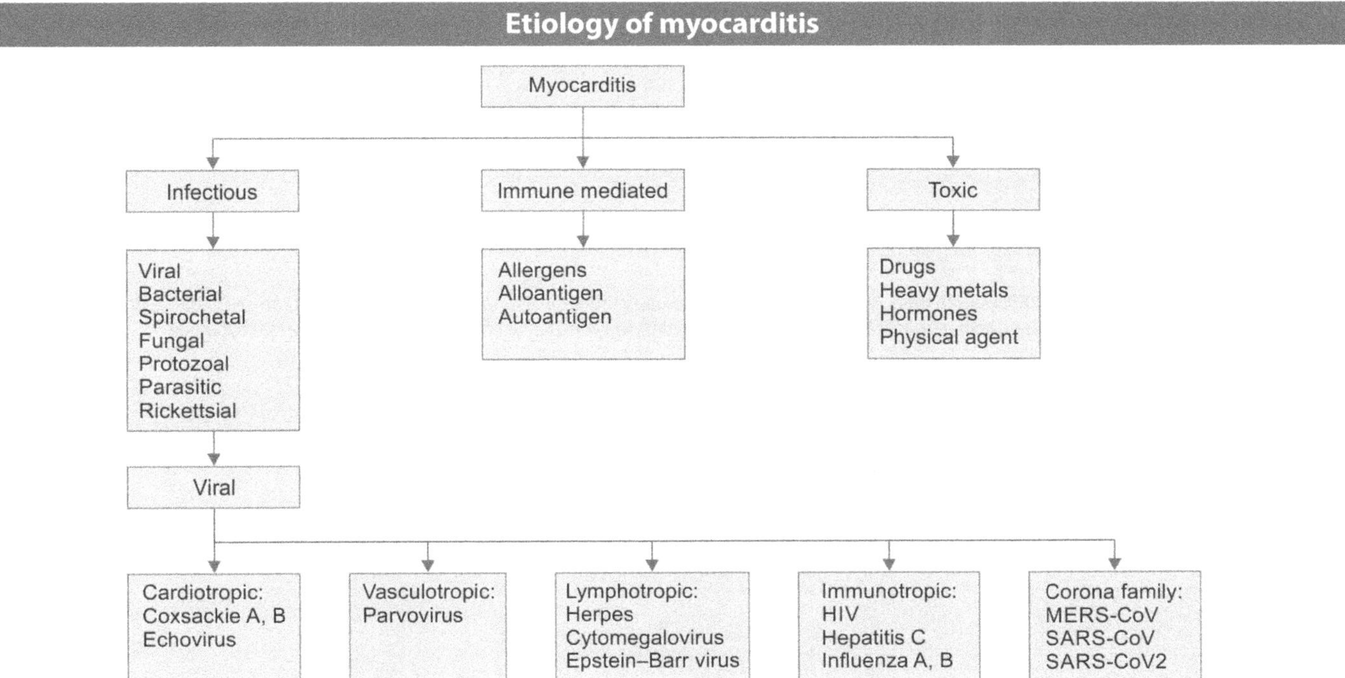

(HIV: human immunodeficiency virus; MERS-CoV: Middle East respiratory syndrome-related coronavirus; SARS-CoV: severe acute respiratory syndrome-associated coronavirus)

Diagnostic criteria[3]

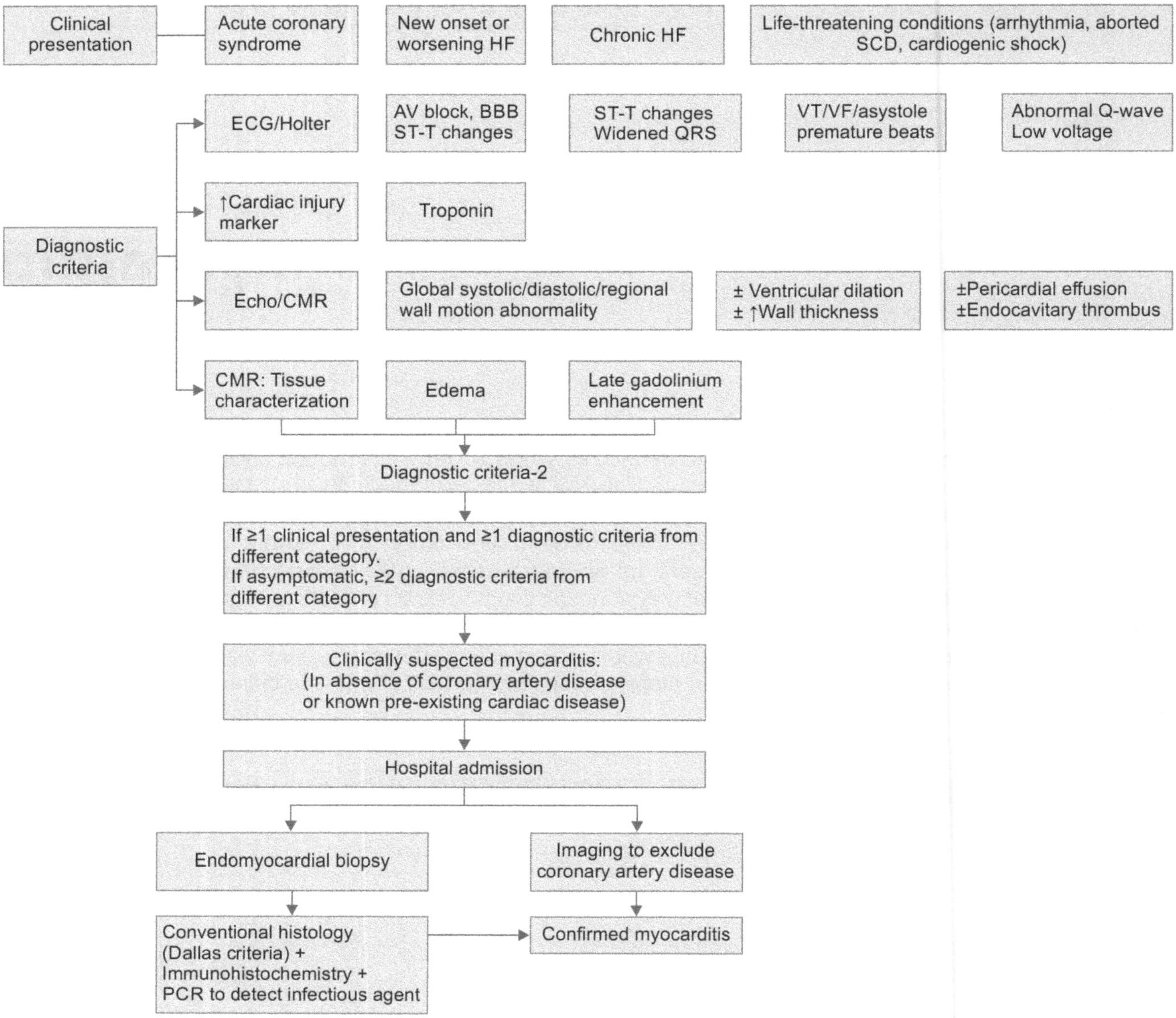

| Clinical presentation | Acute coronary syndrome | New onset or worsening HF | Chronic HF | Life-threatening conditions (arrhythmia, aborted SCD, cardiogenic shock) |

Diagnostic criteria

- **ECG/Holter** — AV block, BBB ST-T changes | ST-T changes Widened QRS | VT/VF/asystole premature beats | Abnormal Q-wave Low voltage
- **↑Cardiac injury marker** — Troponin
- **Echo/CMR** — Global systolic/diastolic/regional wall motion abnormality | ± Ventricular dilation ± ↑Wall thickness | ±Pericardial effusion ±Endocavitary thrombus
- **CMR: Tissue characterization** — Edema | Late gadolinium enhancement

Diagnostic criteria-2

If ≥1 clinical presentation and ≥1 diagnostic criteria from different category.
If asymptomatic, ≥2 diagnostic criteria from different category

Clinically suspected myocarditis:
(In absence of coronary artery disease
or known pre-existing cardiac disease)

Hospital admission

- **Endomyocardial biopsy**
  - Conventional histology (Dallas criteria) + Immunohistochemistry + PCR to detect infectious agent → **Confirmed myocarditis**
- **Imaging to exclude coronary artery disease**

(AV: atrioventricular; BBB: bundle branch block; CMR: cardiovascular magnetic resonance; ECG: echocardiogram; HF: heart failure; PCR: polymerase chain reaction; SCD: sudden cardiac death; VF: ventricular fibrillation; VT: ventricular tachycardia)

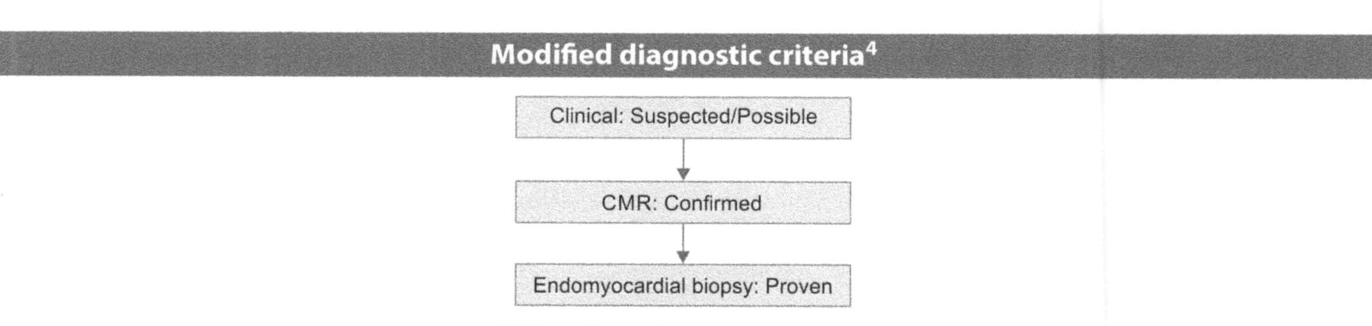

Modified diagnostic criteria[4]

Clinical: Suspected/Possible

↓

CMR: Confirmed

↓

Endomyocardial biopsy: Proven

(CMR: cardiovascular magnetic resonance)

CMR criteria for myocardial inflammation[5]

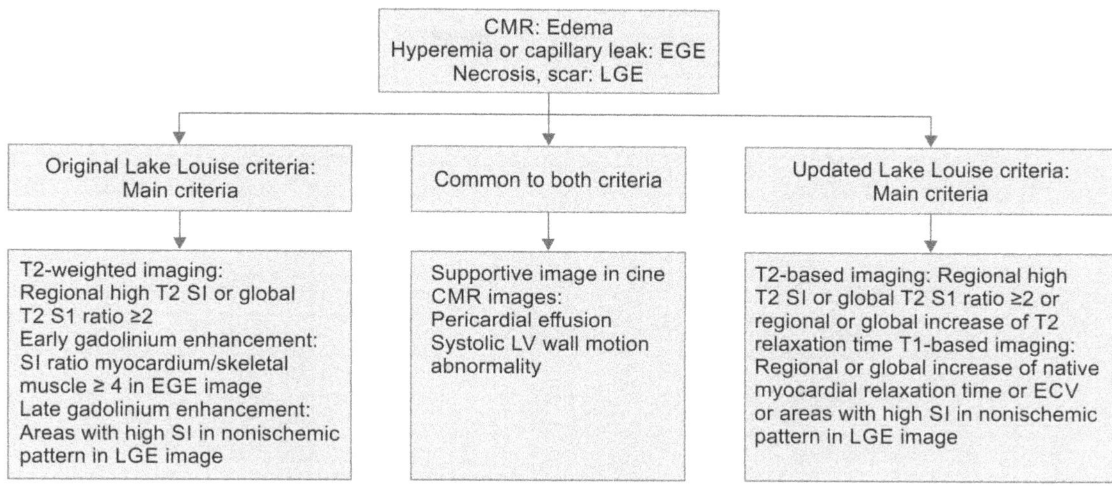

(CMR: cardiovascular magnetic resonance; ECV: extracellular volume; EGE: early gadolinium enhancement; LGE: late gadolinium enhancement)

Dallas criteria for endomyocardial biopsy

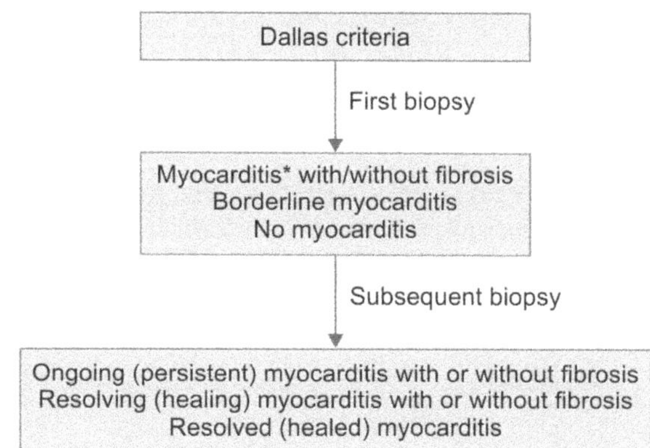

*Definite diagnosis: Lymphocytic, granulocytic, polymorphous, eosinophil, necrotizing eosinophilic, giant cell, granulomatous myocarditis, with or without associated myocyte damage/necrosis.

Classification of myocarditis: Tempo of presentation[6]

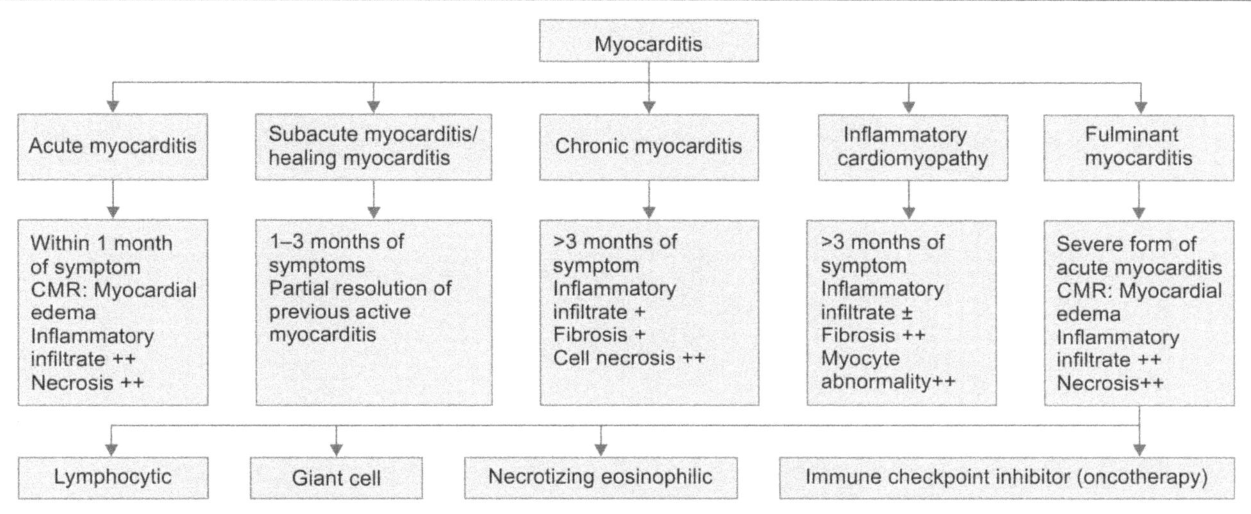

Classification of myocarditis: Myocarditis versus inflammatory cardiomyopathy[6]

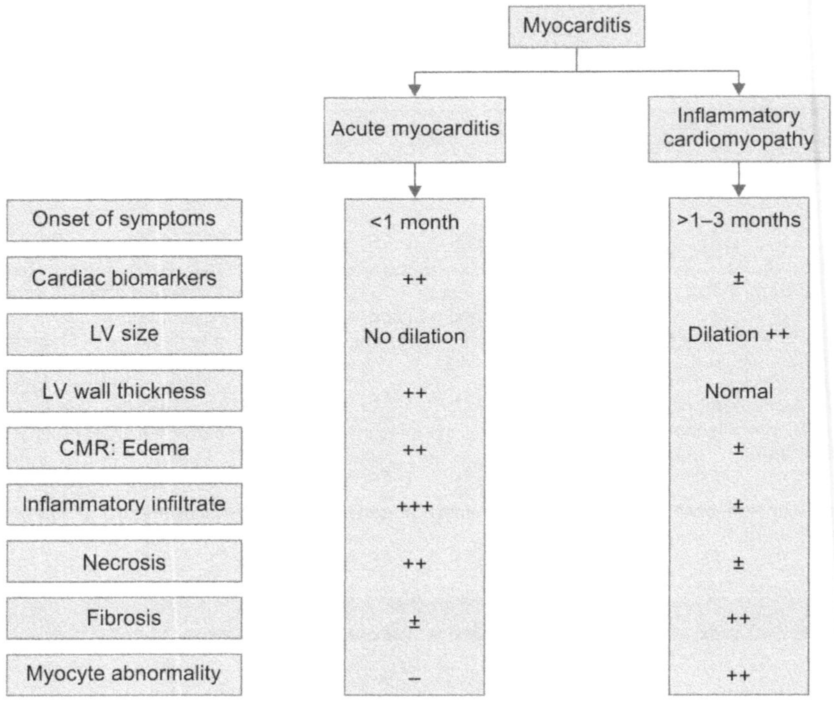

(CMR: cardiovascular magnetic resonance; LV: left ventricular)

Management of myocarditis

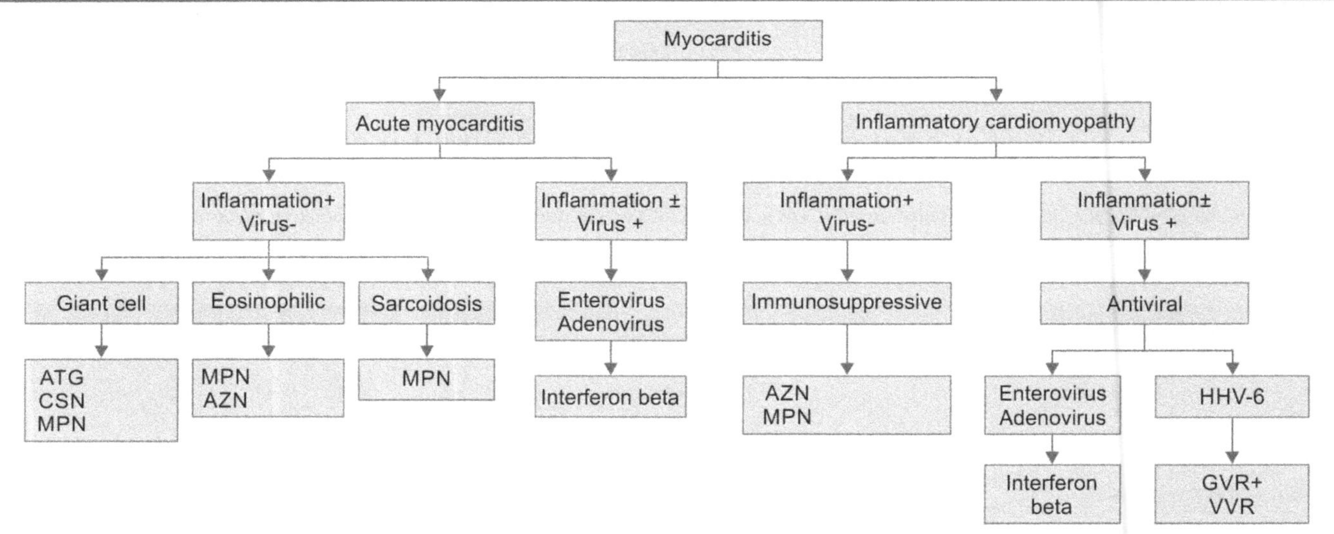

(ATG: antithymoglobulin; AZN: azathioprine; CSN: ciclosporin; GVR: ganciclovir; HHV-6: human herpes virus 6; MPN: methyl prednisolone; VVR: valganciclovir)

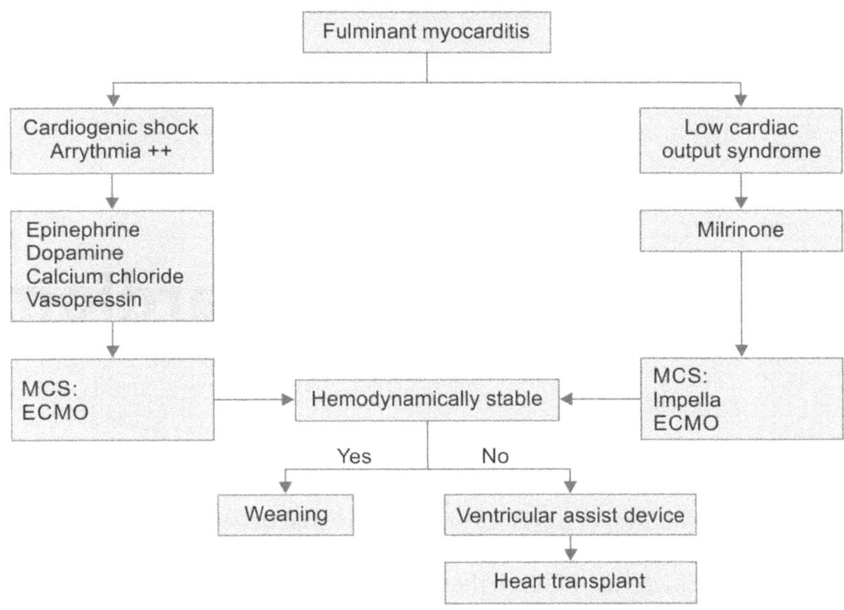

(ECMO: extracorporeal membrane oxygenation; MCS: mechanical circulatory support)

REFERENCES

1. Richardson P, McKenna W, Bristow M, Maisch B, Mautner B, O'Connell J, et al. Report of the 1995 World Health Organization/International Society and Federation of Cardiology Task Force on the Definition and Classification of cardiomyopathies. Circulation. 1996;93:841-2.
2. Ammirati E, Veronese G, Cipriani M, Moroni F, Garascia A, et al. Acute and fulminant myocarditis: a pragmatic clinical approach to diagnosis and treatment. Curr Cardiol Rep. 2018;20:114.
3. Caforio AL, Pankuweit S, Arbustini E, Basso C, Gimeno-Blanes J, Felix SB, et al. Current state of knowledge on aetiology, diagnosis, management, and therapy of myocarditis: a position statement of the European Society of Cardiology Working Group on Myocardial and Pericardial Diseases. Eur Heart J. 2013;34:2636-48.
4. Law YM, Lal AK, Chen S, Čiháková D, Cooper LT Jr, Deshpande S, et al. Diagnosis and Management of Myocarditis in Children A Scientific Statement From the American Heart Association Circulation. 2021;144:e123-e135.
5. Ferreira VM, Schulz-Menger J, Holmvang G, Kramer CM, Carbone I, Sechtem U, et al. Cardiovascular magnetic resonance in nonischemic myocardial inflammation: expert recommendations. J Am Coll Cardiol. 2018;72:3158-76.
6. Ammirati E, Frigerio M, Adler ED, Basso C, Birnie DH, Brambatti M, et al. Management of Acute Myocarditis and Chronic Inflammatory Cardiomyopathy An Expert Consensus Document.Circ Heart Fail. 2020;13:e007405.
7. Kociol RD, Cooper LT, Fank JC, Moslehi JJ, Pang PS, Sabe MA, et al. Recognition and Initial Management of Fulminant Myocarditis: A Scientific Statement From the American Heart Association. Circulation. 2020;141:e69–e92.

CHAPTER 39

Peripartum Cardiomyopathy

INTRODUCTION

Peripartum cardiomyopathy (PPCM) was first defined[1] as heart failure that develops in the last month of pregnancy or up to 5 months postpartum with left ventricular ejection fraction (LVEF) < 45%.[1] Later, the European Society of Cardiology (ESC) in a position statement[2] redefined PPCM as heart failure that occurs toward end of the pregnancy or in the months following delivery in the absence of a preexisting heart disease. The most common time of presentation is the 1st week of pregnancy. 50–80% of patients with PPCM improve within the first 6 months.[3] Anticoagulant is indicated when left ventricular function is severely affected with LVEF < 30–35%.[3] It should be given during late pregnancy and 6–8 weeks postpartum.[4] Vaginal delivery is preferred, as cesarean delivery is associated with a higher incidence of hemorrhage and thromboembolic events.

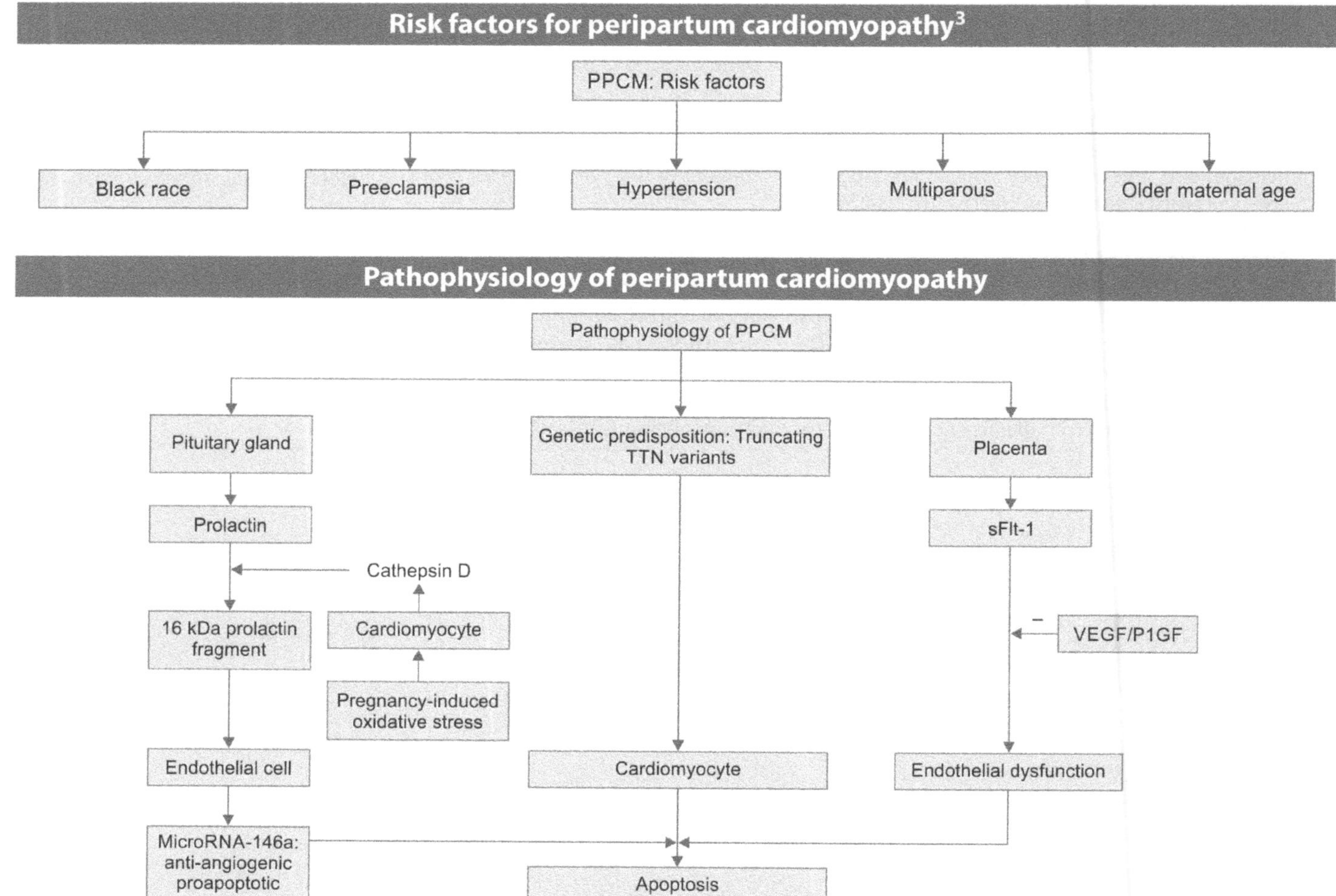

(P1GF: placental growth factor; PPCM: peripartum cardiomyopathy; sFlt-1: soluble fms-like tyrosine kinase-1; TTN: truncating titin; VEGF: vascular endothelial growth factor)

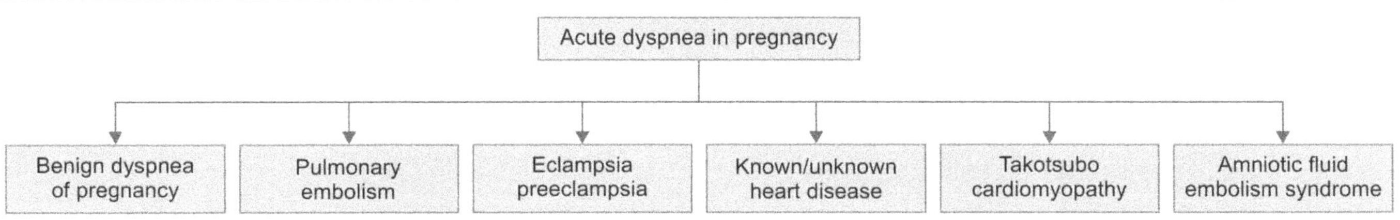

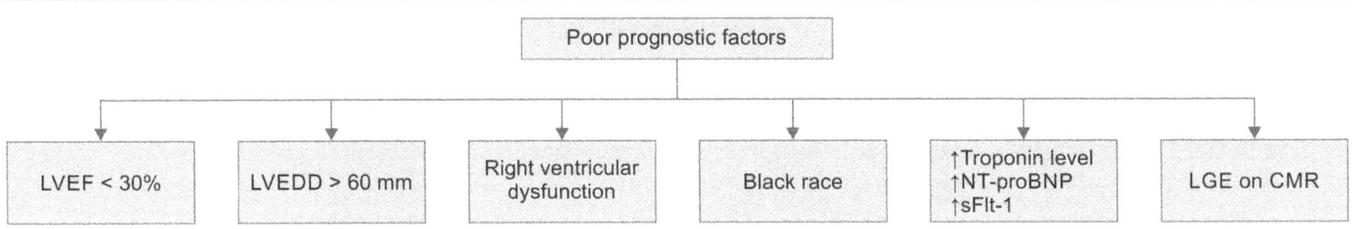

(CMR: cardiovascular magnetic resonance; LGE: late gadolinium enhancement; LVEDD: left ventricular end diastolic diameter; LVEF: left ventricular ejection fraction; NT-porBNP; N-terminal pro-brain natriuretic peptide)

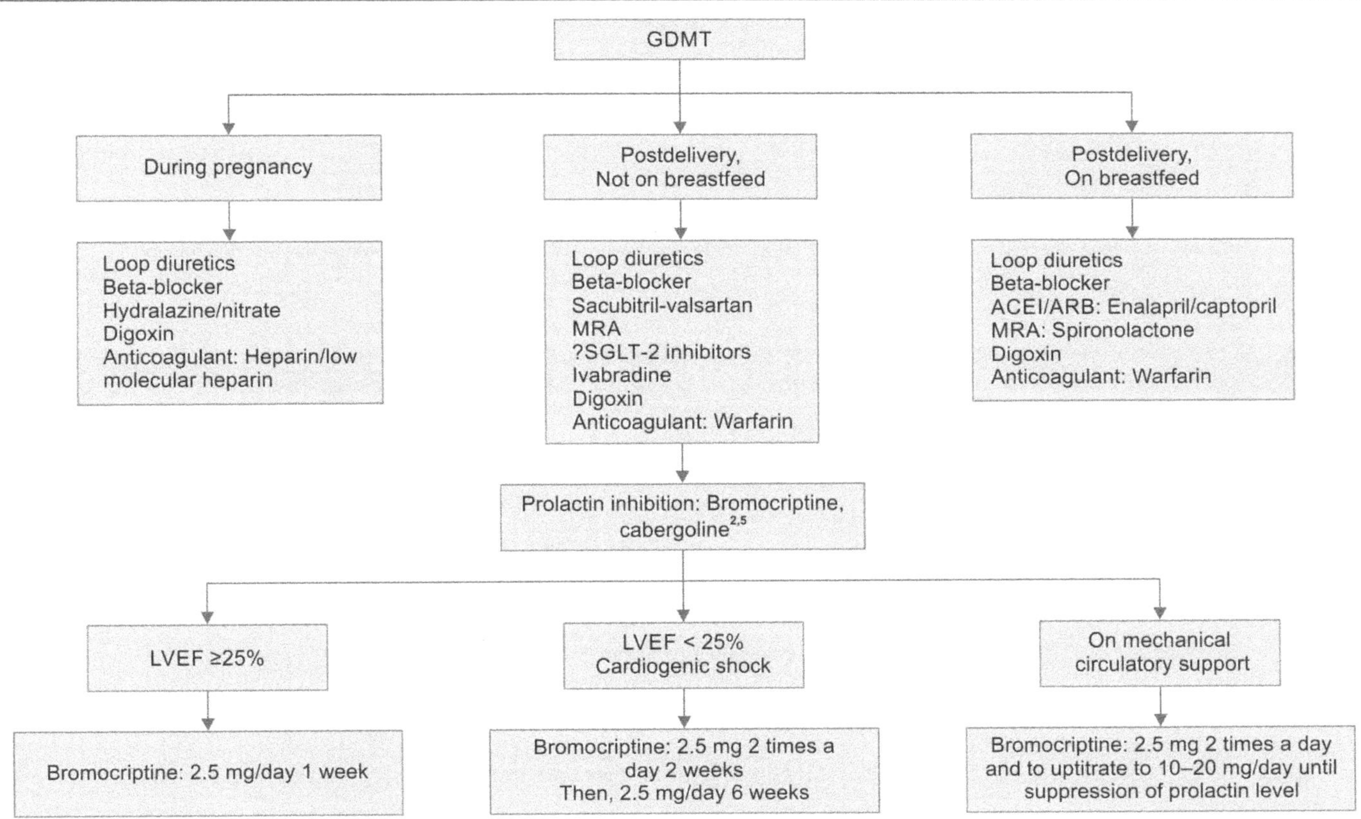

(ACEI: angiotensin-converting enzyme inhibitor; ARB: angiotensin receptor blocker; GDMT: guideline-directed medical therapy; LVEF: left ventricular ejection fraction; MRA: mineralocorticoid receptor antagonist; SGLT-2: sodium-glucose cotransporter-2)

Breastfeeding controversy in peripartum cardiomyopathy

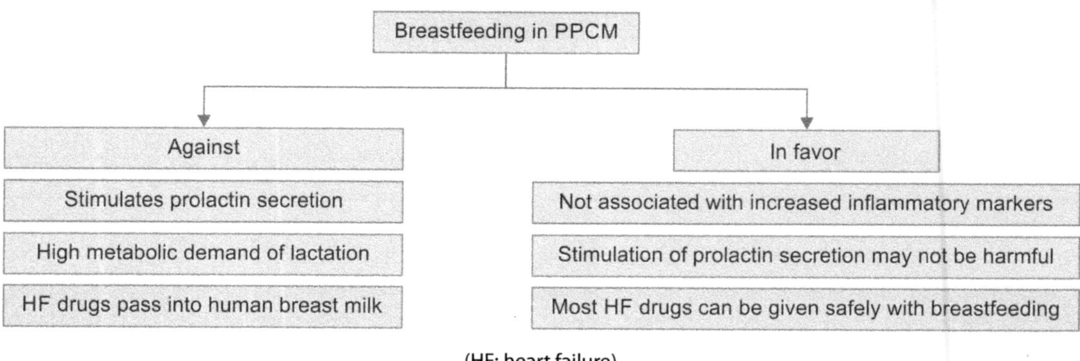

(HF: heart failure)

Device therapy in peripartum cardiomyopathy[2]

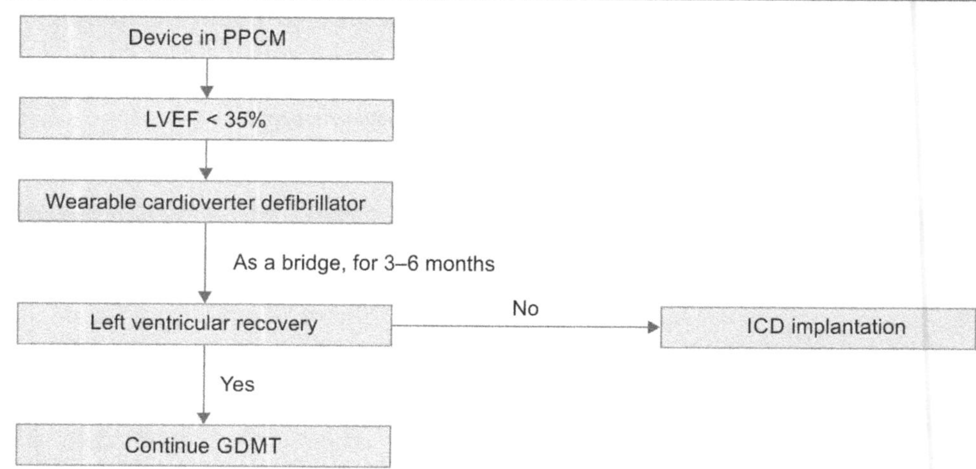

(GDMT: guideline-directed medical therapy; ICD: implantable cardioverter-defibrillator; LVEF: left ventricular ejection fraction)

Duration of guideline-directed medical therapy (GDMT) for heart failure

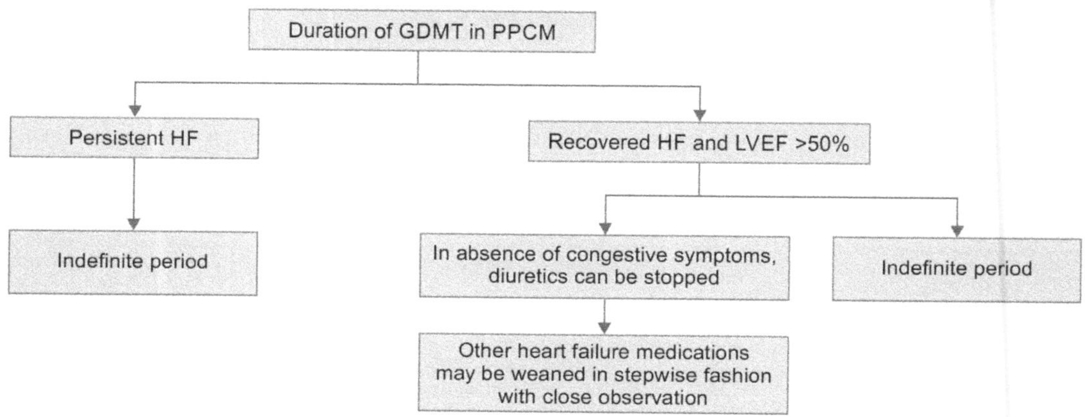

(LVEF: left ventricular ejection fraction; PPCM: peripartum cardiomyopathy)

REFERENCES

1. Pearson GD, Veille JC, Rahimtoola S, Hsia J, Oakley CM, Hosenpud JD, et al. Peripartum cardiomyopathy: National Heart, Lung, and Blood Institute and Office of Rare Diseases (National Institutes of Health) workshop recommendations and review. JAMA. 2000;283:1183-8.
2. Bauersachs J, König T, van der Meer P, Petrie MC, Hilfiker-Kleiner D, Mbakwem A, et al. Pathophysiology, diagnosis and management of peripartum cardiomyopathy: a position statement from the Heart Failure Association of the European Society of Cardiology Study Group on peripartum cardiomyopathy. Eur J Heart Fail. 2019;21:827-43.
3. Honigberg MC, Givertz MM. Peripartum cardiomyopathy. BMJ. 2019;364:k5287.
4. Arany Z, Elkayam U. Peripartum Cardiomyopathy. Circulation. 2016;133:1397-409.
5. Sieweke JT, Pfeffer TJ, Berliner D, Koenig T, Hallbaum M, Napp LC, et al. Cardiogenic shock complicating peripartum cardiomyopathy: importance of early left ventricular unloading and bromocriptine therapy. Eur Heart J Acute Cardiovasc Care. 2020;9(2):173-82.

CHAPTER 40

Arrhythmogenic Right Ventricular Cardiomyopathy

INTRODUCTION

As mentioned earlier, arrhythmogenic cardiomyopathy (ACM) is an inherited disease of heart muscle which is progressively replaced by fibrofatty tissue, and which may act as a substrate for malignant ventricular arrhythmia and sudden cardiac death regardless of the severity of ventricular dysfunction.[1] The original description, in relation to right ventricle, is arrhythmogenic right ventricular cardiomyopathy/dysplasia (ARVC/D) which is a genetic disease of right ventricle involving the mutation of genes coding protein of desmosomes, which are intercellular structures attaching myocytes. Detached myocytes die and replaced by fibrofatty tissue which extends from epicardium to endocardium. This process of replacement fibrosis remains restricted to the "triangle of dysplasia" of the right ventricle, bounded by the anterior part of infundibulum, the apex, and the infero–posterior wall. ARVC-causing mutations have been identified in genes encoding five desmosome proteins, namely plakoglobin, desmoplakin, plakophilin-2, desmoglein-2, and desmocollin-2. ACM is familial in more than 50% of cases, typically inherited as an autosomal dominant disorder. The most common age of presentation is between second and fourth decade.

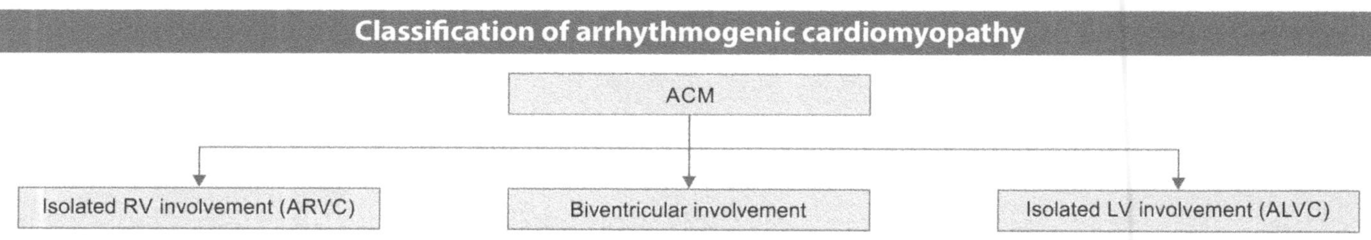

(ACM: arrhythmogenic cardiomyopathy; ALVC: arrhythmogenic left ventricular cardiomyopathy; ARVC: arrhythmogenic right ventricular cardiomyopathy; LV: left ventricular; RV: right ventricular)

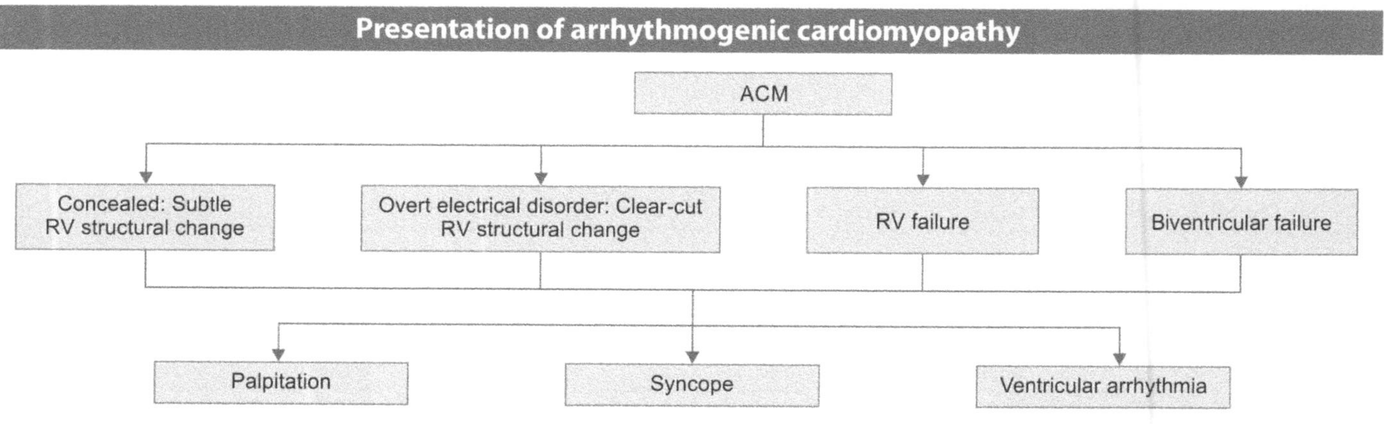

(ACM: arrhythmogenic cardiomyopathy; RV: right ventricular)

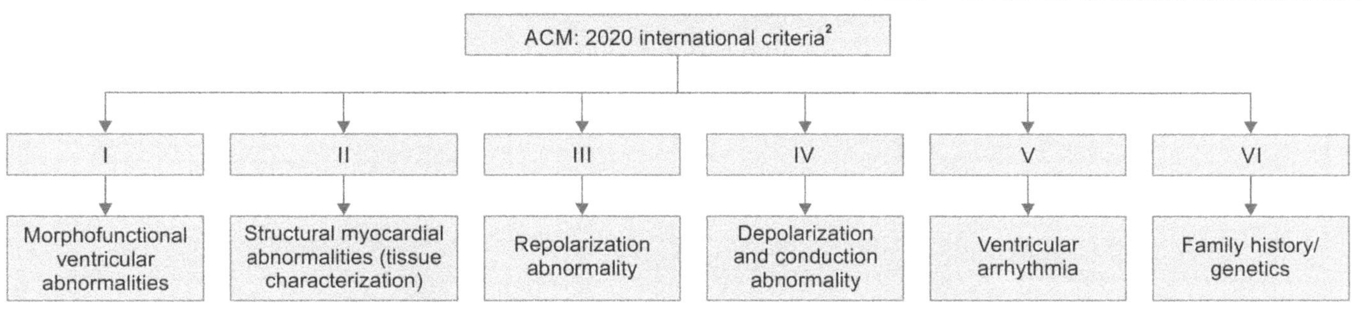

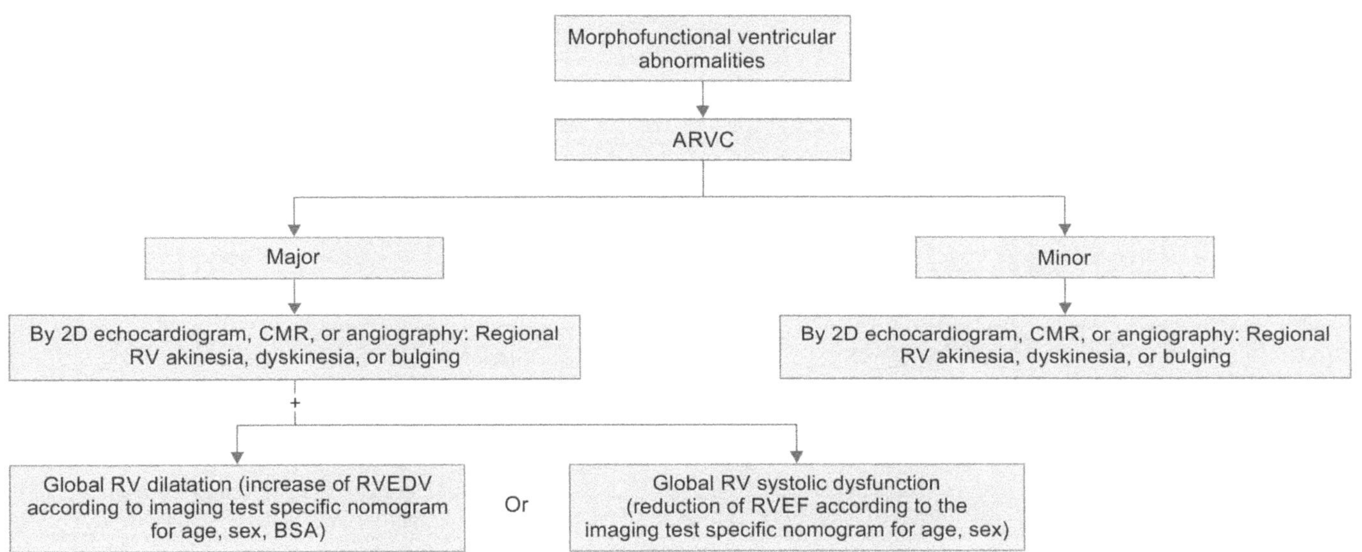

(ARVC: arrhythmogenic right ventricular cardiomyopathy; BSA: body surface area; CMR: cardiovascular magnetic resonance; RV: right ventricular; RVEDV: right ventricular end-diastolic volume; RVEF: right ventricular ejection fraction)

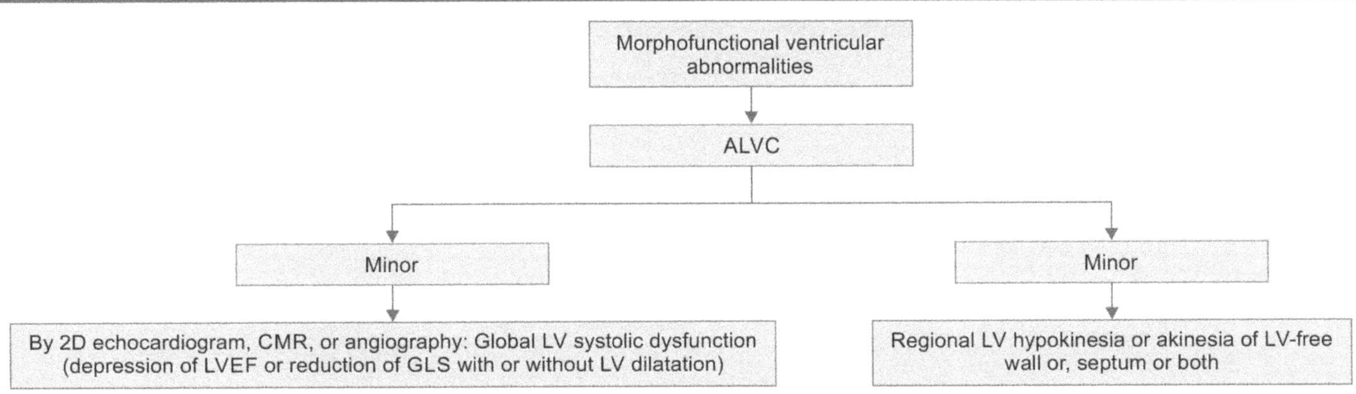

(ALVC: arrhythmogenic left ventricular cardiomyopathy; CMR: cardiovascular magnetic resonance; GLS: global longitudinal strain; LV: left ventricular; LVEF: left ventricular ejection fraction)

Padua criteria (structural)

Structural myocardial abnormalities

ARVC

Major

Transmural LGE ≥1 RV regions (inlet, outlet, and apex in two orthogonal views)

Major

By EBM: Fibrous replacement of myocardium in ≥1 sample with or without fatty tissue

ALVC

Major

LVLGE ≥1 bull's eye segments of free wall, septum, or both

(ALVC: arrhythmogenic left ventricular cardiomyopathy; ARVC: arrhythmogenic right ventricular cardiomyopathy; EBM: evidence-based medicine; LGE: late gadolinium enhancement; LVLGE: left ventricular late gadolinium enhancement)

Padua criteria (repolarization)

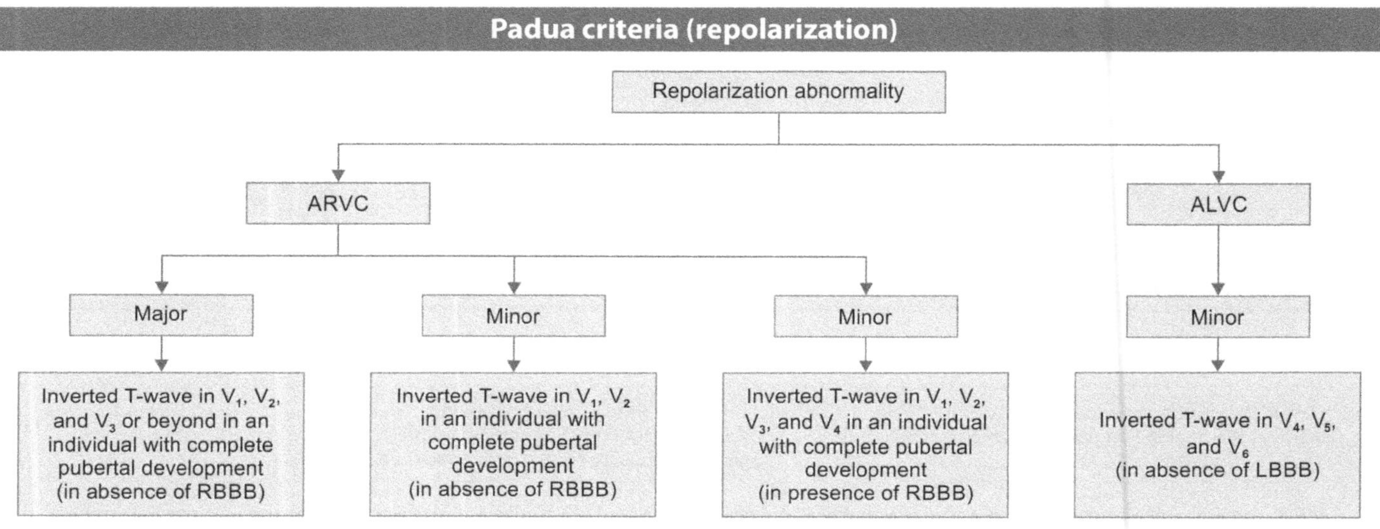

(ALVC: arrhythmogenic left ventricular cardiomyopathy; ARVC: arrhythmogenic right ventricular cardiomyopathy; LBBB: right bundle branch block; RBBB: right bundle branch block)

Padua criteria (depolarization)

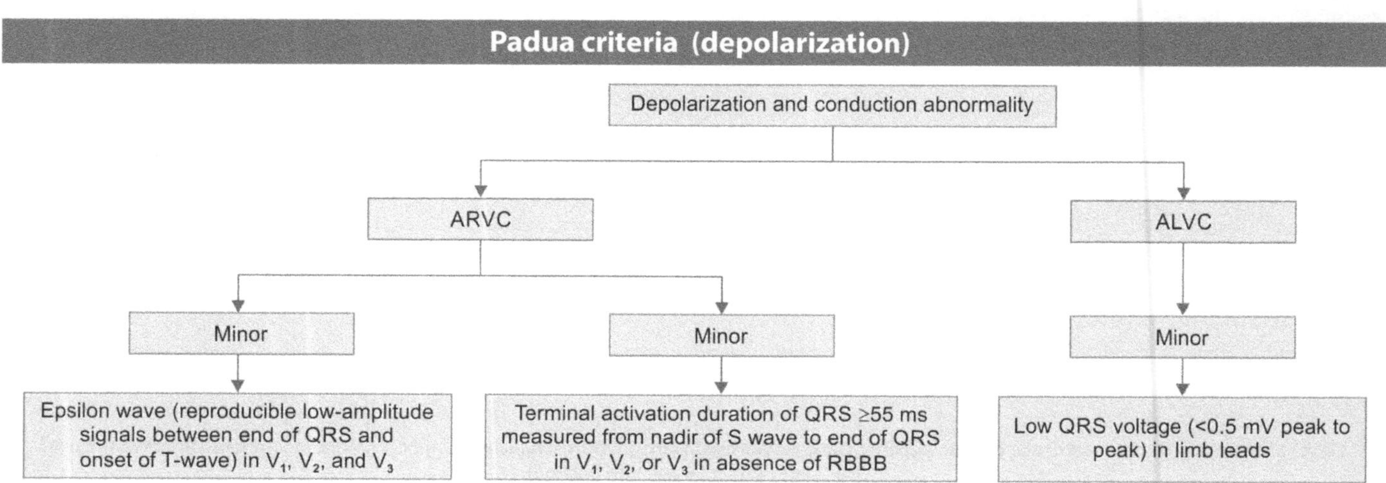

(ALVC: arrhythmogenic left ventricular cardiomyopathy; ARVC: arrhythmogenic right ventricular cardiomyopathy; RBBB: right bundle branch block)

Padua criteria (arrhythmia)

(ALVC: arrhythmogenic left ventricular cardiomyopathy; ARVC: arrhythmogenic right ventricular cardiomyopathy; LBBB: right bundle branch block; RBBB: right bundle branch block; RVOT: right ventricular outflow tract; VPB: ventricular premature beats; VT: ventricular)

Padua criteria (genetic)

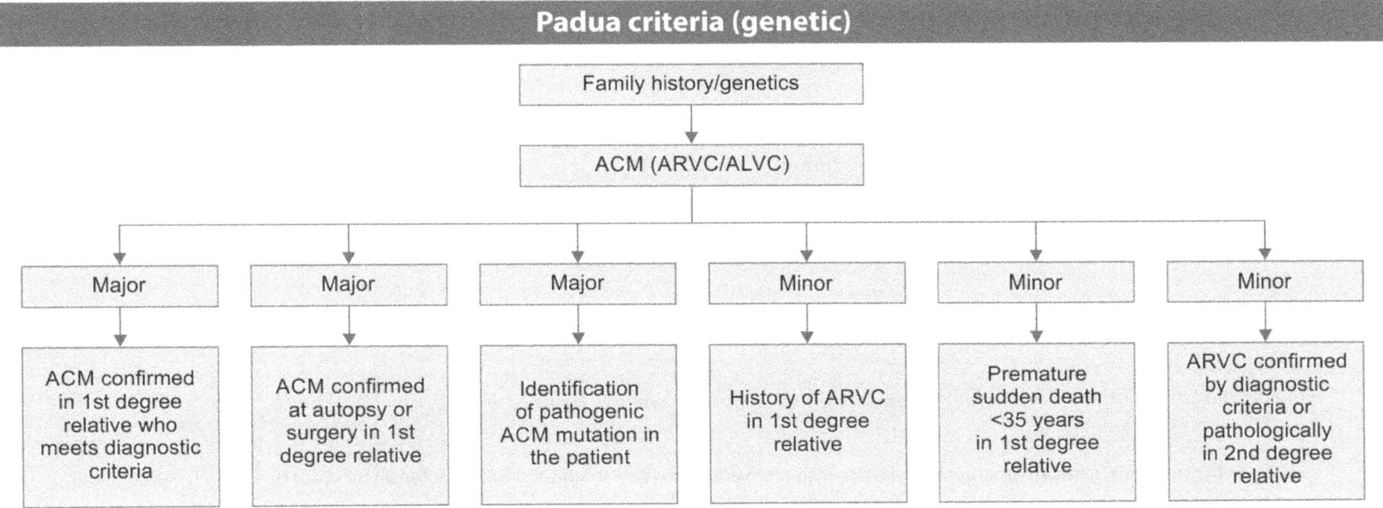

(ACM: arrhythmogenic cardiomyopathy; ARVC: arrhythmogenic right ventricular cardiomyopathy)

Padua criteria (conclusion)

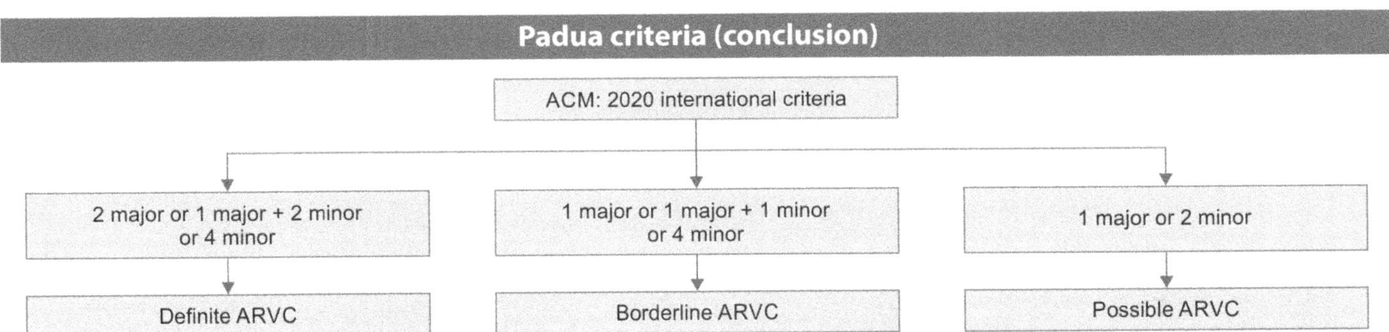

*≥1 morphofunctional and/or structural criteria, either major or minor needed for each degree of diagnosis.

Extrapolating PADUA criteria for ALVC

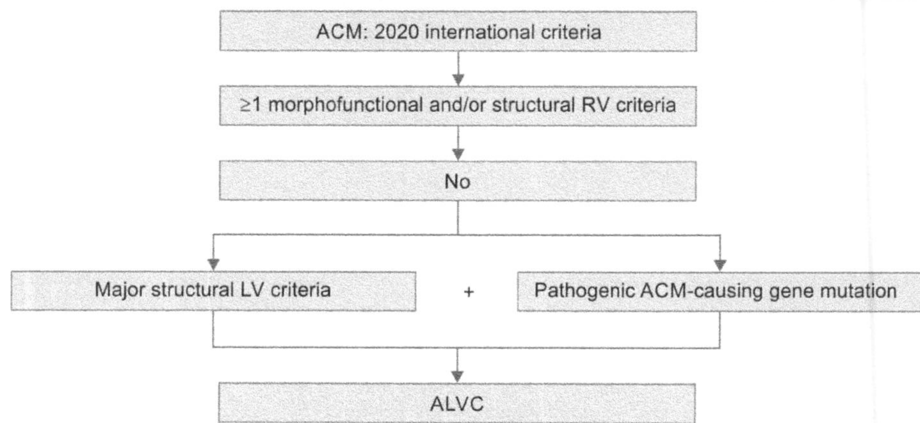

(ACM: arrhythmogenic cardiomyopathy; ALVC: arrhythmogenic left ventricular cardiomyopathy; LV: left ventricular)

Management of arrhythmogenic cardiomyopathy

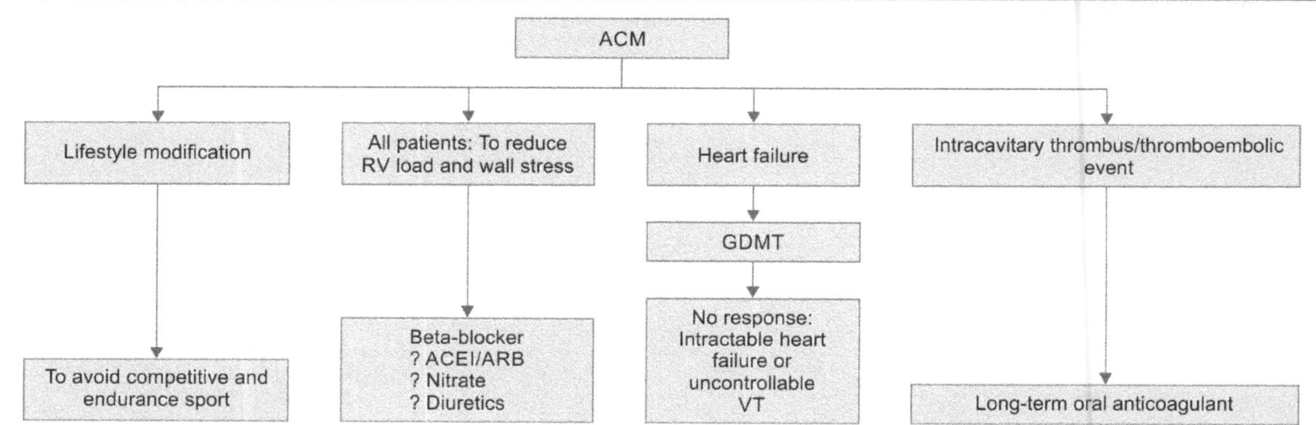

(ACM: arrhythmogenic cardiomyopathy; ACEI: angiotensin-converting enzyme inhibitor; ARB: angiotensin receptor blocker; VT: ventricular)

Risk stratification for sudden cardiac death[2]

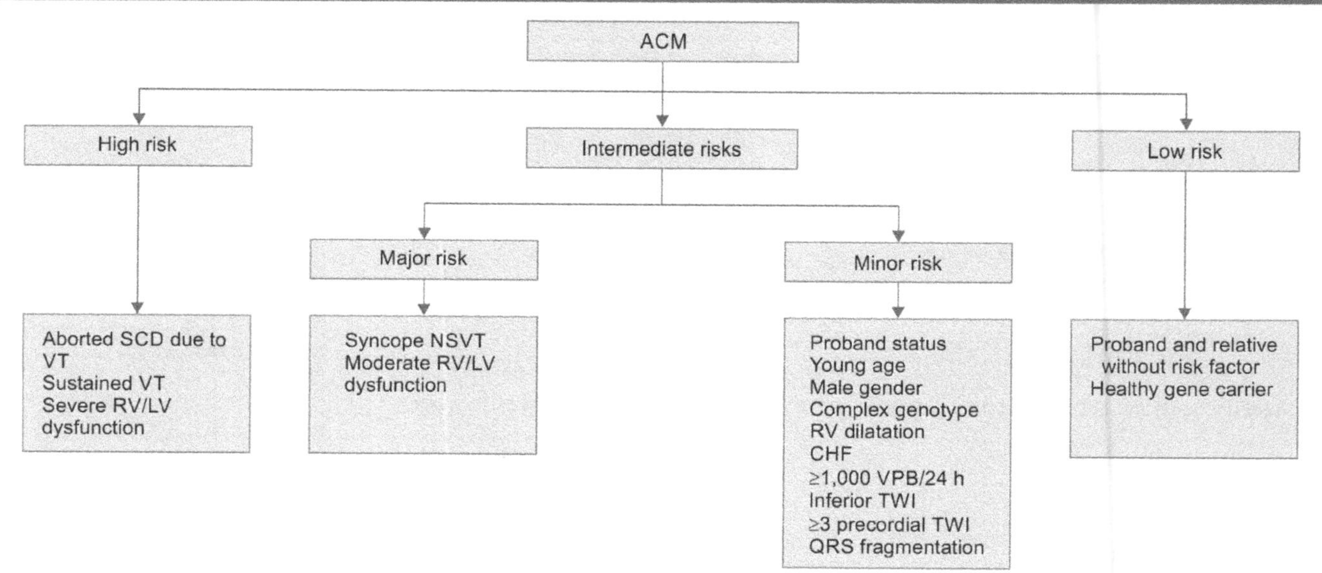

(ACM: arrhythmogenic cardiomyopathy; CHF: chronic heart failure; LV: left ventricular; NSVT: nonsustained ventricular tachycardia; RV: right ventricular; SCD: sudden cardiac death; TWI: T wave inversion; VBT: ventricular premature beats; VT: ventricular)

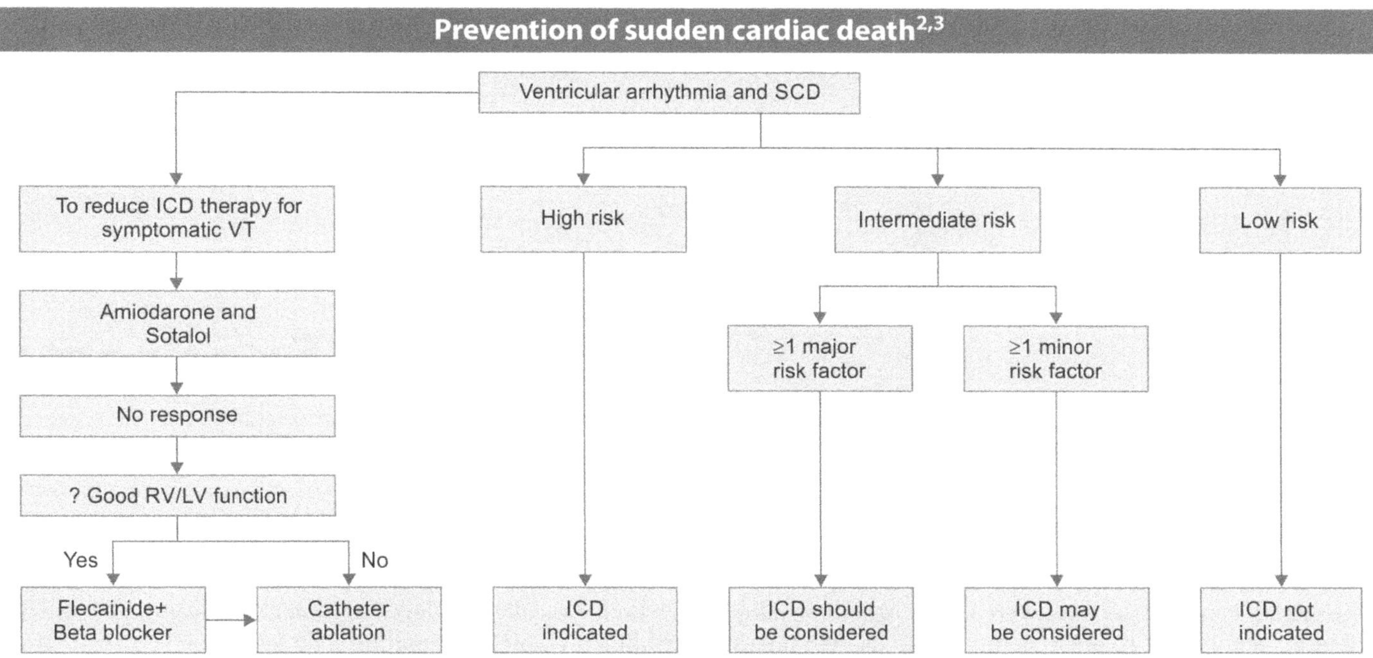

(ICD: implantable cardioverter-defibrillators; LV: left ventricular; RV: right ventricular; SCD: sudden cardiac death)

REFERENCES

1. Towbin JA, McKenna WJ, Abrams DJ, Ackerman MJ, Calkins H, Darrieux FCC, et al. 2019 HRS expert consensus statement on evaluation, risk stratification, and management of arrhythmogenic cardiomyopathy. Heart Rhythm. 2019;16:e373-e407.
2. Corrado D, Perazzolo Marra M, Zorzi A, Beffagna G, Cipriani A, Lazzari MD, et al. Diagnosis of arrhythmogenic cardiomyopathy: the Padua criteria. Int J Cardiol. 2020;319:106-14.
3. Wallace R, Calkins H. Risk stratification in Arrhythmogenic cardiomyopathy. AER. 2021;10:26-32.

CHAPTER 41

Takotsubo Syndrome

INTRODUCTION

Takotsubo syndrome (TTS) is an acute cardiac syndrome presenting as characteristic left ventricular regional wall motion abnormality leading to acute severe left ventricular dysfunction which typically recovers spontaneously over days or weeks. The term "takotsubo" refers to octopus trap used in Japan resembling the apical ballooning seen in the left ventriculogram of patients with TTS. TTS is also known as stress cardiomyopathy or broken heart syndrome, because acute mental or strenuous physical stress usually precipitates the event. However, in 20% of cases, there may not be any history of stress. Other names for this syndrome are apical ballooning syndrome, Takotsubo cardiomyopathy, happy heart syndrome, etc. TTS is classified as both primary and acquired cardiomyopathy by American Heart Association (AHA) and as unclassified cardiomyopathy by the European Society of Cardiology (ESC). Up to 2% of patients presenting as suspected acute coronary syndrome have been identified with TTS; 90% of patients are postmenopausal women.[1]

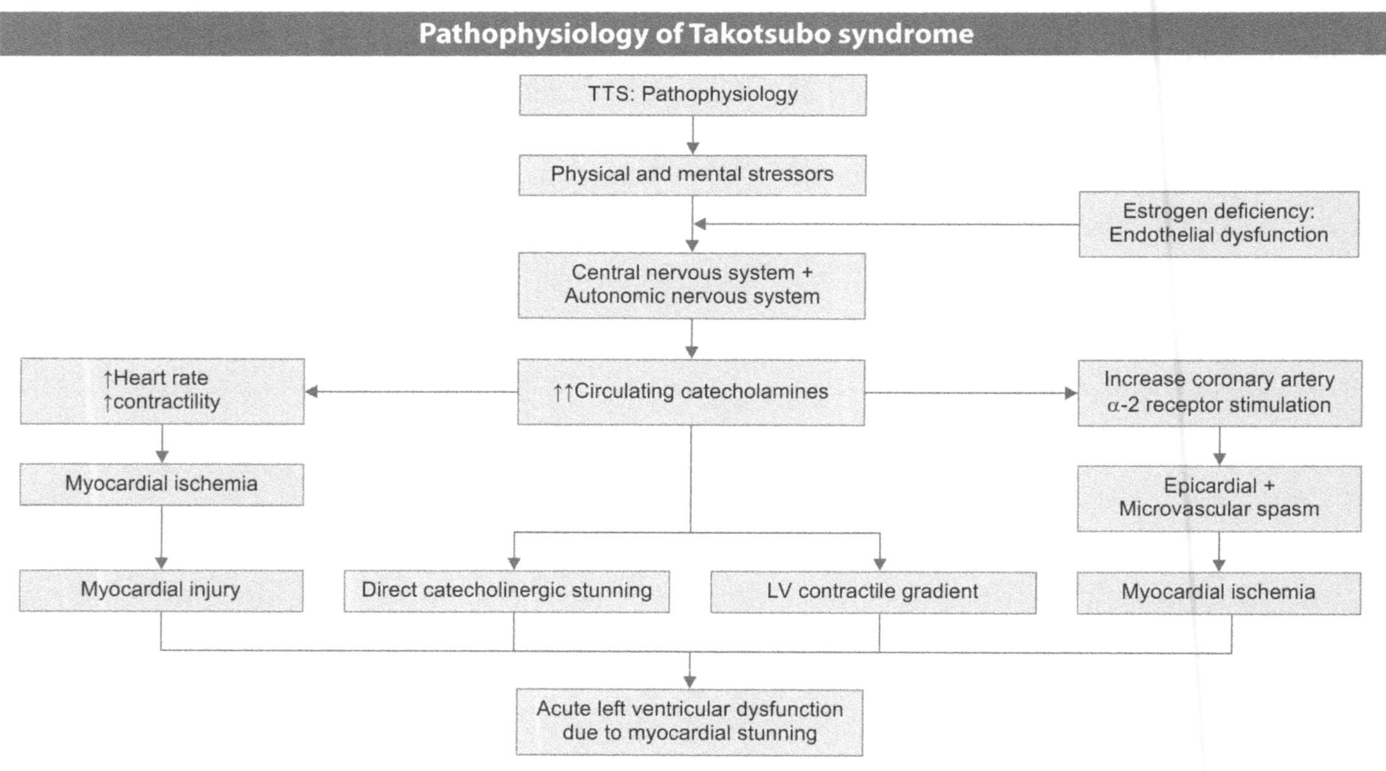

(LV: left ventricular; TTS: Takotsubo syndrome)

Takotsubo syndrome: Sympatho-adrenal mechanism

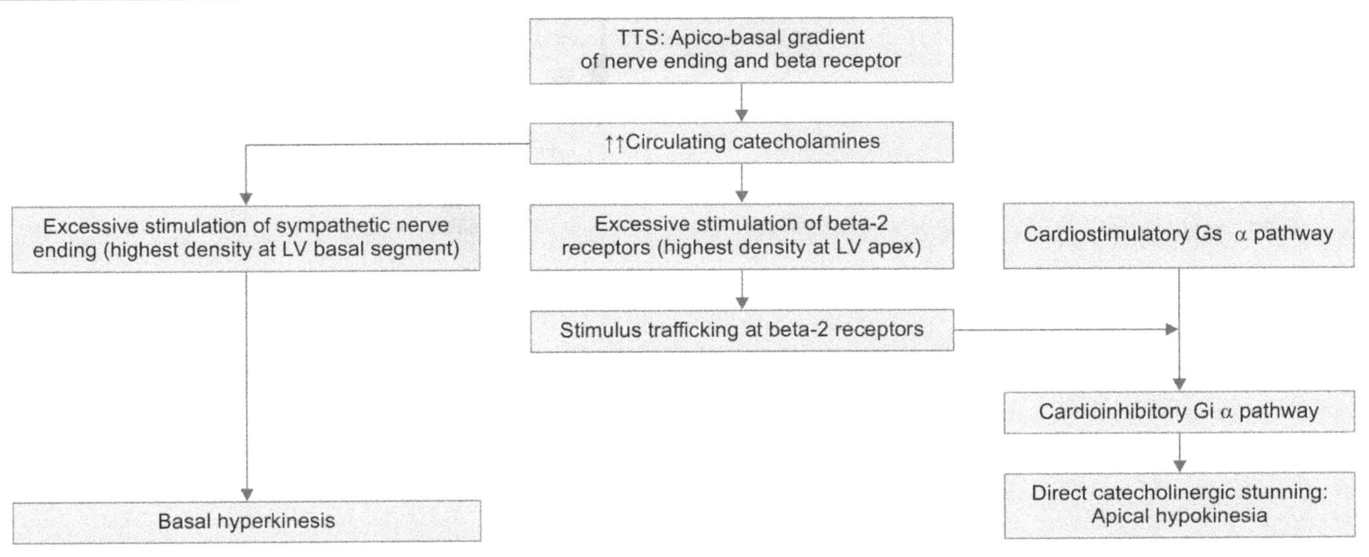

Subtypes of Takotsubo syndrome (TTS)

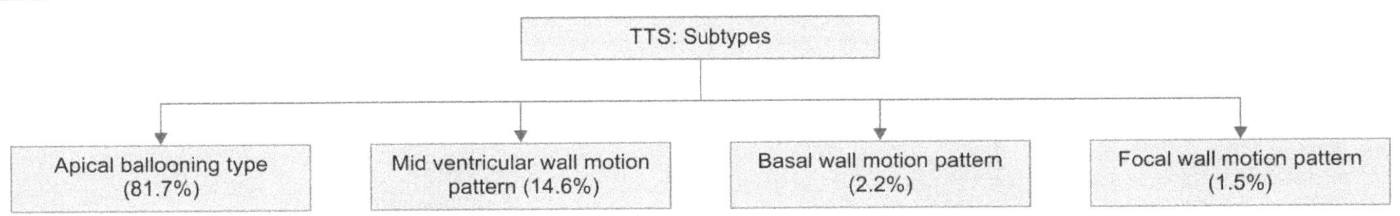

Diagnostic criteria of Takotsubo syndrome (TTS)

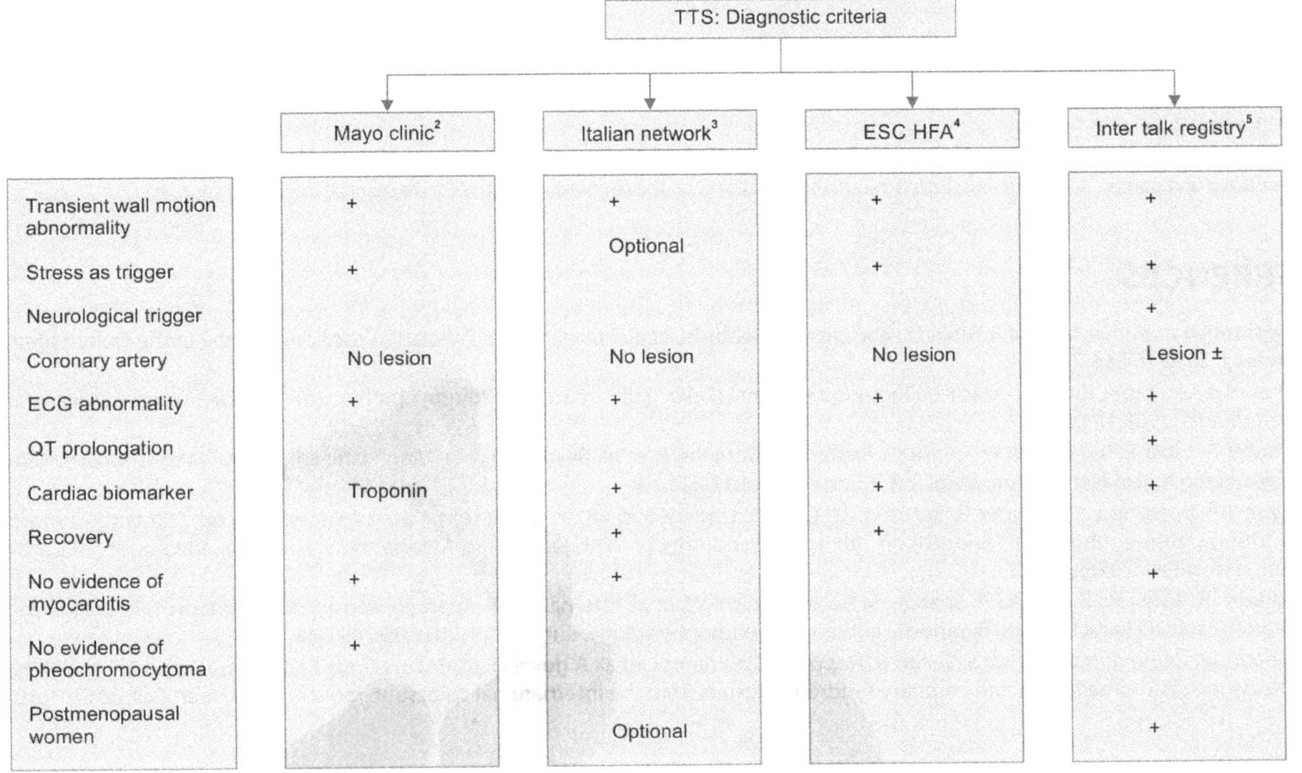

	Mayo clinic[2]	Italian network[3]	ESC HFA[4]	Inter talk registry[5]
Transient wall motion abnormality	+	+	+	+
Stress as trigger	+	Optional	+	+
Neurological trigger				+
Coronary artery	No lesion	No lesion	No lesion	Lesion ±
ECG abnormality	+	+	+	+
QT prolongation				+
Cardiac biomarker	Troponin	+	+	+
Recovery		+	+	
No evidence of myocarditis	+	+		+
No evidence of pheochromocytoma	+			
Postmenopausal women		Optional		+

(ESC: European Society of Cardiology; HFA: heart failure association)

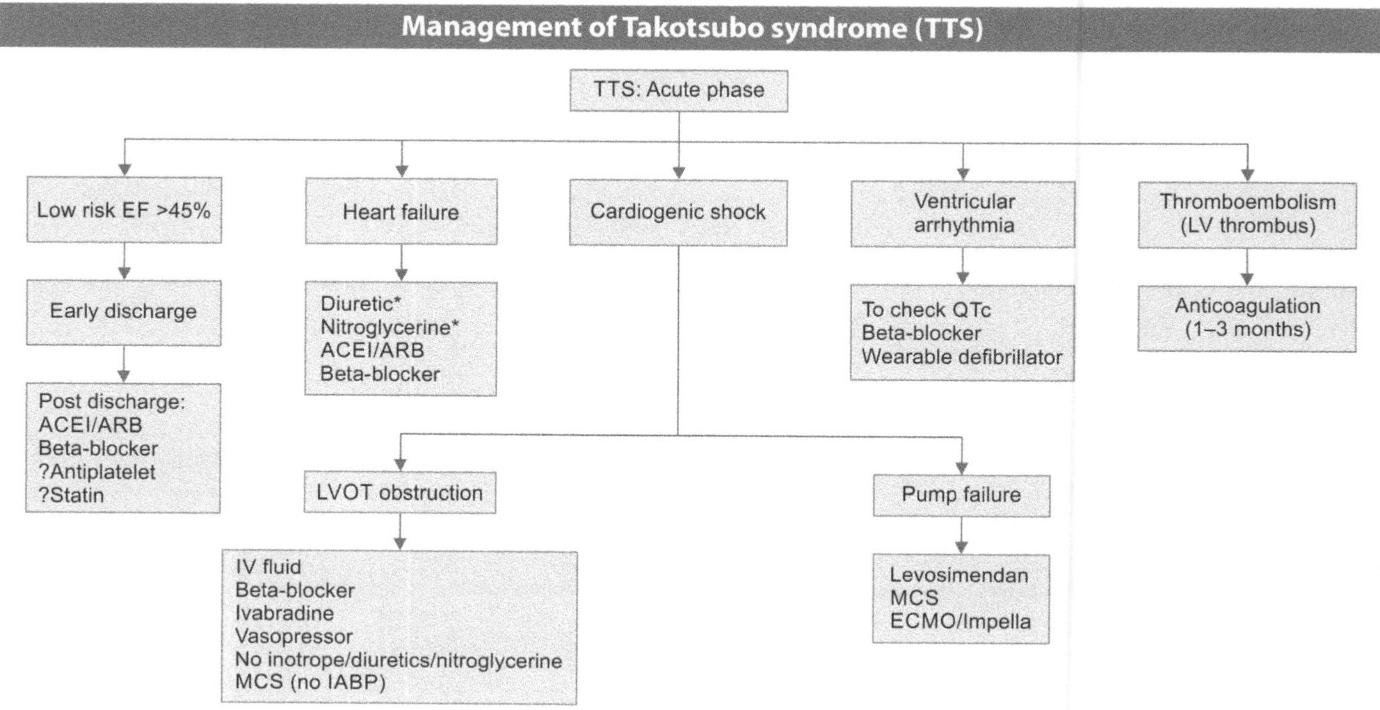

*When patients with a score ≥50 are diagnosed as TTS, then the diagnosis is correct in 95% of cases.

*No LVOT obstruction.

(ACEI: angiotensin-converting enzyme inhibitor; ARB: angiotensin receptor blocker; ECMO: extracorporeal membrane oxygenation; EF: ejection fraction; IABP: intra-aortic balloon pumps; IV: intravenous; LV: left ventricular; LVOT: left ventricular outflow tract; MCS: mechanical circulatory support)

REFERENCES

1. Deshmukh A, Kumar G, Pant S, Rihal C, Murugiah K, Mehta JL, et al. Prevalence of Takotsubo cardiomyopathy in the United States. Am Heart J. 2012;164:66-71.

2. Prasad A, Lerman A, Rihal CS. Apical ballooning syndrome (Tako-Tsubo or stress cardiomyopathy): a mimic of acute myocardial infarction. Am Heart J. 2008;155:408-17.

3. Parodi G, Citro R, Bellandi B, Provenza G, Marrani M, Bossone E, et al. Revised clinical diagnostic criteria for Tako-tsubosyndrome: the Tako-tsubo Italian Network proposal. Int J Cardiol. 2014;172:282-3.

4. Lyon AR, Bossone E, Schneider B, Sechtem U, Citro R, Underwood SR, et al. Current state of knowledge on Takotsubo syndrome: a position statement from the Taskforce on Takotsubo Syndrome of the Heart Failure Association of the European Society of Cardiology. Eur J Heart Fail. 2016;18:8-27.

5. Ghadri JR, Wittstein IS, Prasad A, Sharkey S, Dote K, Akashi YJ, et al. International expert consensus document on Takotsubo syndrome (Part I): clinical characteristics, diagnostic criteria, and pathophysiology. Eur Heart J. 2018;39:2032-46.

6. Ghadri JR, Cammann VL, Jurisic S, Seifert B, Napp LC, Diekmann J, et al. A novel clinical score (InterTAK diagnostic score) to differentiate takotsubo syndrome from acute coronary syndrome: results from the international takotsubo registry. Eur J Heart Fail. 2017;19:1036-42.

CHAPTER 42

Noncompaction Cardiomyopathy

INTRODUCTION

Noncompaction cardiomyopathy (NCCM) is a heterogeneous cardiomyopathy characterized by multiple myocardial trabeculation and deep intertrabecular recesses. NCCM is classified by the American Heart Association (AHA) as genetic cardiomyopathy, whereas the European Society of Cardiology (ESC) and World Health Organization (WHO) classify it as familial/genetic unclassified cardiomyopathy. NCCM has been described with different terminologies including left ventricular noncompaction (LVNC), left ventricular hypertrabeculation (LVHT), spongy myocardium, fetal myocardium, etc. NCCM is more common in children. In some pediatric registry, it is as high as 9.2% of primary cardiomyopathy, i.e., third most common type of cardiomyopathy after dilated cardiomyopathy (DCM) and hypertrophic cardiomyopathy (HCM).[1] Familial occurrence is found in up to 40% of cases as an autosomal genetic disorder resulting in intrauterine arrest of normal ventricular trabecular maturation and compaction. Barth syndrome is an X-linked disease associated with DCM, HCM, neutropenia, and NCCM. There is also an additional nonembryogenic-acquired hypothesis supported by its development in sickle cell anemia and chronic renal failure.

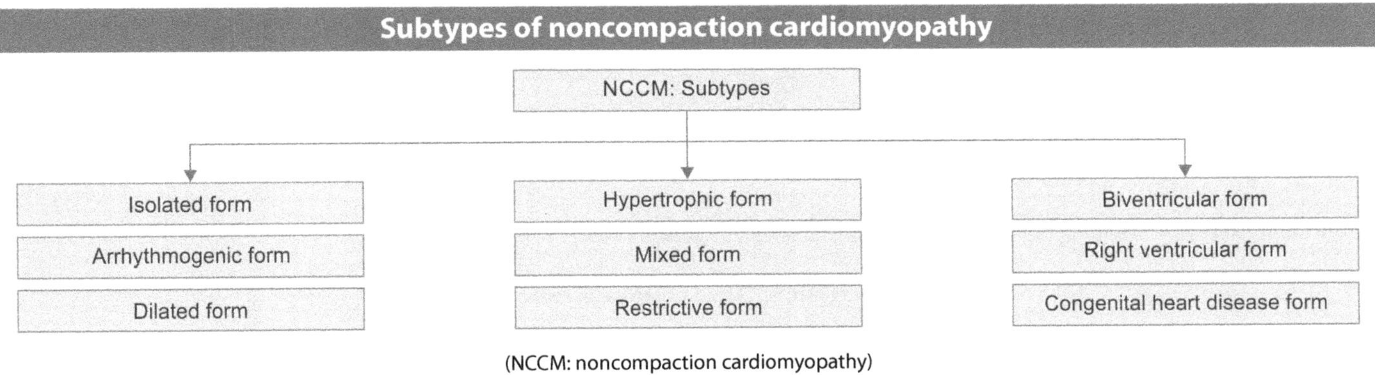

(NCCM: noncompaction cardiomyopathy)

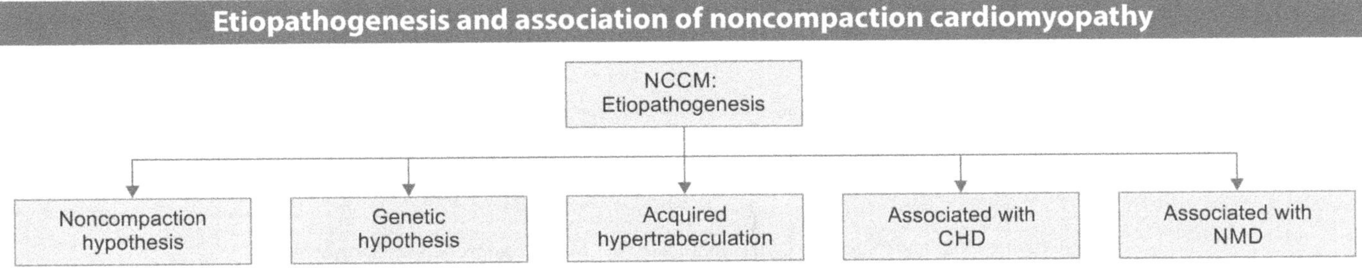

(CHD: congenital heart disease; NCCM: noncompaction cardiomyopathy; NMD: neuromuscular disease)

Clinical presentation of noncompaction cardiomyopathy[2]

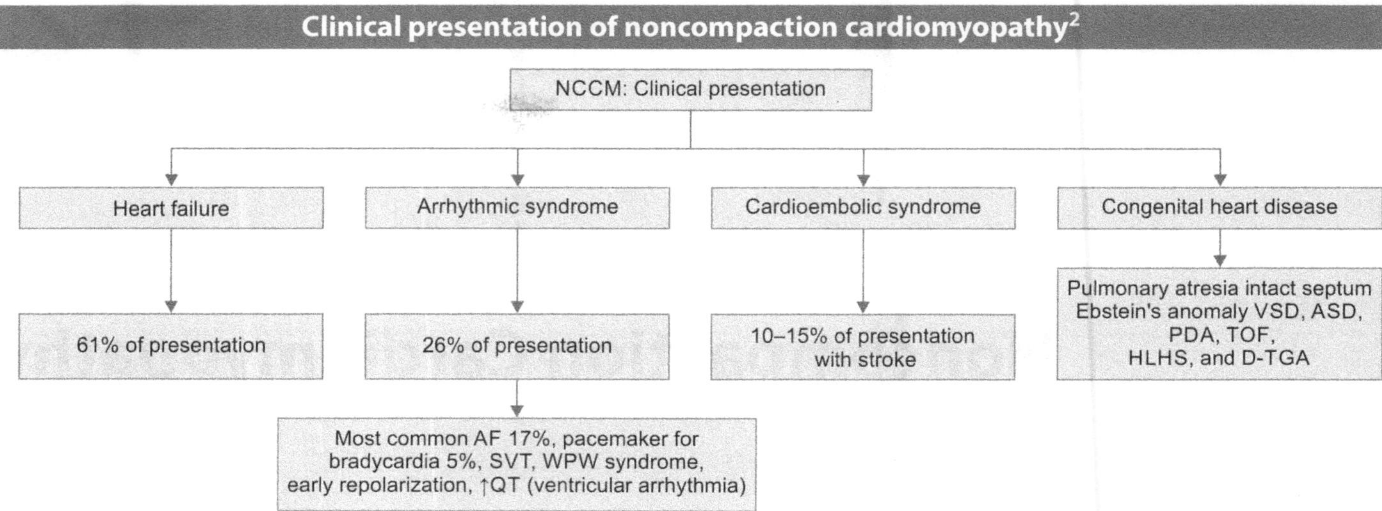

(AF: atrial fibrillation; ASD: atrial septal defect; D-TGA: dextro-transposition of the great arteries; HLHS: hypoplastic left heart syndrome; NCCM: noncompaction cardiomyopathy; PDA: patent ductus arteriosus; SVT: supraventricular tachycardia; TOF: tetralogy of Fallot; VSD: ventricular septal defect; WPW: Wolff–Parkinson–White)

Echocardiographic criteria of noncompaction cardiomyopathy

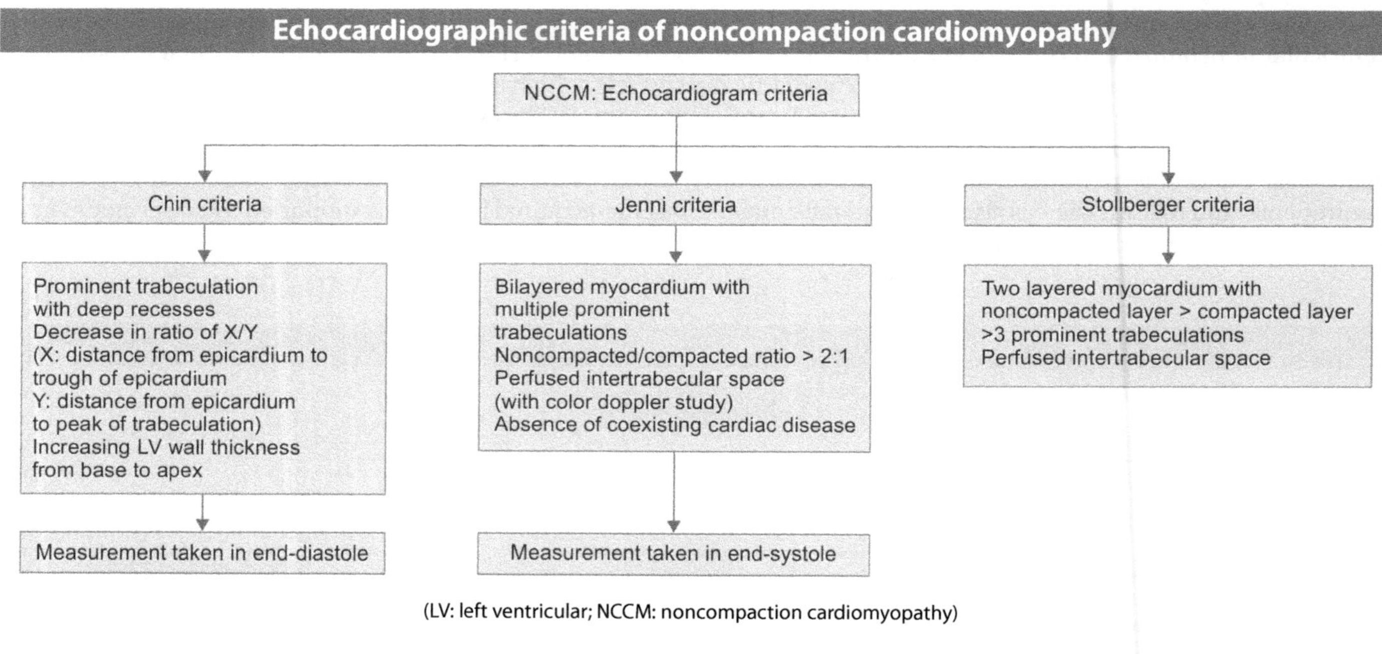

(LV: left ventricular; NCCM: noncompaction cardiomyopathy)

CMR criteria of noncompaction cardiomyopathy

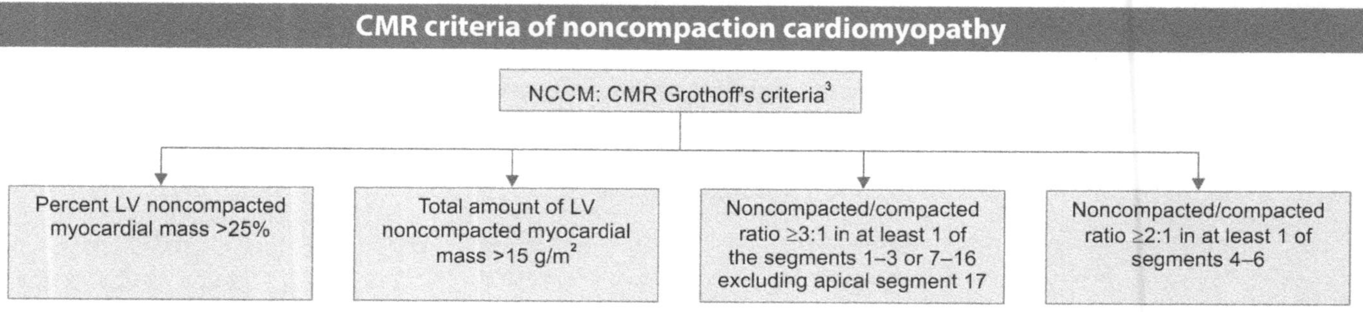

(CMR: cardiac magnetic resonance; LV: left ventricular; NCCM: noncompaction cardiomyopathy)

Diagnostic criteria of noncompaction cardiomyopathy

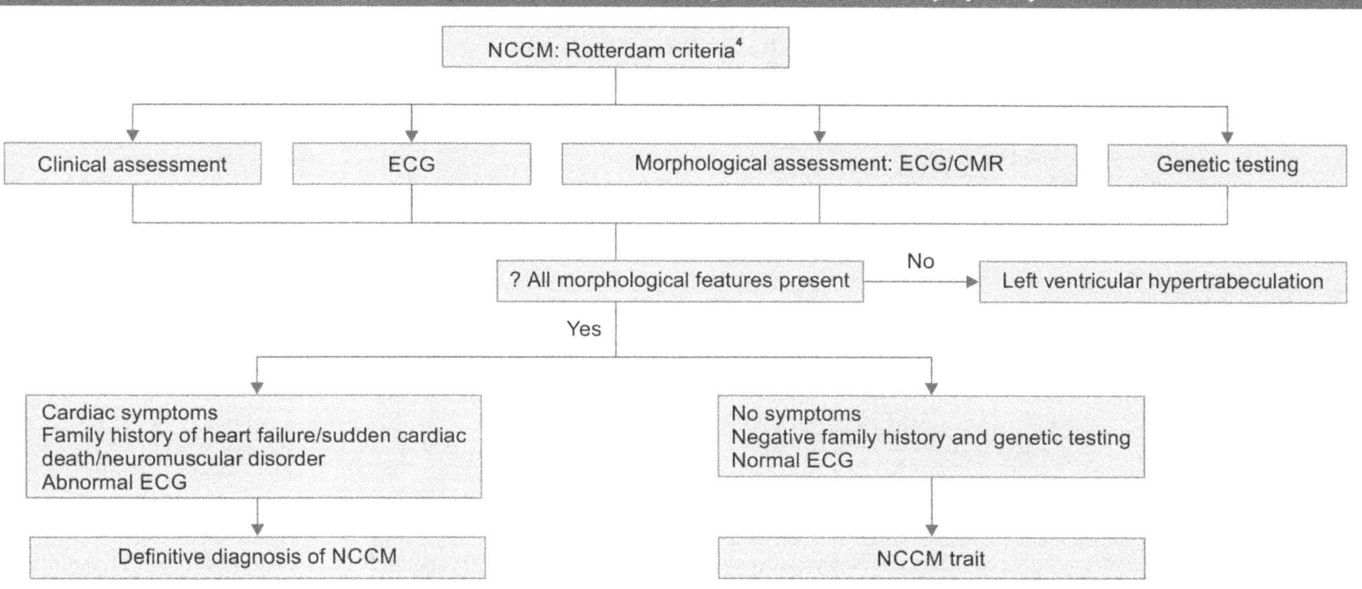

(CMR: cardiac magnetic resonance; ECG: electrocardiogram; NCCM: noncompaction cardiomyopathy)

Management of noncompacted cardiomyopathy

(?: indicating doubtful role; AF: atrial fibrillation; GDMT: guideline-directed medical therapy; LV: left ventricular; NCCM: noncompaction cardiomyopathy; NMD: neuromuscular disease; NOAC: non-vitamin K antagonists oral anticoagulant; VKA: vitamin K antagonist)

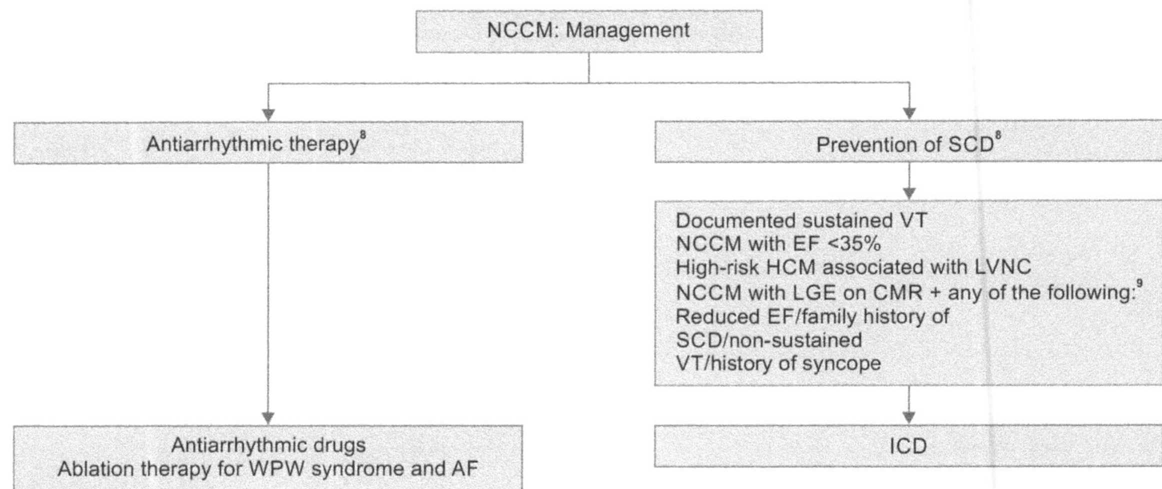

(AF: atrial fibrillation; CMR: cardiac magnetic resonance; EF: ejection fraction; HCM: hypertrophic cardiomyopathy; LGE: late gadollinium enhancement; LV: left ventricular; LVNC: left ventricular noncompaction cardiomyopathy; NCCM: noncompaction cardiomyopathy; SCD: sudden cardiac death; VT: ventricular tachycardia; WPW: Wolff–Parkinson–White)

REFERENCES

1. Jefferies JL, Wilkinson JD, Sleeper LA, Colan SD, Lu M, Pahl E, et al. Cardiomyopathy Phenotypes and Outcomes for Children with Left Ventricular Myocardial Noncompaction: Results From the Pediatric Cardiomyopathy Registry. J Card Fail. 2015;21:877-84.

2. Engberding R, Stöllberger C, Schneider B, Nothnagel D, Fehske W, Gerecke BJ. Heart failure in noncompaction cardiomyopathy—Data from the German noncompaction registry (ALKK). Circulation. 2012;126:A14769.

3. Grothoff M, Pachowsky M, Hoffmann J, Posch M, Klaassen S, Lehmkuhl L, et al. Value of cardiovascular MR in diagnosing left ventricular non-compaction cardiomyopathy and in discriminating between other cardiomyopathies. Eur Radiol. 2012;22:2699-709.

4. Soliman OI, McGhie J, ten Cate FJ, Paelinck BP, Caliskan K. Multimodality imaging, diagnostic challenges and proposed diagnostic algorithm for noncompaction cardiomyopathy. In: Caliskan K, Soliman OI, ten Cate FJ (Eds). Noncompaction Cardiomyopathy. Cham: Springer International Publishing; 2019. pp. 17-40.

5. Engberding R, Stöllberger C, Ong P, Yelbuz TM, Gerecke BJ, Breithardt G. Isolated Non-Compaction Cardiomyopathy. Dtsch Aerztebl Int. 2010;107:206-13.

6. Finsterer J, Stollberger C, Towben JA. Left ventricular noncompaction cardiomyopathy: cardiac, neuromuscular, and genetic factors. Nat Rev Cardiol. 2017;14:224-37.

7. Li J, Franke J, Pribe-Wolferts R, Meder B, Ehlermann P, Mereles D, et al. Effects of β-blocker therapy on electrocardiographic and echocardiographic characteristics of left ventricular noncompaction. Clin Res Cardiol. 2015;104:241-49.

8. Al Khatib SM, Stevenson WG, Ackerman MJ, Bryant WJ, Callans DJ, Curtis AB, et al. AHA/ACC/HRS Guideline for Management of Patients with Ventricular Arrhythmias and the Prevention of Sudden Cardiac Death: Executive Summary: A Report of the American College of Cardiology/American Heart Association Task Force on Clinical Practice Guidelines and the Heart Rhythm Society. Heart Rhythm. 2018;1510: e190-e252.

9. Bennett CE, Freudenberger R. The current approach to diagnosis and management of left ventricular noncompaction cardiomyopathy: review of the literature. Cardiol Res Pract. 2016;2016:5172308.

Infective and Autoimmune Disease

CHAPTER 43

Rheumatic Fever: Approach

INTRODUCTION

Acute rheumatic fever (ARF) is a systemic inflammatory autoimmune disease that follows throat infection with Lancefield group A β-hemolytic streptococci [group A *Streptococcus pyogenes* (GAS)]. ARF is believed to involve the triad of a genetically susceptible individual, infection with a rheumatogenic strain of GAS, and a host immune response. Among β-hemolytic streptococci, GAS, most commonly, has been related to human infection. Usually, GAS pharyngitis may lead to rheumatic fever. Occasionally, GAS skin infection can lead to rheumatic fever in certain population, such as Aboriginal communities of Central and Northern Australia.[1]

Only 0.3–3% of individuals affected by streptococcal pharyngitis may develop ARF; host factor including a genetic factor may be the determinable factor. Most studies[2] have shown an association of human leukocyte antigen (HLA) with ARF. *DR7* and *HLAB5* are the most common alleles. In Indian context, important association is between *HLA A33, DR2, DR3*, and ARF.

The prevalence of rheumatic heart disease (RHD) is highest in Samoa in Hawaii and reported to be 77.7 per 1,000. Aboriginal population, Maori in New Zealand, South and Central Asia, and Sub-Saharan Africa have also a high prevalence rate. Crowding, hygiene practice, carrier of rheumatogenic strains, and genetic predispositions are the presumptions of this ethnic susceptibility.

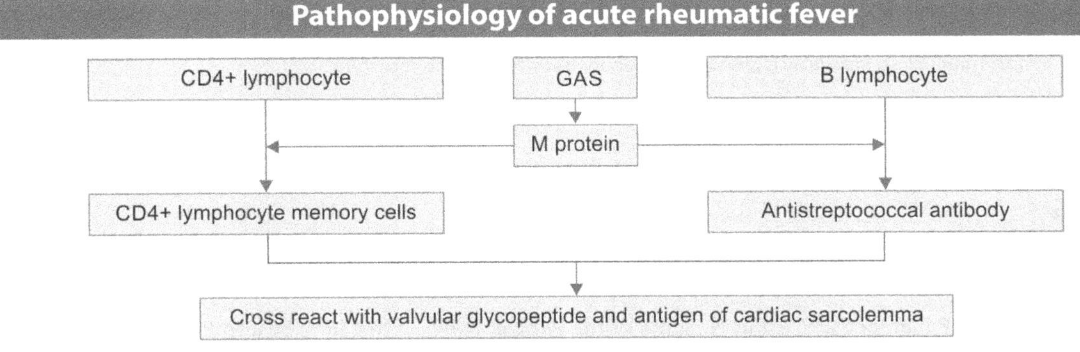

(GAS: group A *Streptococcus pyogenes*)

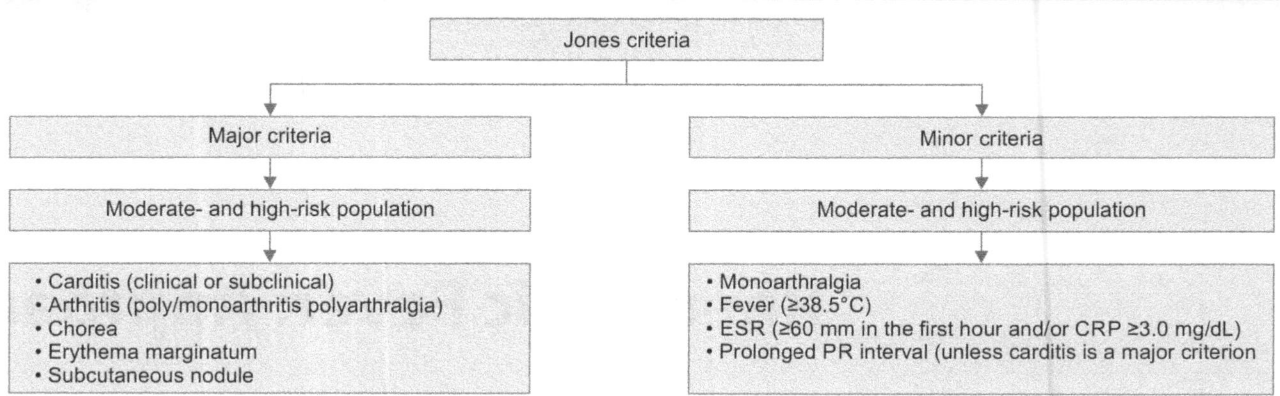

Notes: In low-risk population, major criteria arthritis means polyarthritis and minor criteria arthralgia means polyarthralgia.

Low-risk populations are those with ARF incidence ≤2 per 100,000 school-aged children or all-age rheumatic heart disease prevalence of ≤1 per 1,000 population per year.

To diagnose ARF, there must be two major criteria and one minor criterion or one major and two minor criteria in the presence of preceding GAS infection.

To diagnose recurrent rheumatic fever, there must be two major criteria and one minor criterion or one major and two minor criteria or three minor criteria in the presence of preceding GAS infection.

(CRP: C-reactive protein; ESR: erythrocyte sedimentation rate)

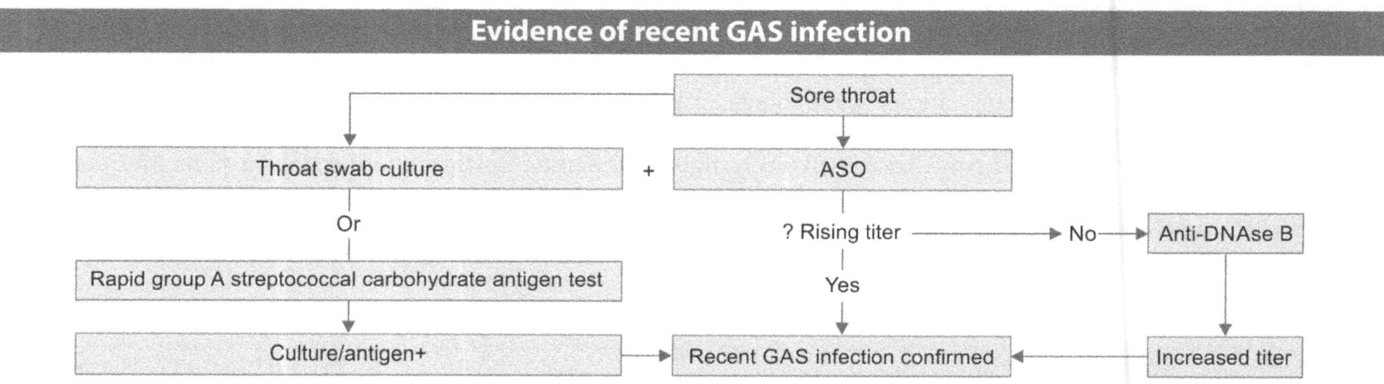

Notes: When done both ASO and anti-DNase, specificity is raised to 90% and sensitivity is near cent percent[4]

(Anti-DNAse: anti-deoxyribonuclease B; ASO: antistreptolysin O; GAS: group A *Streptococcus pyogenes*)

REFERENCES

1. McDonald M, Currie BJ, Carapetis JR. Acute rheumatic fever: a chink in the chain that links the heart to the throat? Lancet Infect Dis. 2004;4(4):240-5.
2. Bryant PA, Robins-Browne R, Carapetis JR, Curtis N. Some of the People, Some of the Time Susceptibility to Acute Rheumatic Fever. Circulation. 2009;119:742-53.
3. Gewitz MH, Baltimore RS, Tani LY, Sable CA, Shulman ST, Carapetis J, et al. American Heart Association Committee on Rheumatic Fever, Endocarditis, and Kawasaki Disease of the Council on Cardiovascular Disease in the Young. Revision of the Jones criteria for the diagnosis of acute rheumatic fever in the era of Doppler echocardiography: a scientific statement from the American Heart Association. Circulation. 2015;131:1806-18.
4. Wannamaker LW, Ayoub EM. Antibody titers in acute rheumatic fever. Circulation. 1960;21:598-614.

CHAPTER 44

Acute Rheumatic Fever: Management

INTRODUCTION

Management of acute rheumatic fever (ARF) includes the management of the indexed episode of rheumatic fever and secondary prevention. Considering the worldwide huge burden of rheumatic heart disease, primordial and primary preventions are also very important issues in management program of rheumatic fever.

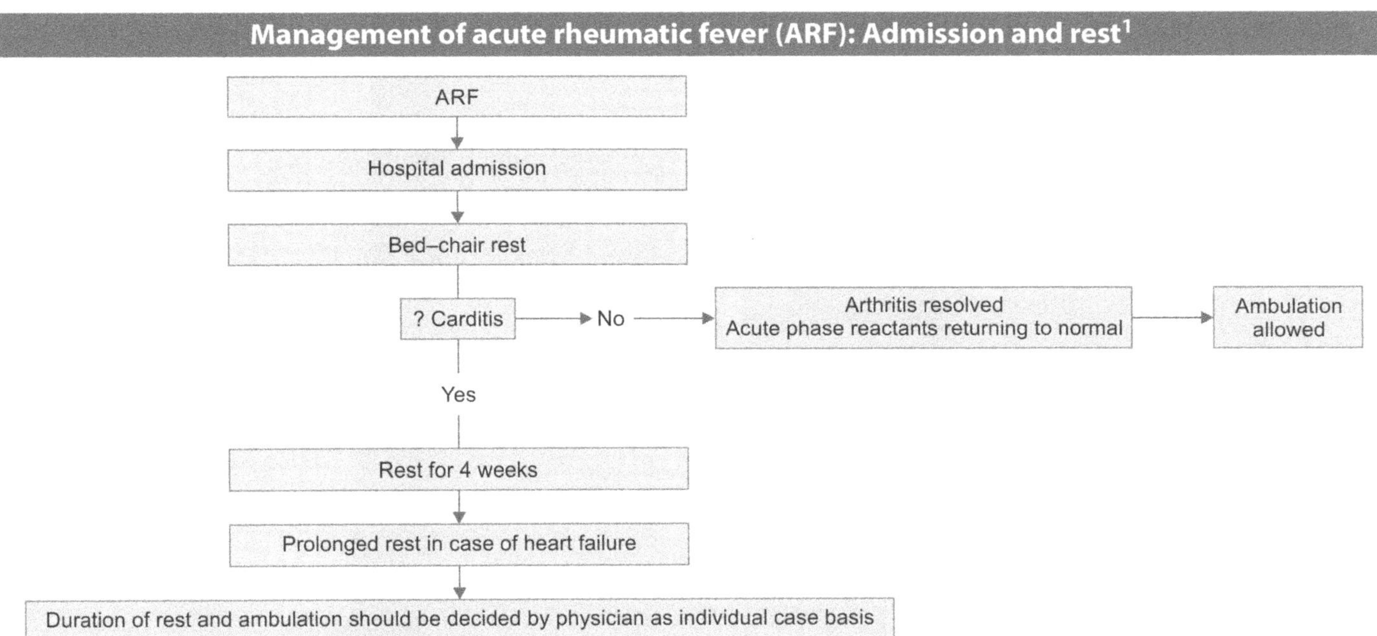

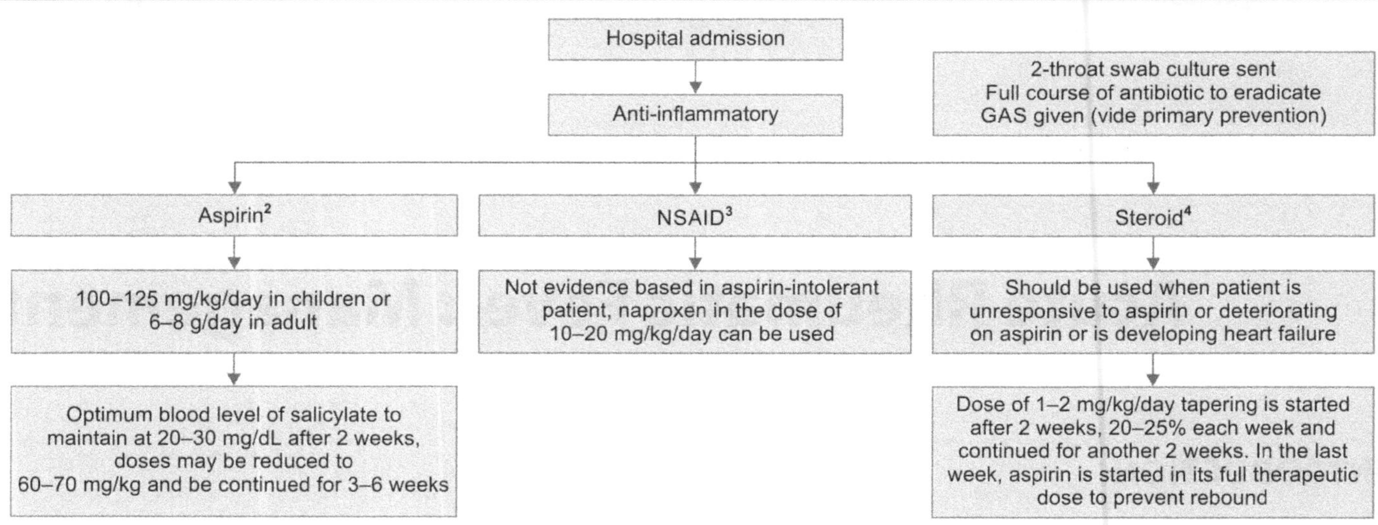

(GAS: group A *Streptococcus pyogenes*; NSAID: nonsteroidal anti-inflammatory drugs)

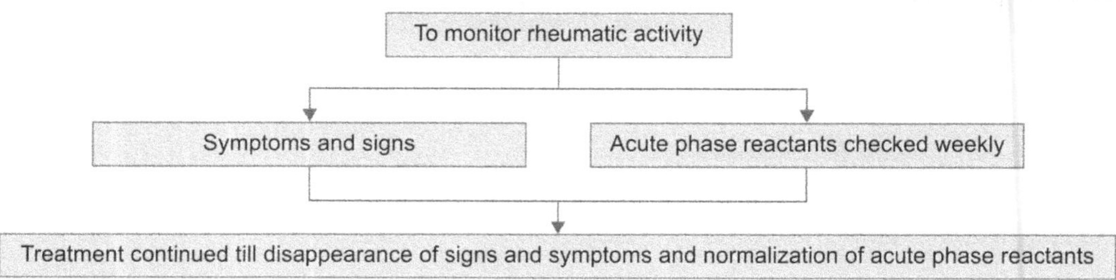

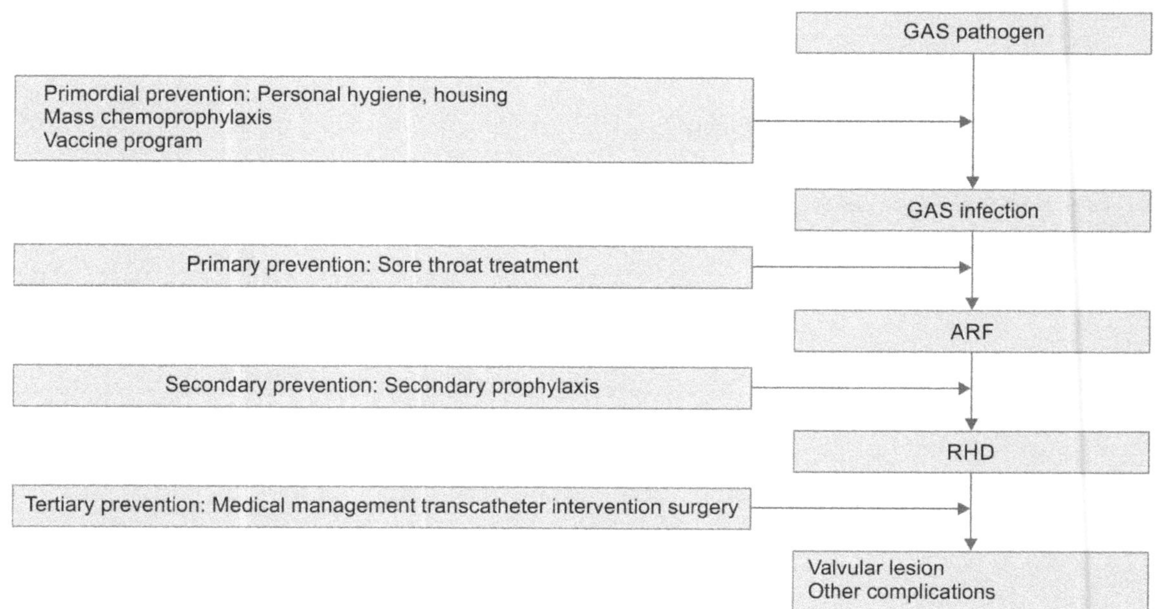

(GAS: group A *Streptococcus pyogenes*; RHD: rheumatic heart disease)

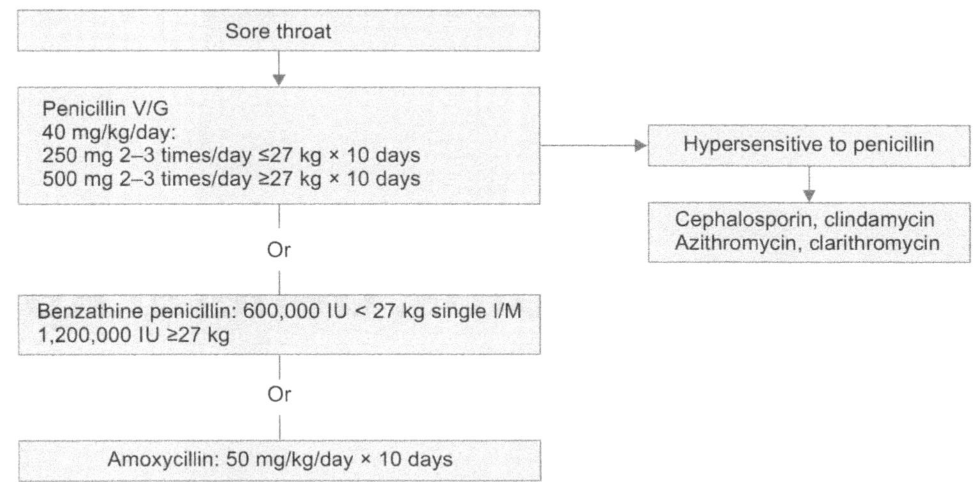

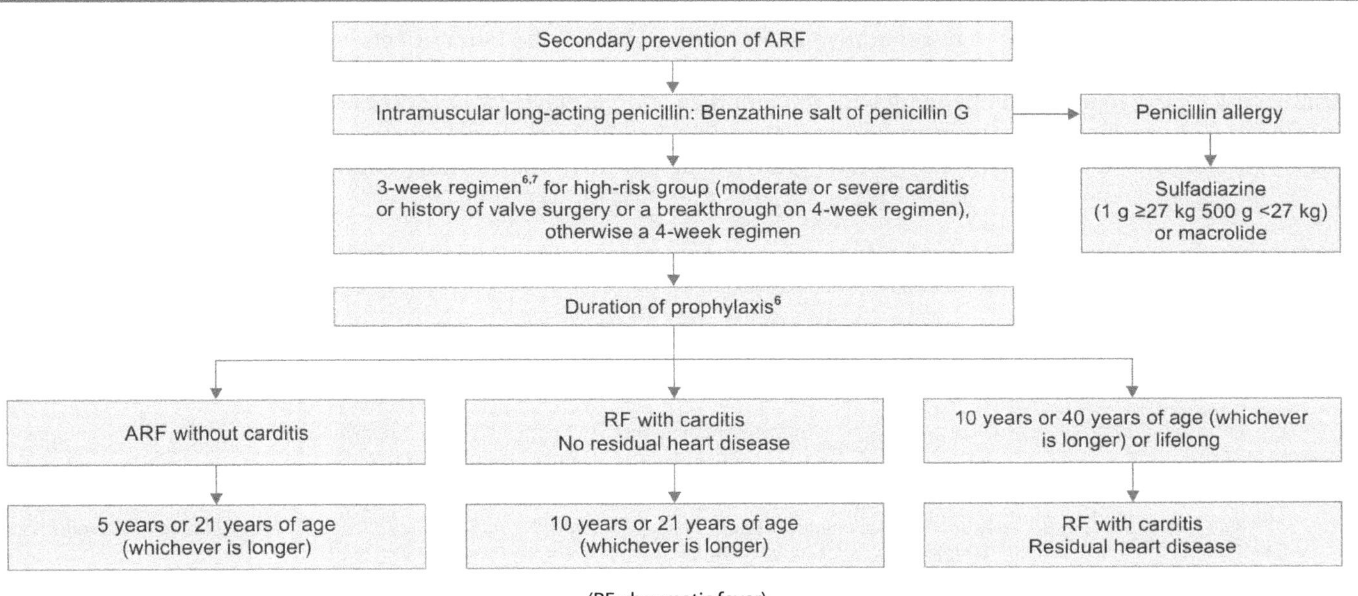

REFERENCES

1. Silva NA, Pereira BA. Acute rheumatic fever: still a challenge. Rheumatic Disease Clinic of North America, 1997;23(3):545-68.
2. Thatai D, Turi ZG. Current guidelines for the treatment of patients with rheumatic fever. Drugs. 1999;57(4):545-55.
3. Uziel Y, Hashkes PJ, Kassem E, Padeh S, Goldman R, Wolach B. The use of naproxen in the treatment of children with rheumatic fever. Journal Pediatr. 2000;137:269-71.
4. World Health Organization. Rheumatic fever and rheumatic heart disease. Report of a WHO Expert Committee. WHO Technical Report Series, No. 764. Geneva: World Health Organization; 1988.
5. Gerber MA, Baltimore RS, Eaton CB, Gewitz M, Rowley AH, Shulman ST, et al. Prevention of Rheumatic Fever and Diagnosis and Treatment of Acute Streptococcal Pharyngitis: a scientific statement from the American Heart Association Rheumatic Fever, Endocarditis, and Kawasaki Disease Committee of the Council on Cardiovascular Disease in the Young, the Interdisciplinary Council on Functional Genomics and Translational Biology, and the Interdisciplinary Council on Quality of Care and Outcomes Research: endorsed by the American Academy of Pediatrics. Circulation. 2009;119:1541-51.
6. National Heart Foundation of Australia (RF/RHD guideline development working group) and the Cardiac Society of Australia and New Zealand. Diagnosis and management of acute rheumatic fever and rheumatic heart disease in Australia - an evidence-based review; 2006.
7. Gewitz MH, Baltimore RS, Tanil LY, et al. Revisions of the Jones criteria for the diagnosis of acute rheumatic fever in the era of Doppler echocardiography: A scientific statement from the American Heart Association. Circulation 2015;131:1806-18.

CHAPTER 45

Infective Endocarditis: General Approach

INTRODUCTION

Infective endocarditis (IE) is a relatively rare life-threatening disease with an incidence ranging from 1.5 to 11.6 cases per 100,000 person-year.[1] There is a change in the disease profile of IE. Median age has been shifted from less than 30 years to more than 50 years over a century. This is due to multiple factors. First, as predisposing heart disease has changed from rheumatic heart disease (RHD) to degenerative heart disease (DHD), the latter affects older people. Second, the age of population has increased gradually. Last, the emergence of health contact-associated IE affects the elderly more. The causative infective agent is also changing with the emergence of *Staphylococcus aureus* replacing the Viridians group of streptococci. Echocardiogram is the most important imaging. Sensitivity to detect vegetation for native valve and prosthetic valve is 70% and 50% for transthoracic echocardiogram and 96% and 92% for transesophageal echocardiogram, respectively.

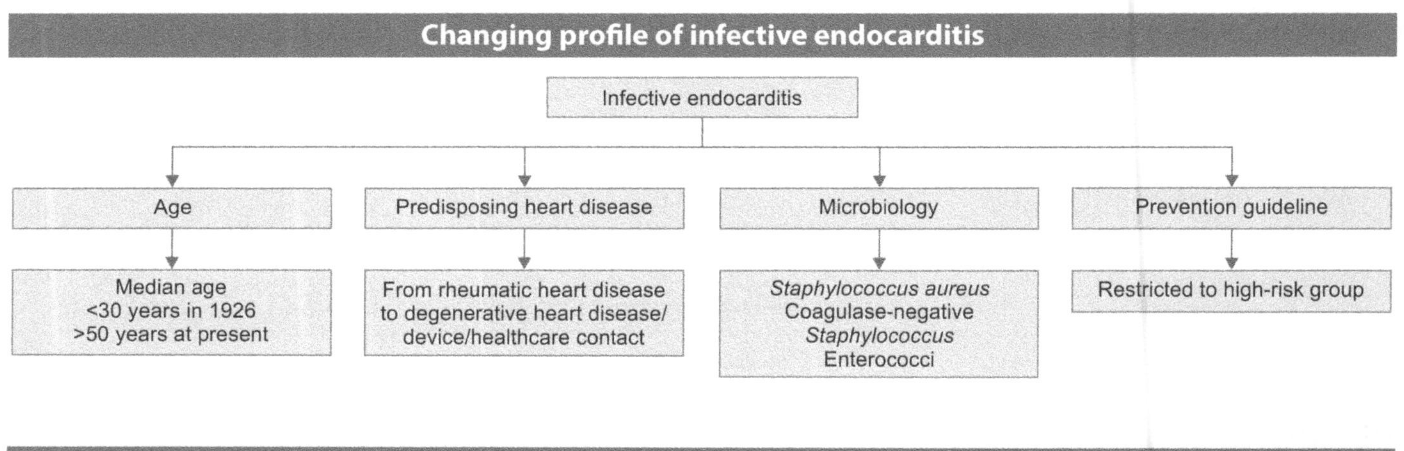

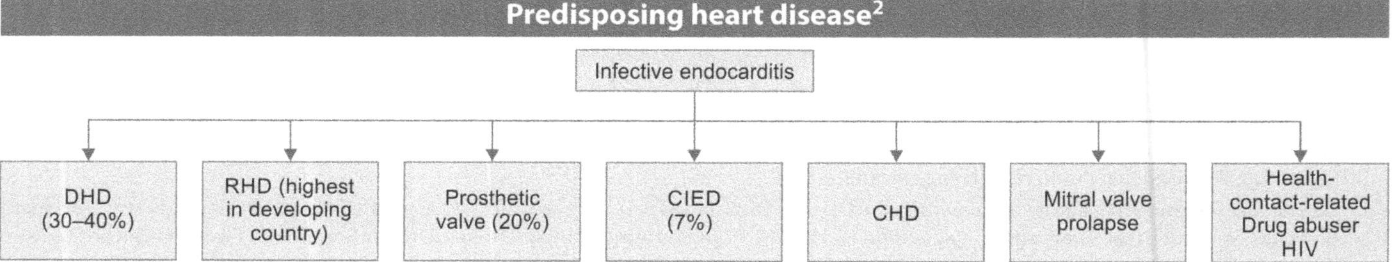

(CHD: congenital heart disease; CIED: cardiac implantable electronic device; DHD: degenerative heart disease; HIV: human immunodeficiency virus; RHD: rheumatic heart disease)

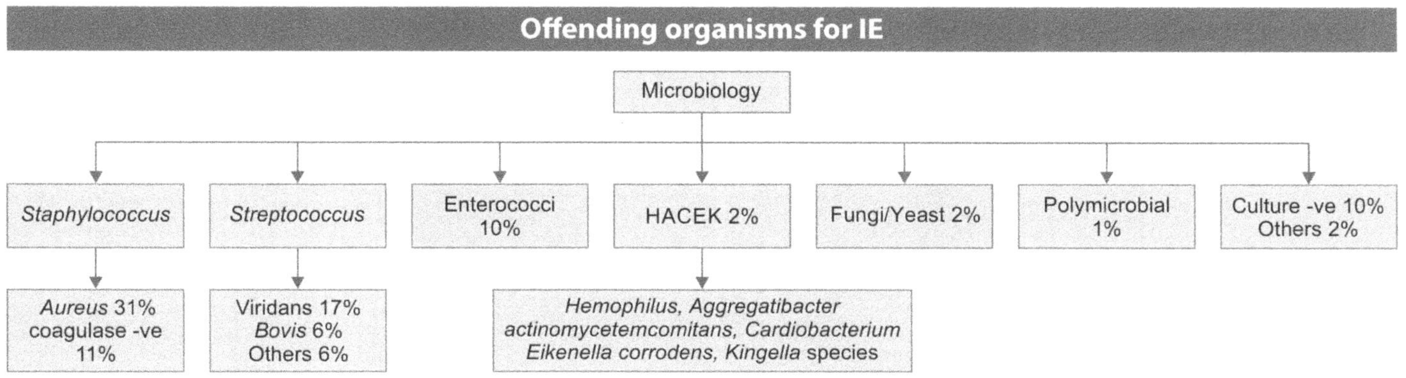

(IE: infective endocarditis; PCR: polymerase chain reaction)

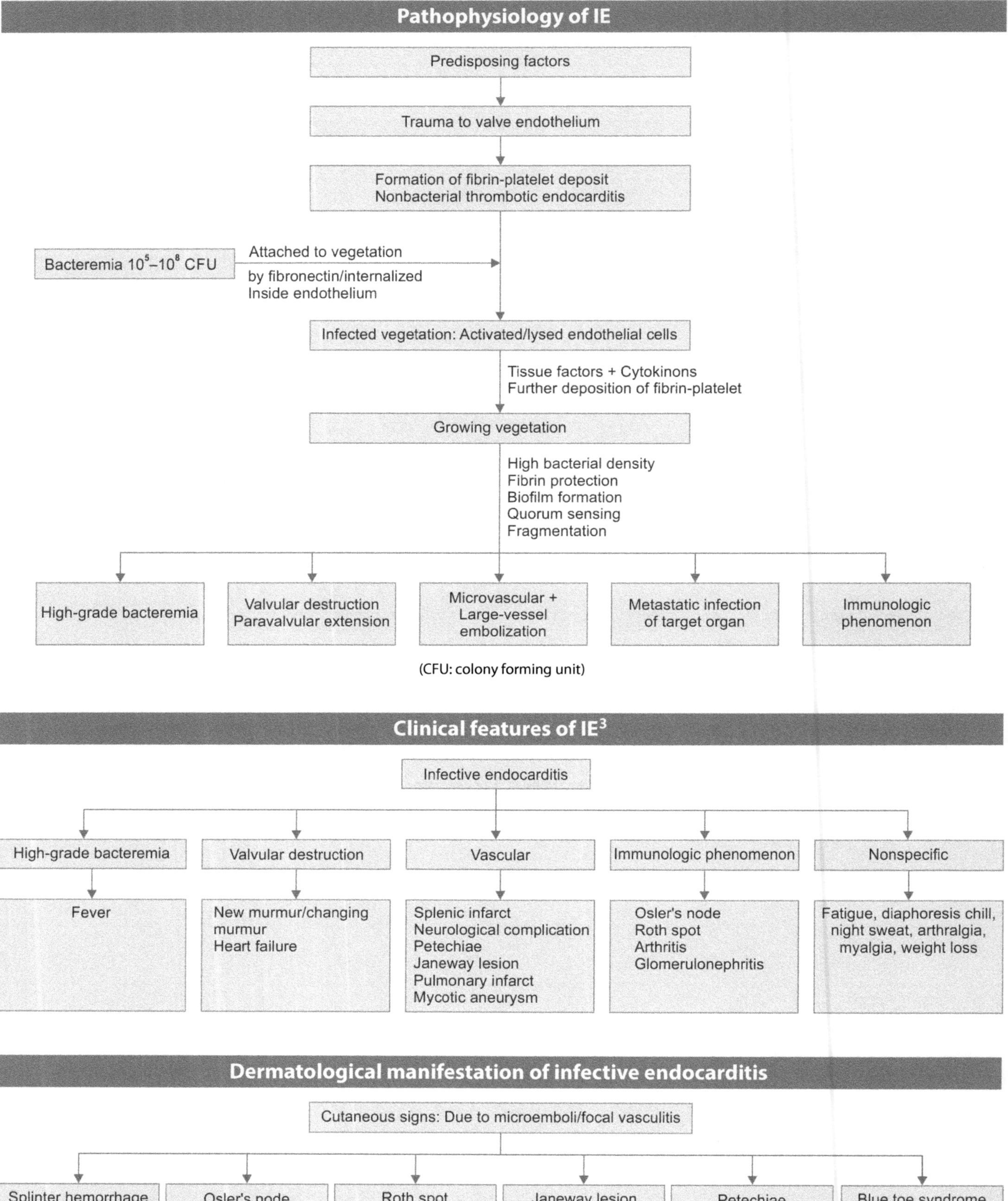

Notes: Splinter hemorrhage: 1–2 mm brown streak under the finger or toenails, in the proximal nailbeds; Osler's node: red, tender, indurated lesions on palm and soles, 2–15 mm in size; Janeway lesion: nontender, erythematous macules on palm and sole; petechiae: appear in crops on buccal mucosa, soft palate and extremities; blue toe syndrome: tender, cyanotic toes and digits due to embolization of fragmented vegetation).

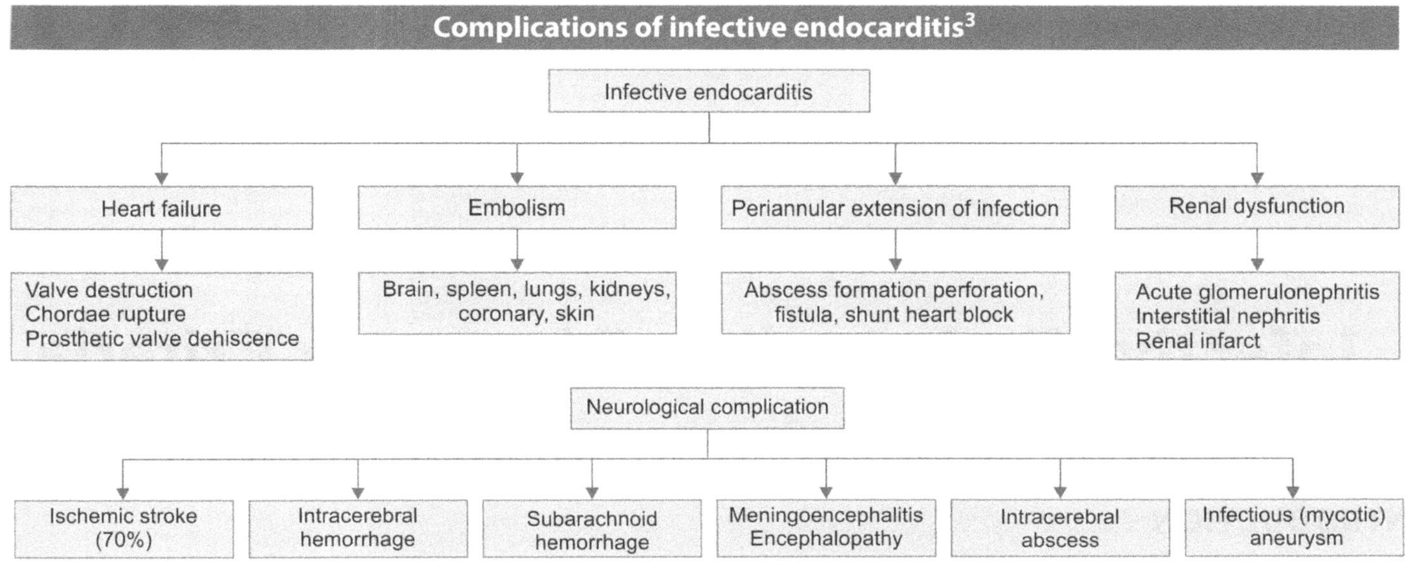

REFERENCES

1. Bin Abdulhak AA, Baddour LM, Erwin PJ, Hoen B, Chu VH, Mensah GA, et al. Global and regional burden of infective endocarditis, 1990–2010: a systematic review of the literature. Glob Heart. 2014;9:131-43.
2. Murdoch DR, Corey GR, Hoen B, Miró JM, Fowler VG Jr, Bayer AS, et al. Clinical presentation, etiology, and outcome of infective endocarditis in the 21st century: the International Collaboration on Endocarditis-Prospective Cohort study. Arch Intern Med. 2009;169:463-73.
3. Habib G, Lancellotti P, Antunes MG, Bongiorni G, Casalta JP, Del Zotti F, et al. 2015 ESC guidelines for the management of infective endocarditis. Eur Heart J. 2015;36:3075-128.

Infective Endocarditis: Diagnostic Criteria

INTRODUCTION

There are three pods in the diagnosis of infective endocarditis, namely clinical features, blood culture, and echocardiogram. Imaging other than echocardiogram namely nuclear imaging and cardiac CT are emerging as important diagnostic tools in infective endocarditis of native valve and more specifically of prosthetic valve.

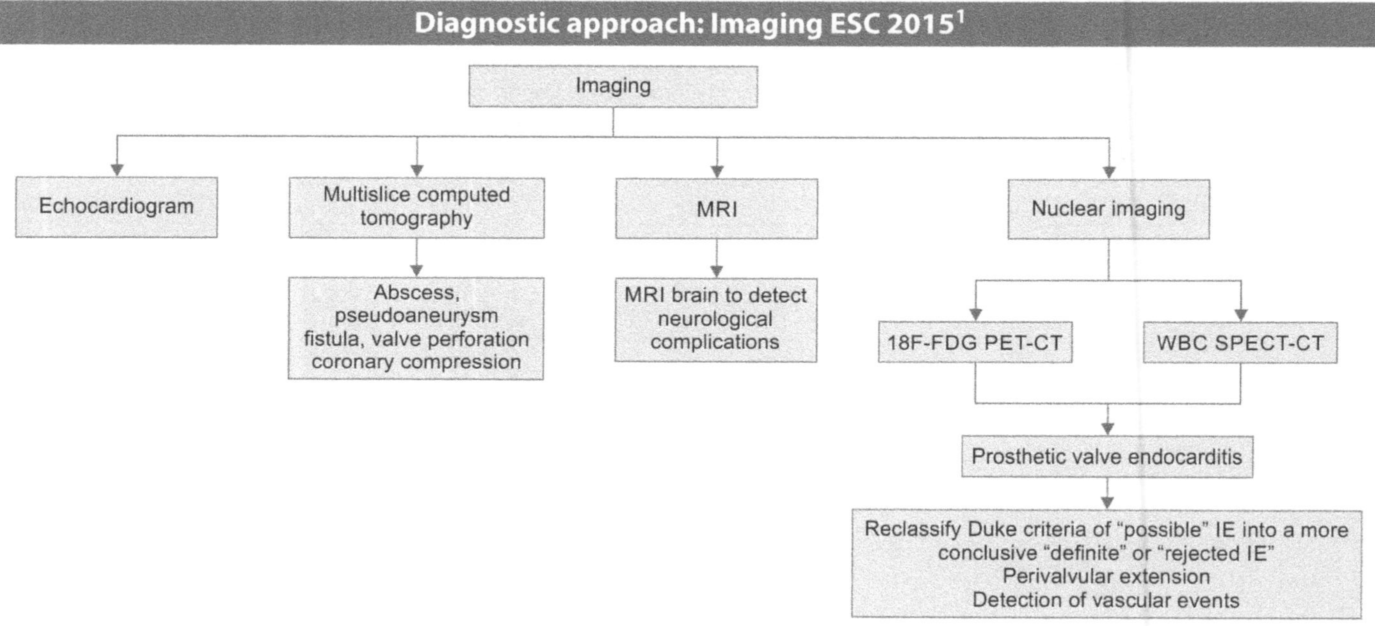

(ESC: European Society of Cardiology; 18F-FDG: 18F-fluorodeoxyglucose; IE: infective endocarditis; MRI: magnetic resonance imaging; PET-CT: positron emission tomography-computed tomography; SPECT-CT: single-photon emission computed tomography; WBC: white blood cell)

Diagnostic approach: Echocardiogram ESC 2015[1]

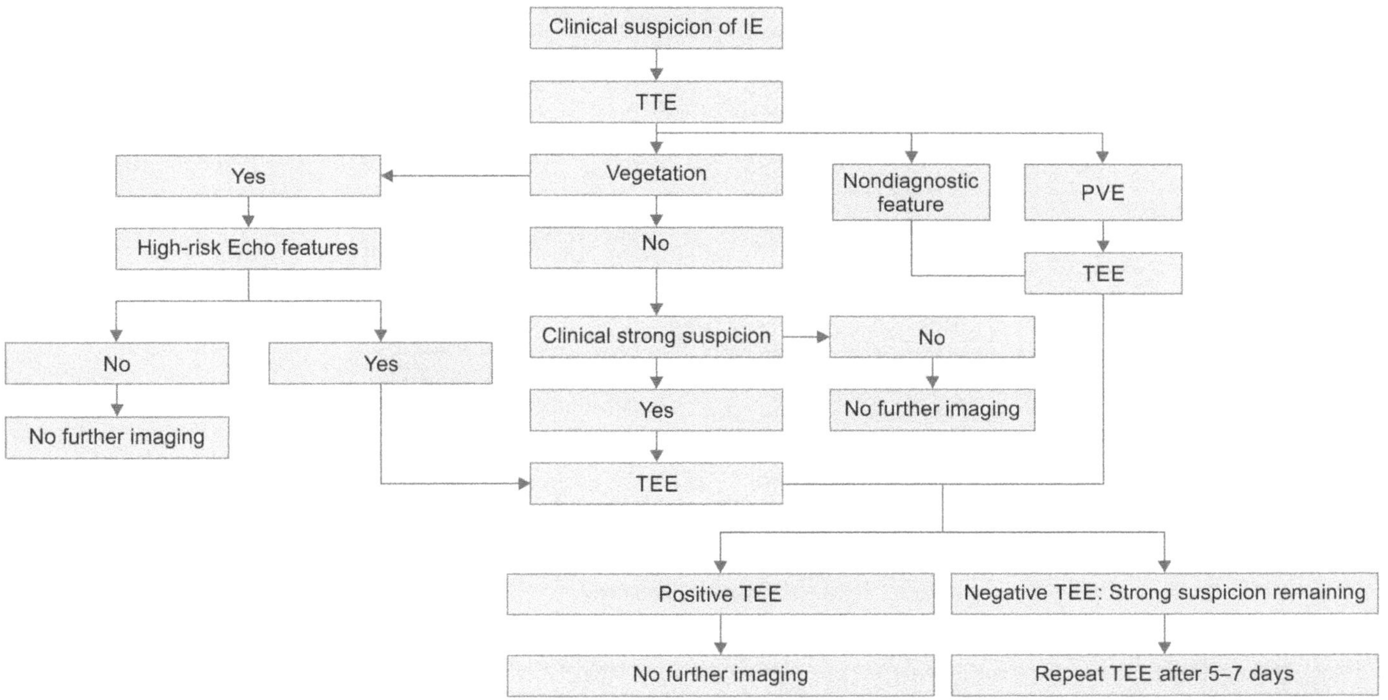

(ESC: European Society of Cardiology; IE: infective endocarditis; PVE: prosthetic valve endocarditis; TEE: transesophageal echocardiogram; TTE: transthoracic echocardiogram)

Diagnostic approach: Microbiological test ESC 2015[1]

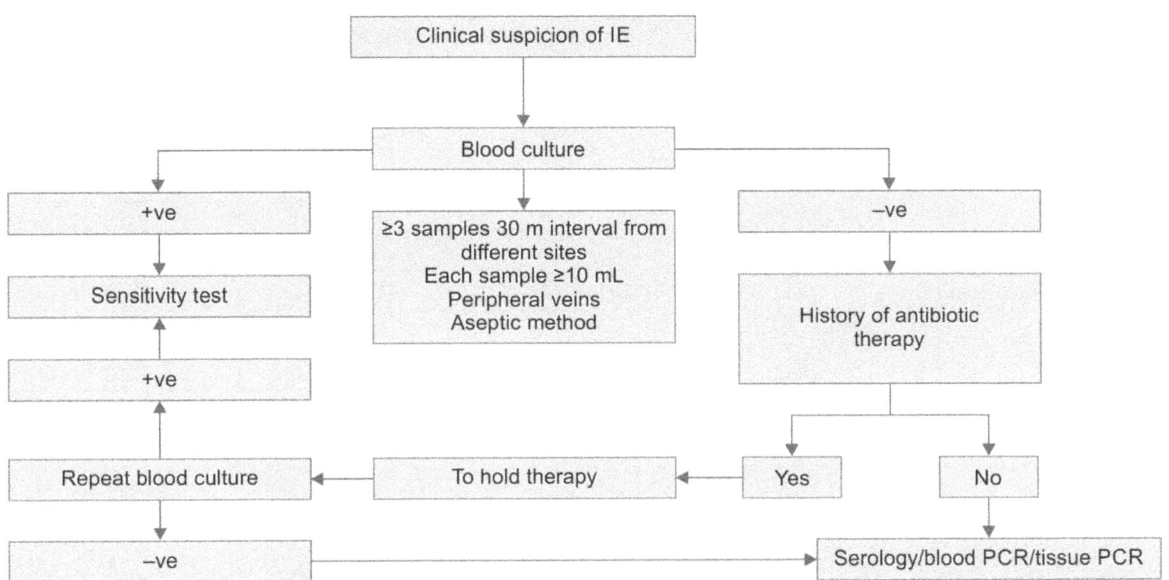

(IE: infective endocarditis; PCR: polymerase chain reaction)

Diagnostic criteria: von Reyn criteria[2]

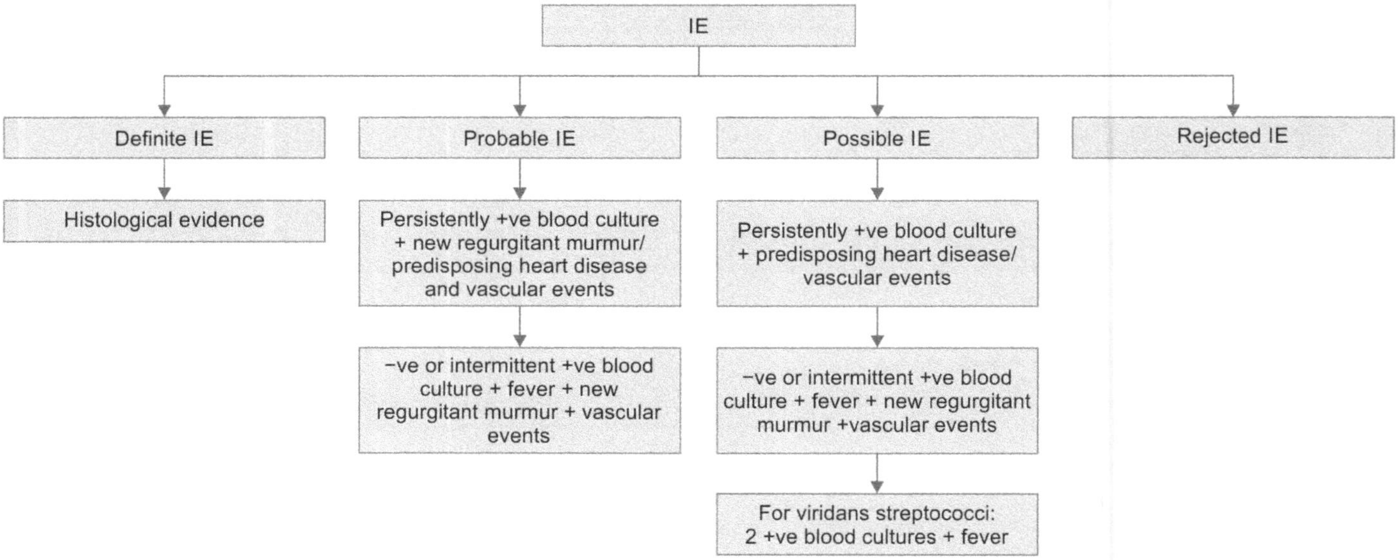

IE

- **Definite IE**
  - Histological evidence

- **Probable IE**
  - Persistently +ve blood culture + new regurgitant murmur/ predisposing heart disease and vascular events
  - −ve or intermittent +ve blood culture + fever + new regurgitant murmur + vascular events

- **Possible IE**
  - Persistently +ve blood culture + predisposing heart disease/ vascular events
  - −ve or intermittent +ve blood culture + fever + new regurgitant murmur +vascular events
  - For viridans streptococci: 2 +ve blood cultures + fever

- **Rejected IE**

(IE: infective endocarditis)

Diagnostic criteria: Modified Duke criteria[3]

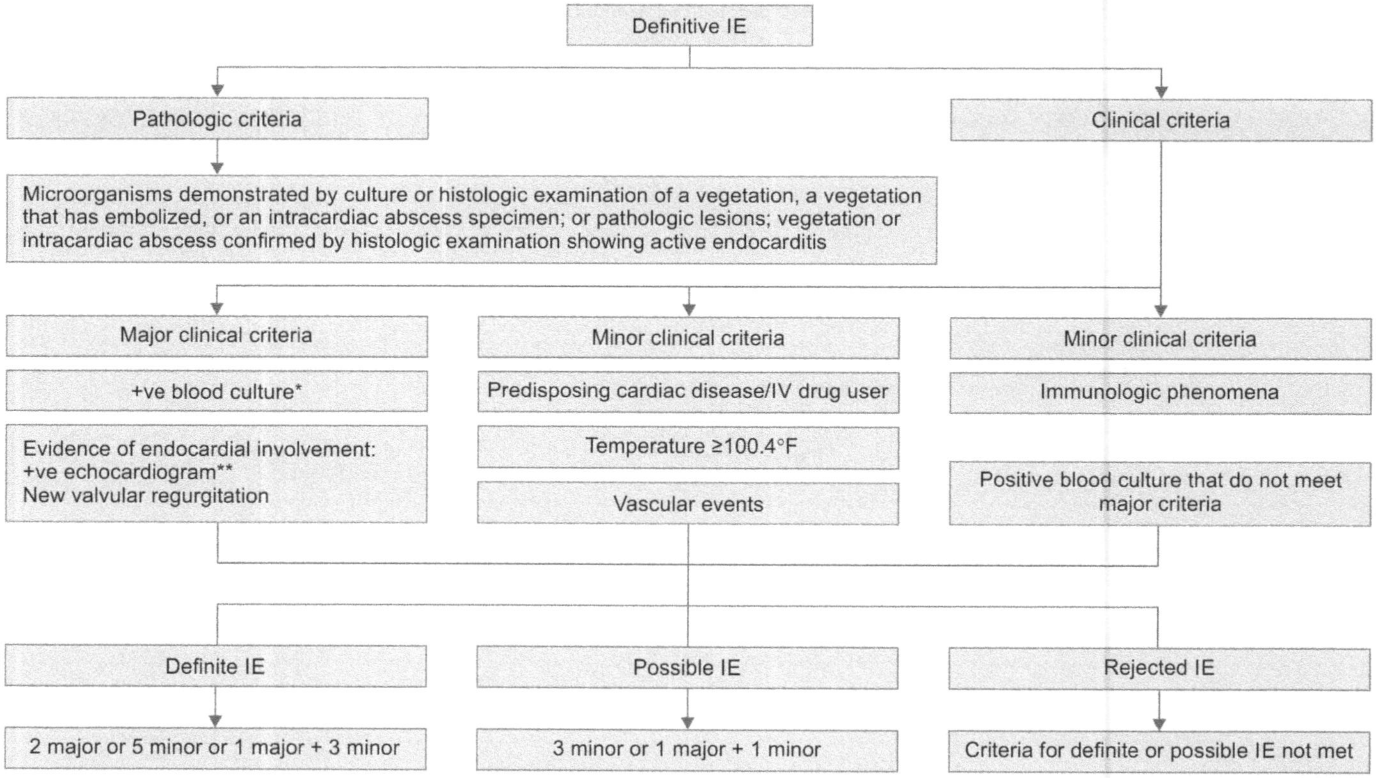

Definitive IE

- **Pathologic criteria**
  - Microorganisms demonstrated by culture or histologic examination of a vegetation, a vegetation that has embolized, or an intracardiac abscess specimen; or pathologic lesions; vegetation or intracardiac abscess confirmed by histologic examination showing active endocarditis

- **Clinical criteria**

Major clinical criteria
- +ve blood culture*
- Evidence of endocardial involvement: +ve echocardiogram** New valvular regurgitation

Minor clinical criteria
- Predisposing cardiac disease/IV drug user
- Temperature ≥100.4°F
- Vascular events

Minor clinical criteria
- Immunologic phenomena
- Positive blood culture that do not meet major criteria

- **Definite IE**
  - 2 major or 5 minor or 1 major + 3 minor

- **Possible IE**
  - 3 minor or 1 major + 1 minor

- **Rejected IE**
  - Criteria for definite or possible IE not met

*Positive blood culture: Typical microorganisms consistent with IE from two separate blood cultures: Viridans streptococci, *Streptococcus bovis*, HACEK group, *Staphylococcus aureus*; or community-acquired enterococci, in the absence of a primary focus; or microorganisms consistent with IE from persistently positive blood cultures, defined as follows: ≥2 positive cultures of blood samples drawn ≥12 h apart; or all of 3 or a majority of ≥4 separate cultures of blood (with first and last sample drawn at least 1 h apart) or single positive blood culture for *Coxiella burnetii* or antiphase I IgG antibody titer >1:800.
**Oscillating intracardiac mass on valve or supporting structures, in the path of regurgitant jets, or on implanted material in the absence of an alternative anatomic explanation; or abscess; or new partial dehiscence of prosthetic valve

(IE: infective endocarditis; IV: intravenous)

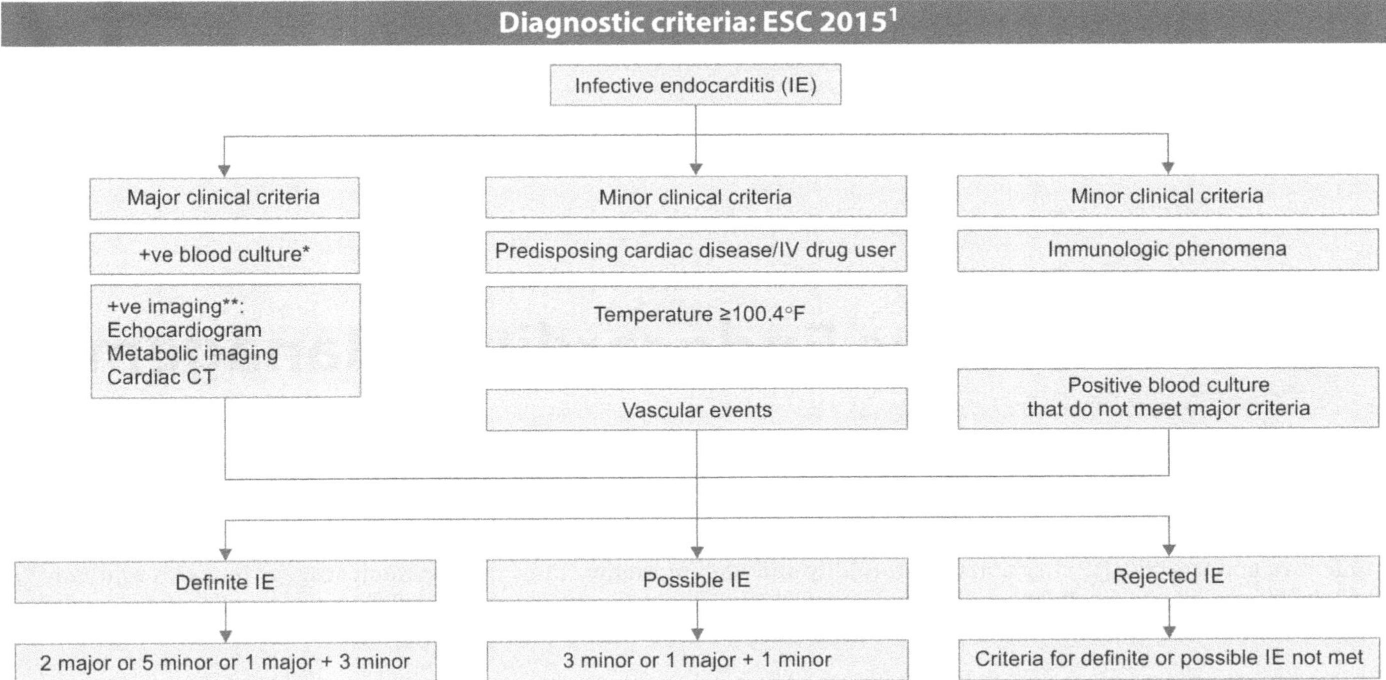

Positive blood culture: Typical microorganisms consistent with IE from 2 separate blood cultures: Viridans streptococci, *Streptococcus bovis*, HACEK group, *Staphylococcus aureus*; or community-acquired enterococci, in the absence of a primary focus; or microorganisms consistent with IE from persistently positive blood cultures, defined as follows: ≥2 positive cultures of blood samples drawn >12 h apart; or all of 3 or a majority of ≥4 separate cultures of blood (with first and last sample drawn at least 1 h apart) or single positive blood culture for *Coxiella burnetii* or antiphase I IgG antibody titer >1:800.

**Echocardiogram: Vegetation/abscess/pseudoaneurysm, intracardiac fistula, valvular perforation or aneurysm/new dehiscence of prosthetic valve; metabolic imaging: 18F-FDG PET CT or WBC SPECT CT: abnormal activity around prosthetic valve; cardiac CT: definite paravalvular lesion.

(CT: computed tomography; IV: intravenous)

REFERENCES

1. Habib G, Lancellotti P, Antunes MG, Bongiorni MG, Casalta JP, Del Zotti F, et al. 2015 ESC guidelines for the management of infective endocarditis. Eur Heart J. 2015;36:3075-128.
2. von Reyn CF, Levy BS, Arbeit RD, Friedland G, Crumpacker CS. Infective endocarditis: an analysis based on strict case definitions. Ann Intern Med. 1981;94(part 1):505-18.
3. Li JS, Sexton DJ, Mick N, Nettles R, Fowler VG Jr, Ryan T, et al. Proposed modifications to the Duke criteria for the diagnosis of infective endocarditis. Clin Infect Dis. 2000;30:3338.

CHAPTER 47

Infective Endocarditis: Management

INTRODUCTION

Infective endocarditis (IE) has a major morbidity and high mortality. Thus, management strategy includes aggressive and meticulous medical as well as surgical management. The antibiotic regimen should kill the bacteria, should be continued in terms of weeks and not days and should have intensive doses to ensure adequate drug level.

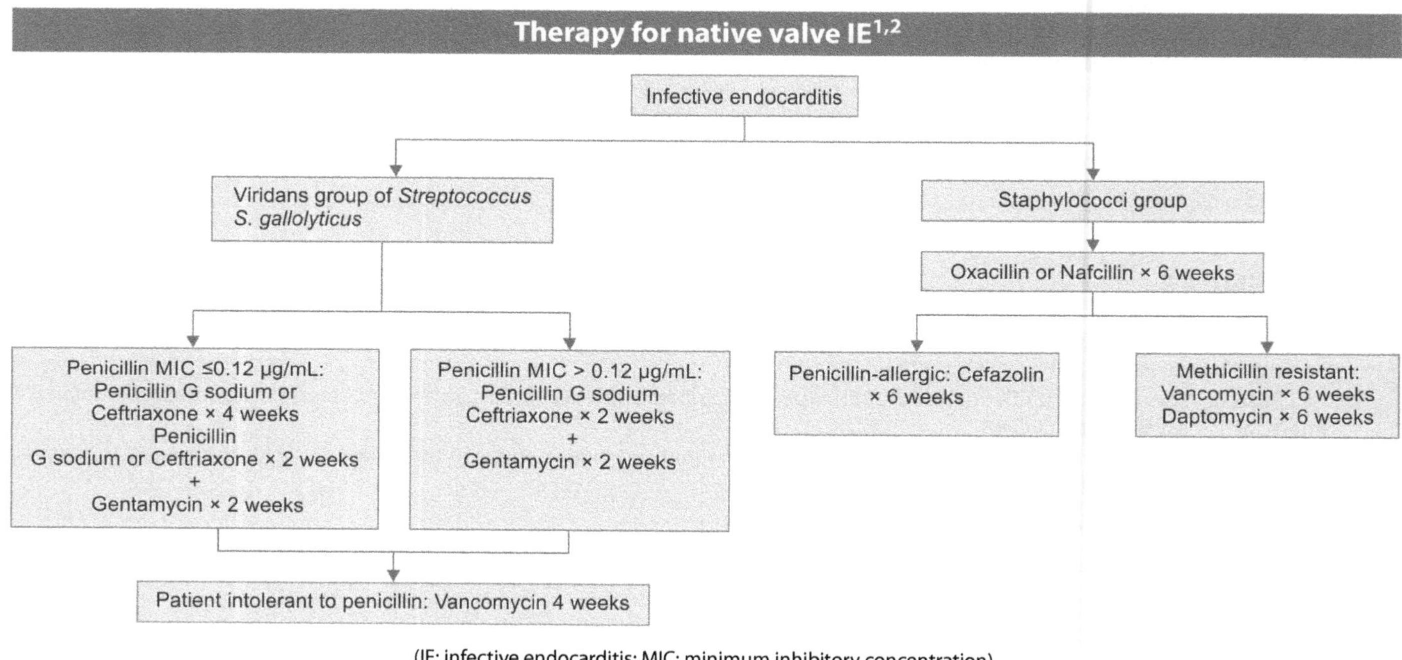

(IE: infective endocarditis; MIC: minimum inhibitory concentration)

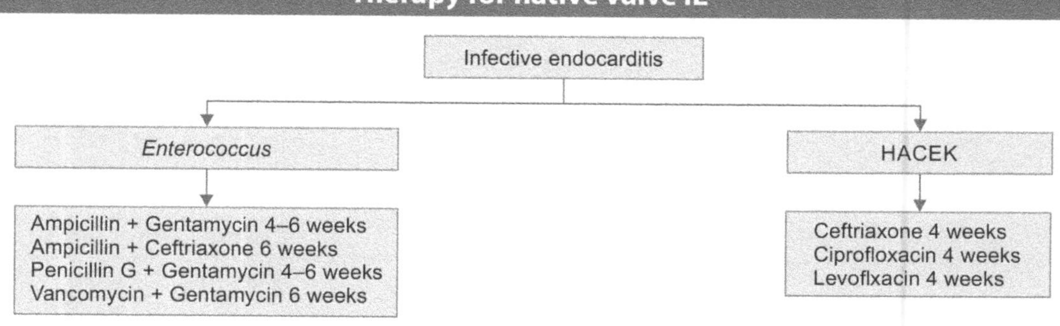

(HACEK: *Hemophilus*, *Aggregatibacter actinomycetemcomitans*, *Cardiobacterium*, *Eikenella corrodens*, *Kingella* species)

Therapy for prosthetic valve endocarditis (PVE)[3]

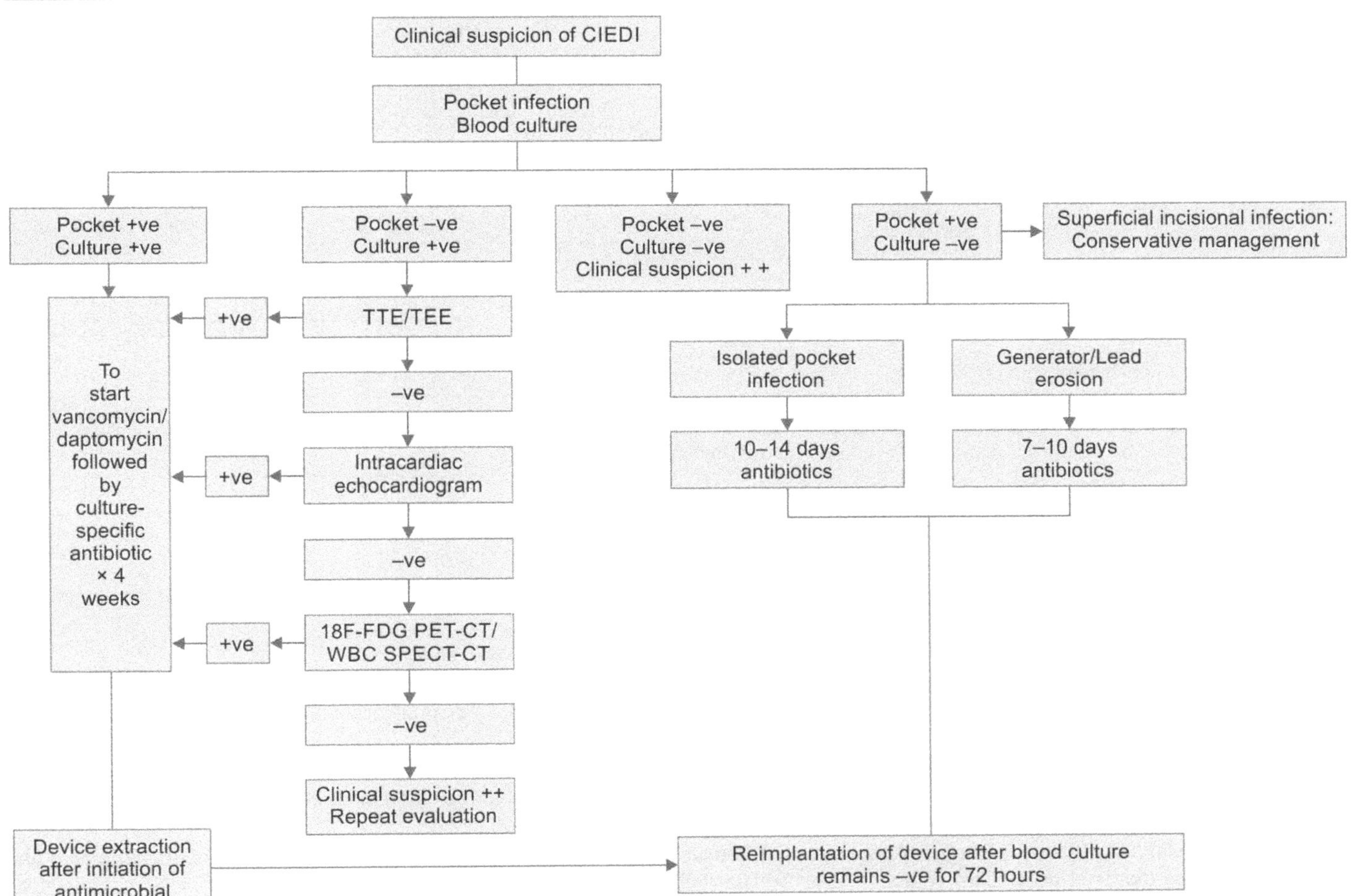

(MIC: minimum inhibitory concentration)

Management for cardiac implantable electronic device infection (CIEDI)[4,5]

(18F-FDG: fluorodeoxyglucose; CIEDI: cardiac implantable electronic device infection; PET-CT: positron emission tomography-computed tomography; SPECT-CT: single-photon emission computed tomography; TEE: transesophageal echocardiogram; TTE: transthoracic echocardiogram; WBC: white blood cell)

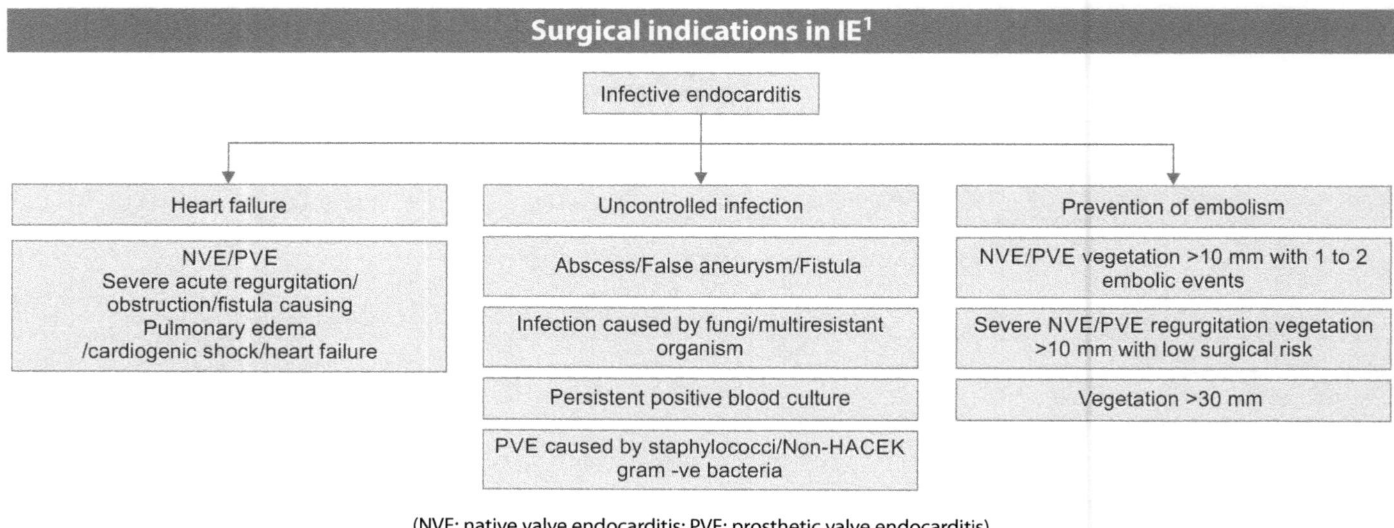

(NVE: native valve endocarditis; PVE: prosthetic valve endocarditis)

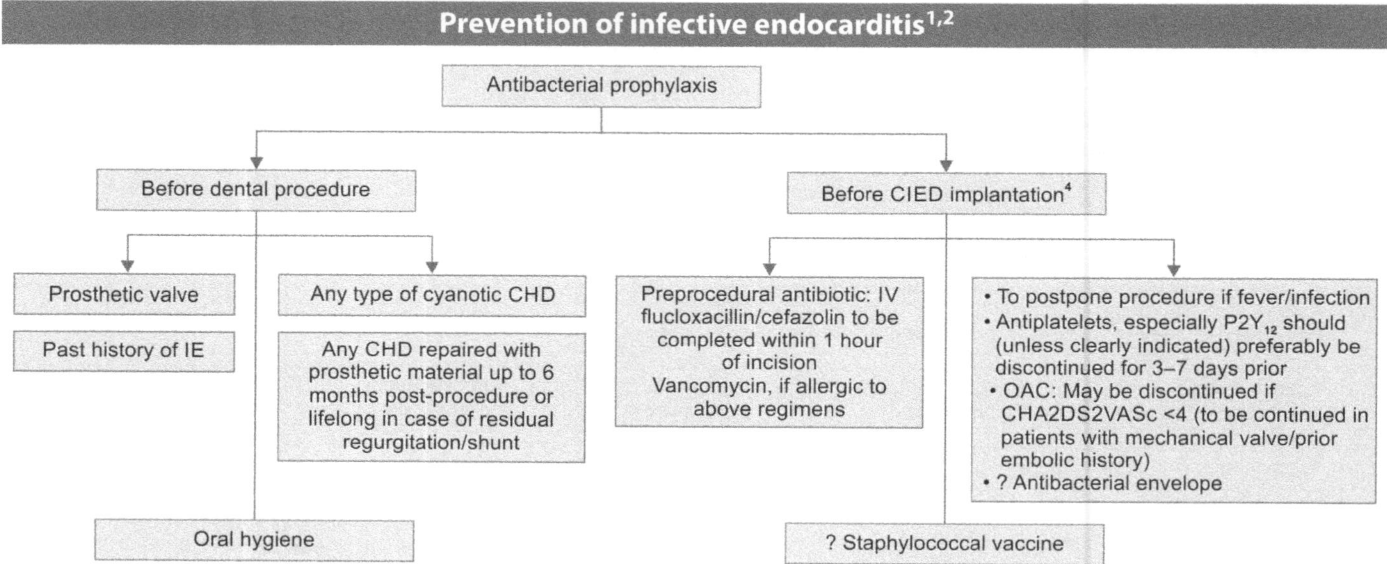

(CIED: cardiac implantable electronic device; CHD: congenital heart disease; IE: infective endocarditis; IV: intravenous; OAC: oral anticoagulant; ?: doubtful effect)

REFERENCES

1. Habib G, Lancellotti P, Antunes MG, Bongiorni MG, Casalta JP, Del Zotti F, et al. 2015 ESC guidelines for the management of infective endocarditis. Eur Heart J. 2015;36:3075-128.
2. Chambers HF, Bayer AS. Native valve infective endocarditis. N Eng J Med. 2020;383:567-76.
3. Baddour LM, Wilson WR, Bayer AS, Fowler VG Jr, Tleyjeh IM, Rybak MJ, et al. Infective endocarditis in adults: diagnosis, antimicrobial therapy, and management of complications. A scientific statement for healthcare personals from the American Heart association. Circulation. 2015;132:1435-86.
4. Blonstrom-Lunquvist C, Traykov V, Erba PA, Burri H, Nielsen JC, Bongiorni MG, et al. European Heart Rhythm Association (EHRA) international consensus document on how to prevent, diagnose, and treat cardiac implantable electronic device infections. Europace. 2020;22:515.
5. Sohail MR, Uslan DZ, Khan AH, Friedman PA, Hayes DL, Wilson WR, et al. Management and outcome of permanent pacemaker and implantable cardioverter-defibrillator infection. J Am Coll Cardiol. 2007;49:1851.

Atrial Fibrillation

Atrial Fibrillation: Basic Approach

INTRODUCTION

Atrial fibrillation (AF) is one of the most common sustained cardiac arrhythmia, associated with significant morbidity and mortality. Its prevalence is increasing and at present ranges from 2 to 4.[1] The prevalence is relatively lower in women and non-Caucasians.

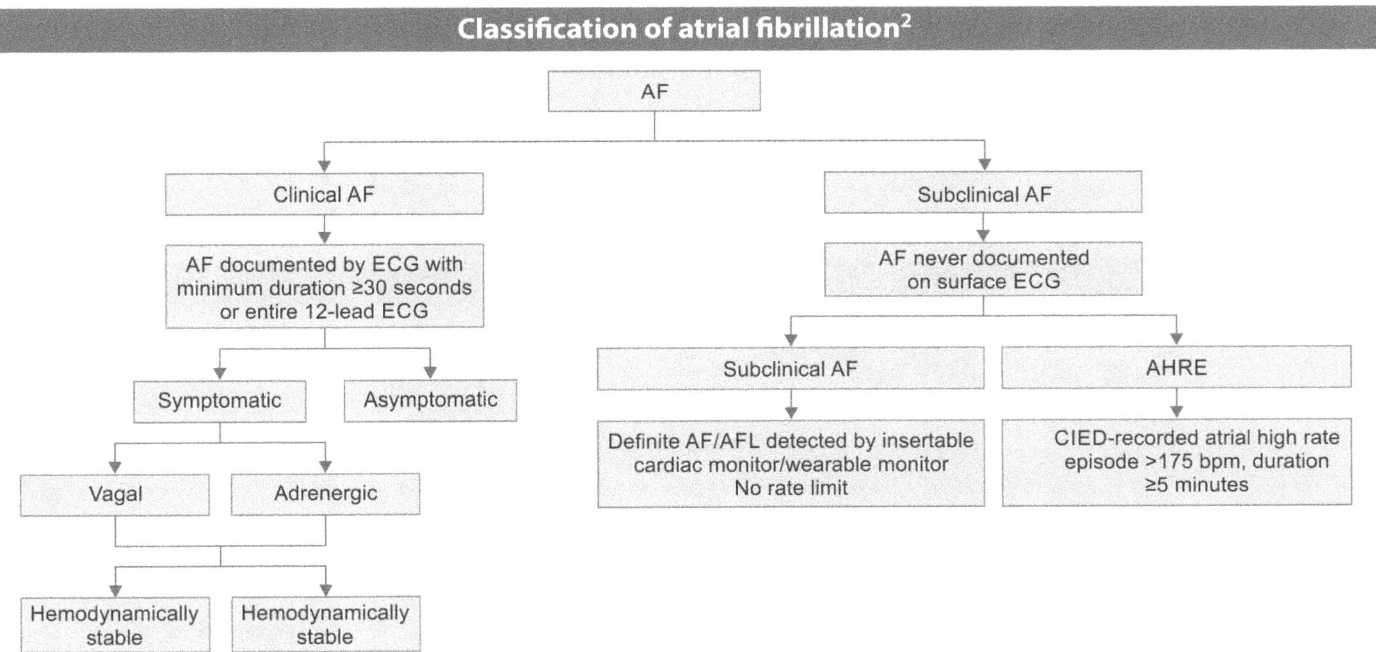

(AF: atrial fibrillation; AFL: atrial flutter; AHRE: atrial high rate episode; CIED: cardiac implantable electronic device; ECG: echocardiogram)

Classification of atrial fibrillation[2]

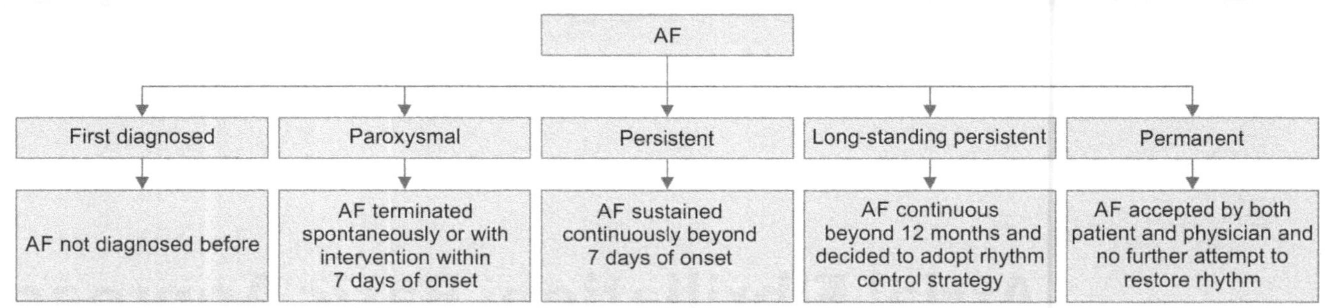

(AF: atrial fibrillation)

Risk factors for atrial fibrillation

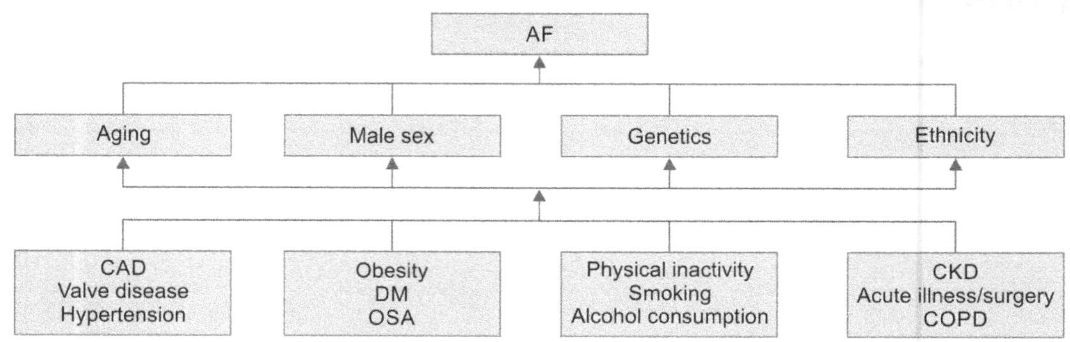

(AF: atrial fibrillation; CAD: coronary artery disease; CKD: chronic kidney disease; COPD: chronic obstructive pulmonary disease; DM: diabetes mellitus; OSA: obstructive sleep apnea)

Mechanism of atrial fibrillation

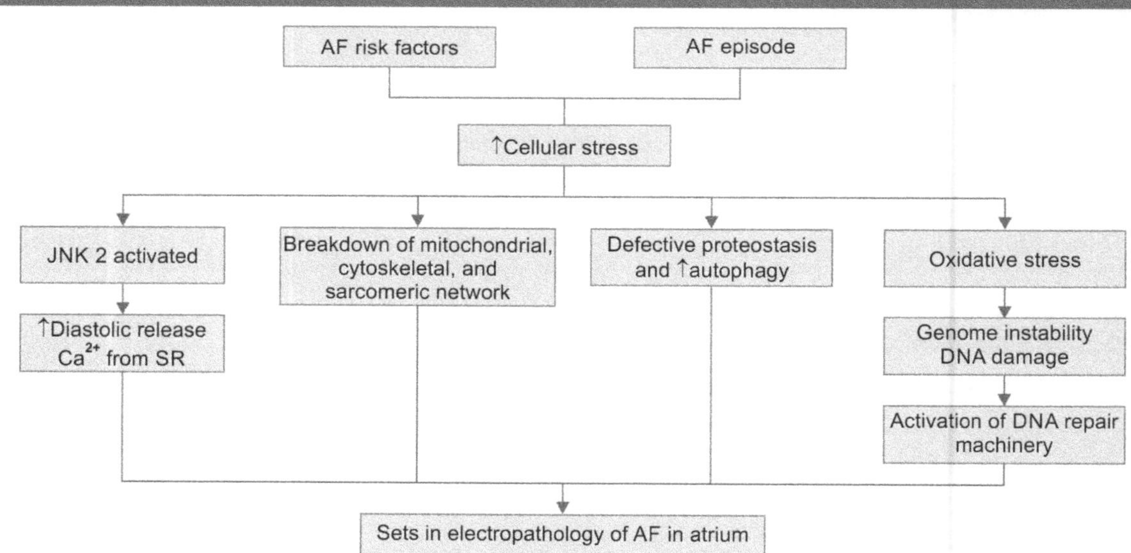

(AF: atrial fibrillation; DNA: deoxyribonucleic acid; JNK: JUN-N terminal kinase; SR: sarcoplasmic reticulum)

European Heart Rhythm Association functional classification of atrial fibrillation[3]

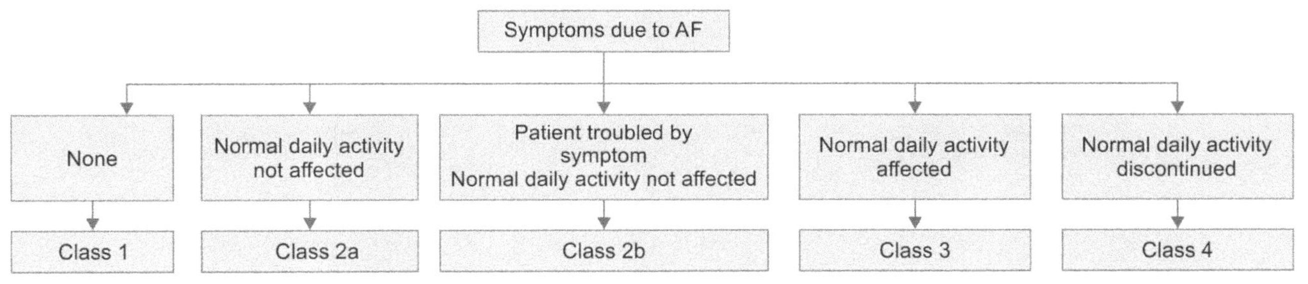

(AF: atrial fibrillation)

How to investigate in atrial fibrillation

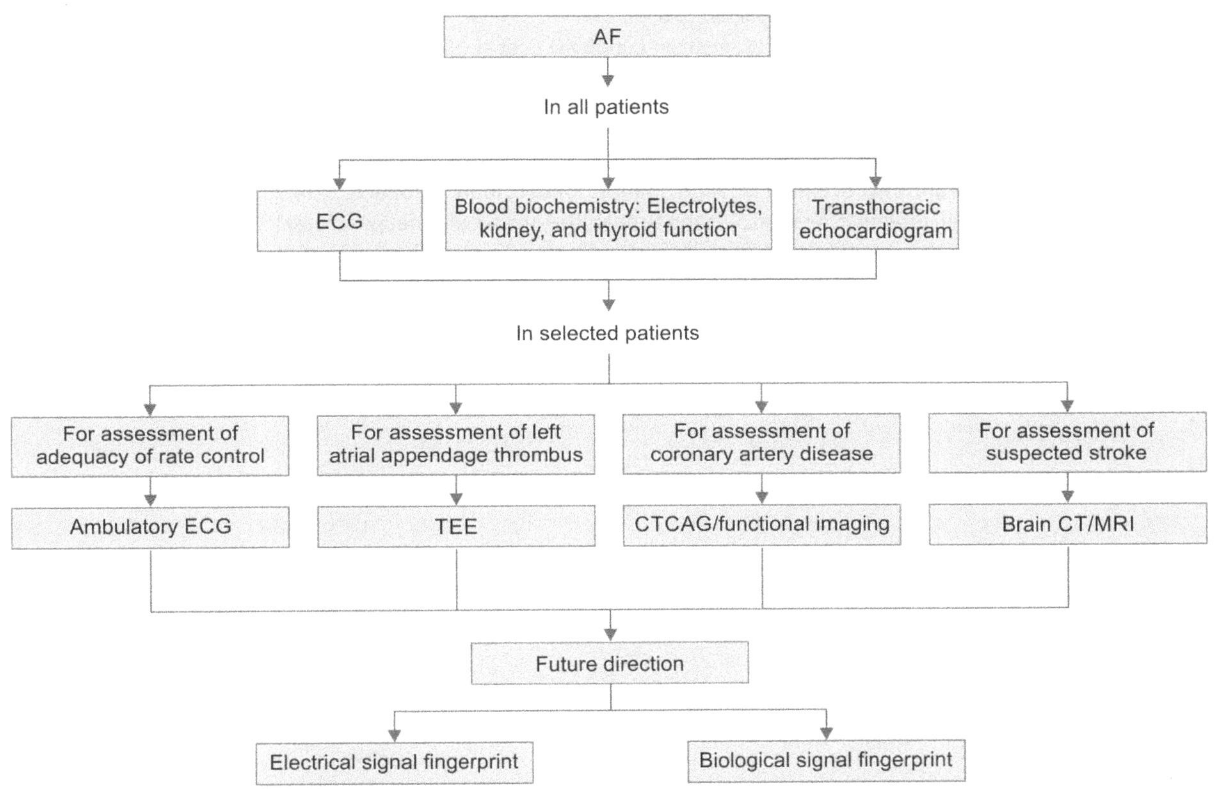

(AF: atrial fibrillation; CT: computed tomography; CTCAG: computed tomography coronary angiogram; ECG: echocardiogram; MRI: magnetic resonance imaging; TEE: transesophageal echocardiogram)

Risk assessment in atrial fibrillation

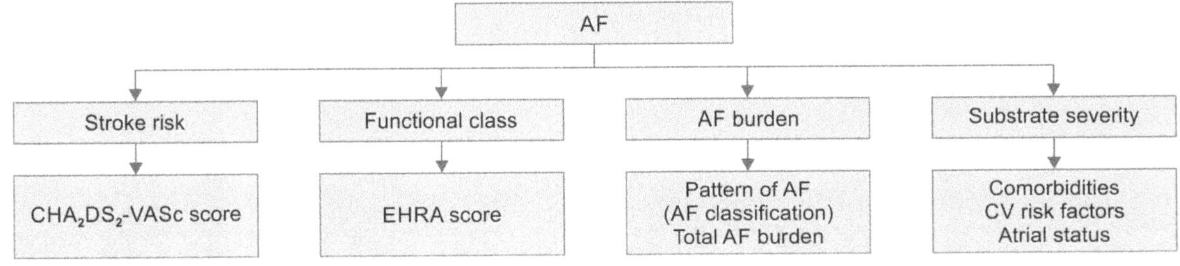

(AF: atrial fibrillation; CV: cardiovascular; EHRA: European Heart Rhythm Association)

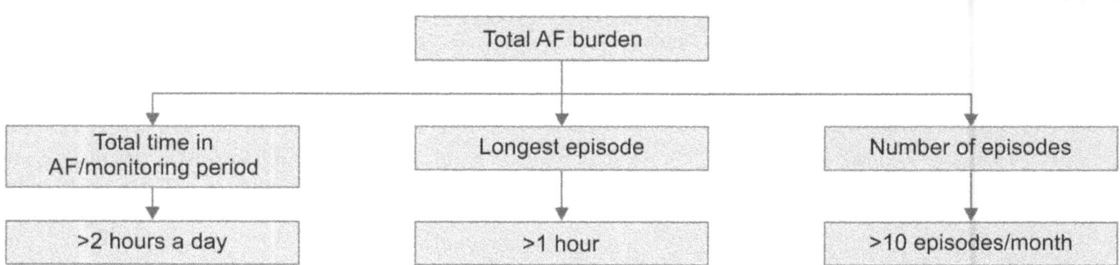

REFERENCES

1. Chamberlain AM, Chang AR, Cheng S, Das SR, Delling FN, Djousse L, et al; American Heart Association Council on Epidemiology and Prevention Statistics Committee and Stroke Statistics Subcommittee. Heart disease and stroke statistics 2019 update: A report from the American Heart Association. Circulation. 2019;139:e56-e528.

2. Hindricks G, Potpara T, Dagres N, Arbelo E, Bax JJ, Blomström-Lundqvist C, et al. 2020 ESC Guidelines for the diagnosis and management of atrial fibrillation developed in collaboration with the European Association for Cardio-Thoracic Surgery (EACTS): The Task Force for the diagnosis and management of atrial fibrillation of the European Society of Cardiology (ESC) Developed with the special contribution of the European Heart Rhythm Association (EHRA) of the ESC. Eur Heart J. 2021;42:373-498.

3. Wynn GJ, Todd DM, Webber M, Bonnett L, McShane J, Kirchhof P, et al. The European Heart Rhythm Association symptom classification for atrial fibrillation: validation and improvement through a simple modification. Europace. 2014;16:965-72.

4. Kochhäuser S, Joza J, Essebag V, Proietti R, Koehler J, Tsang B, et al. The impact of duration of atrial fibrillation recurrences on measures of health-related quality of life and symptoms. Pacing Clin Electrophysiol. 2016;39(2):166-72.

CHAPTER 49

Atrial Fibrillation: Management

INTRODUCTION

Atrial fibrillation (AF) increases stroke rate five times. Thus, stroke prevention is the most important issue in AF management. In the rate versus rhythm control strategy, rhythm control has class IA evidence of indication for symptom and quality of life improvement in symptomatic patients with AF.[1]

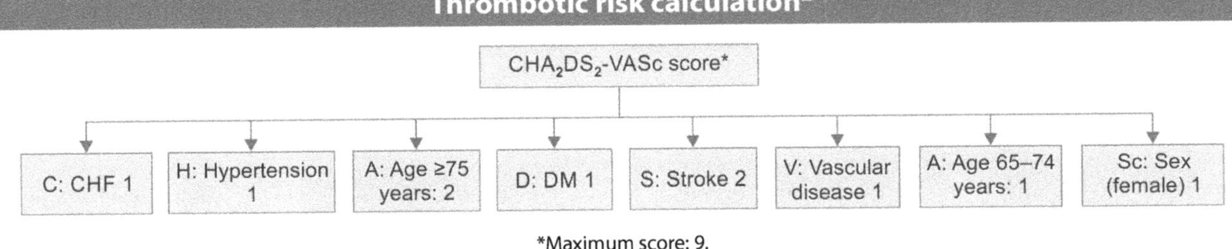

*Maximum score: 9.

(CHF: congestive heart failure; DM: diabetes mellitus)

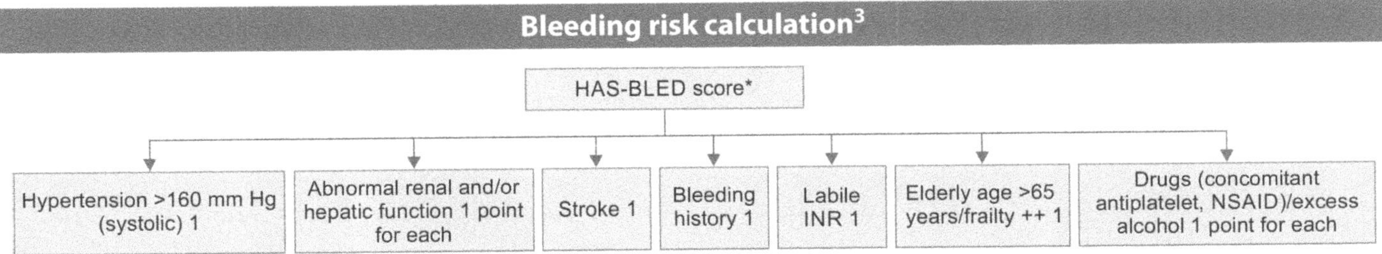

*0–1: low risk; 2–3: moderate risk; 4–5: high risk; >5: very high risk.

(INR: international normalized ratio; NSAID: nonsteroidal anti-inflammatory drug)

Oral anticoagulant to prevent stroke in atrial fibrillation[1]

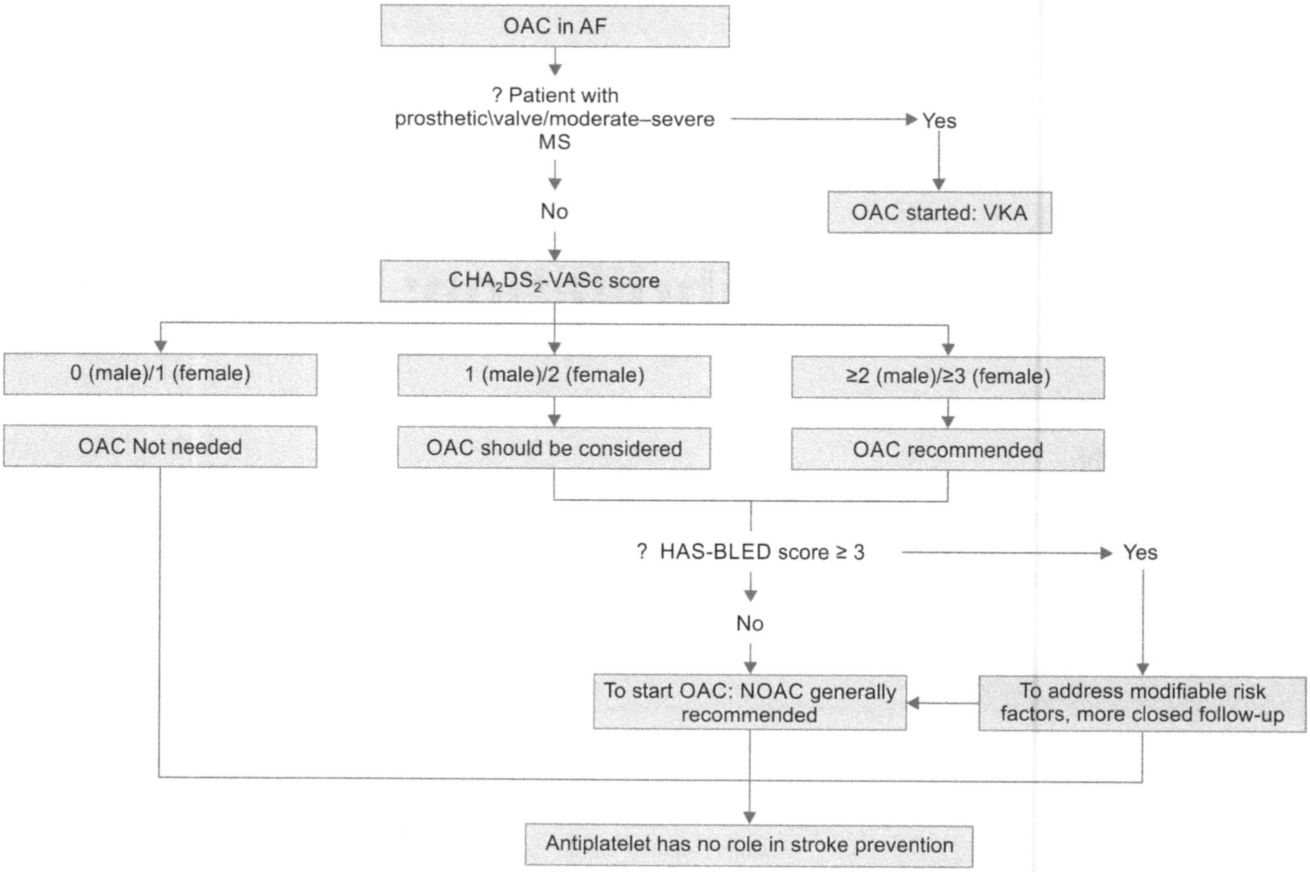

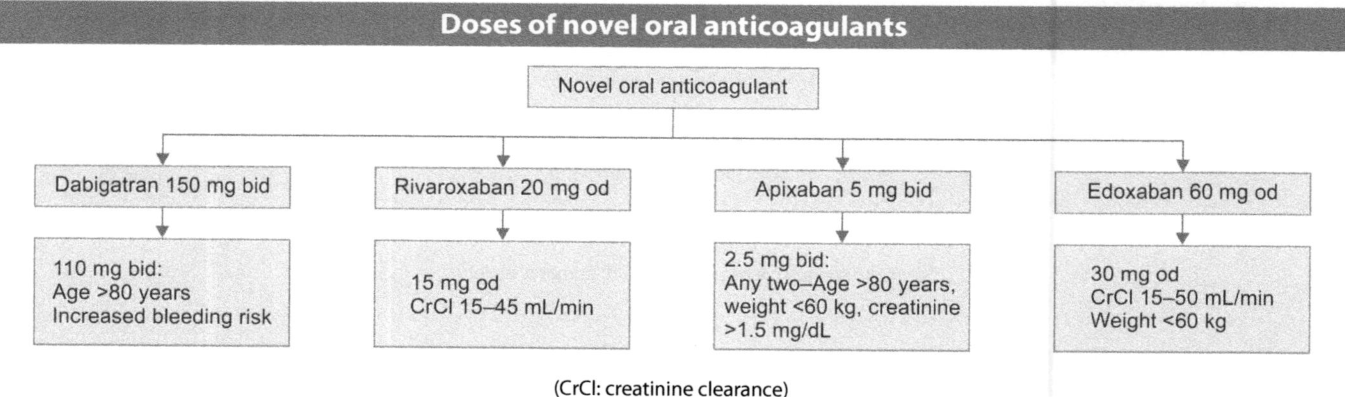

(AF: atrial fibrillation; MS: mitral stenosis; NOAC: novel oral anticoagulant; OAC: oral anticoagulant; VKA: vitamin K antagonist)

Doses of novel oral anticoagulants

Novel oral anticoagulant

Dabigatran 150 mg bid	Rivaroxaban 20 mg od	Apixaban 5 mg bid	Edoxaban 60 mg od
110 mg bid: Age >80 years Increased bleeding risk	15 mg od CrCl 15–45 mL/min	2.5 mg bid: Any two—Age >80 years, weight <60 kg, creatinine >1.5 mg/dL	30 mg od CrCl 15–50 mL/min Weight <60 kg

(CrCl: creatinine clearance)

Rate versus rhythm control in atrial fibrillation

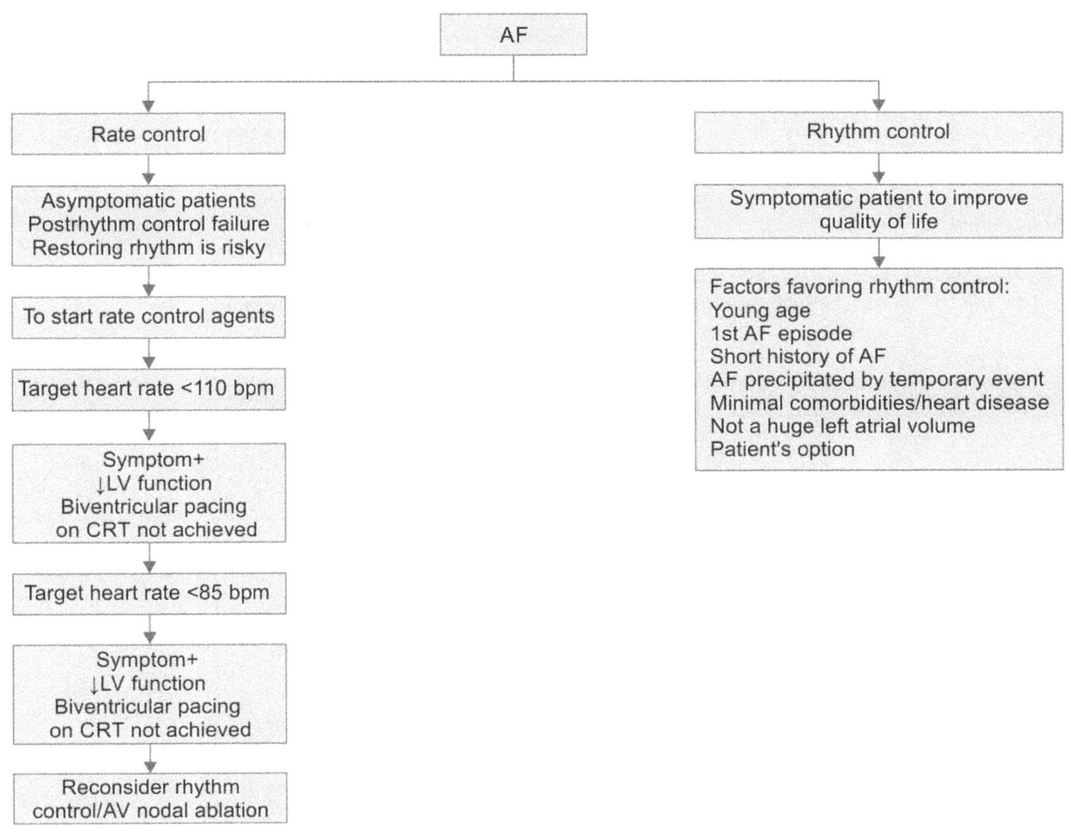

(AF: atrial fibrillation; AV: atrioventricular; CRT: cardiac resynchronization therapy; LV: left ventricular)

Rate and rhythm controlling agents in atrial fibrillation

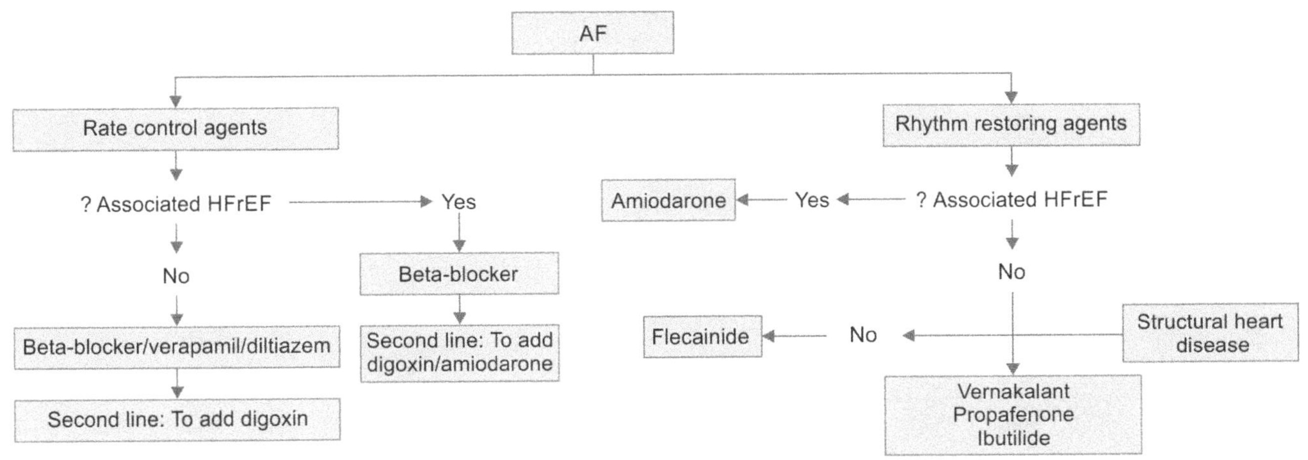

(AF: atrial fibrillation; HFrEF: heart failure with reduced ejection fraction)

Nonarrhythmic drugs with antiarrhythmic property

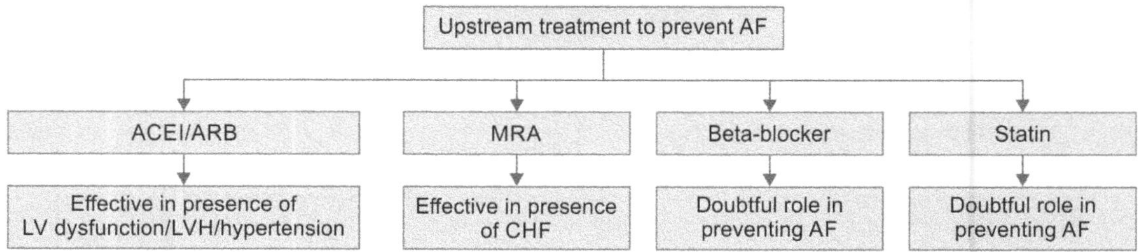

(ACEI: angiotensin-converting enzyme inhibitor; AF: atrial fibrillation; ARB: angiotensin receptor blocker; CHF: congestive heart failure; LV: left ventricular; LVH: left ventricular hypertrophy; MRA: magnetic resonance angiogram)

Catheter ablation in atrial fibrillation[4]

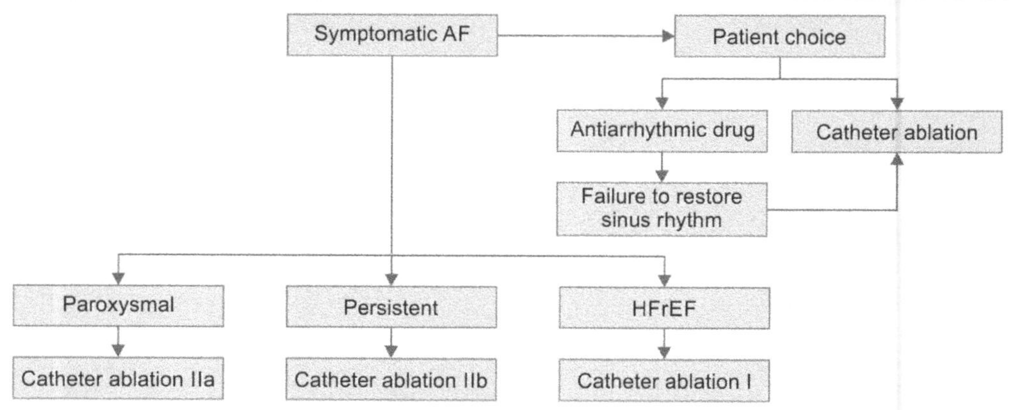

(AF: atrial fibrillation; HFrEF: heart failure with reduced ejection fraction)

Cardioversion in atrial fibrillation[1]

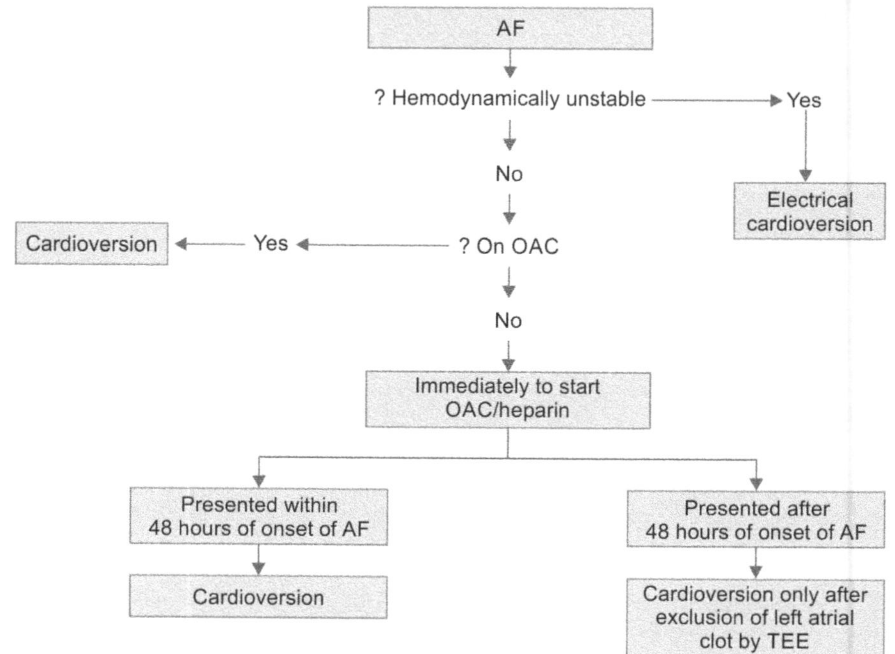

(AF: atrial fibrillation; OAC: oral anticoagulation; TEE: transesophageal echocardiogram)

Long-term antiarrhythmic drug strategy to prevent relapse of atrial fibrillation[1]

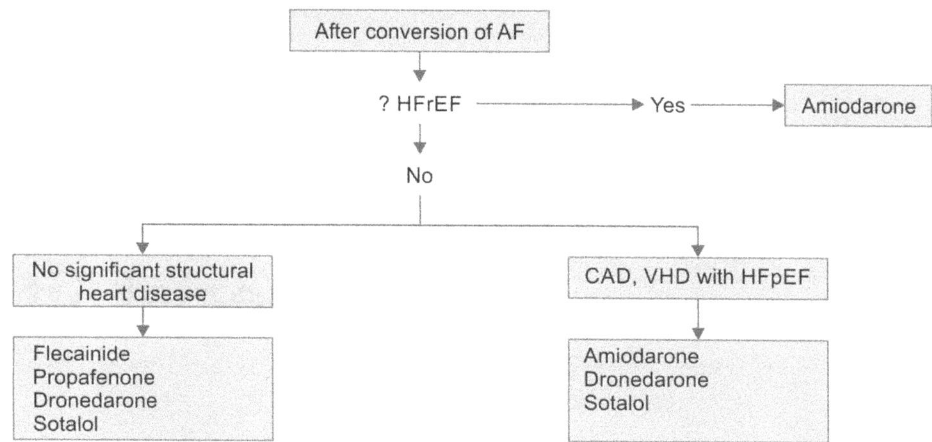

(AF: atrial fibrillation; CAD: coronary artery disease; HFpEF: heart failure with preserved ejection fraction; HFrEF: heart failure with reduced ejection fraction; VHD: valvular heart disease)

Principles of long-term antiarrhythmic drug (AAD) strategy

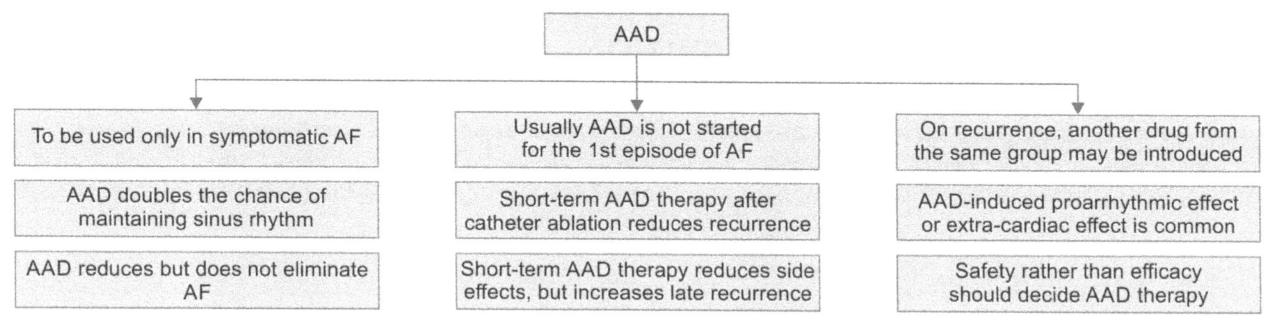

(AAD: antiarrhythmic drug; AF: atrial fibrillation)

REFERENCES

1. Hindrick G, Potpara T, Dagres N, Arbelo E, Bax JJ, Blomström-Lundqvist C, et al. 2020 ESC Guidelines for the diagnosis and management of atrial fibrillation developed in collaboration with the European Association for Cardio-Thoracic Surgery (EACTS): The Task Force for the diagnosis and management of atrial fibrillation of the European Society of Cardiology (ESC) Developed with the special contribution of the European Heart Rhythm Association (EHRA) of the ESC. Eur Heart J. 2021;42:373-498.
2. Lip GY, Nieuwlaat R, Pisters R, Lane DA, Crijns HJ. Refining clinical risk stratification for predicting stroke and thromboembolism in atrial fibrillation using a novel risk factor-based approach: the Euro Heart Survey on atrial fibrillation. Chest. 2010;137(2):263-72.
3. Pisters R, Lane DA, Nieuwlaat R, de Vos CB, Crijns HJ, Lip GY. A novel user- friendly score (HAS-BLED) to assess 1-year risk of major bleeding in patients with atrial fibrillation: the Euro Heart Survey. Chest. 2010;138(5):1093-100.
4. Krittayaphong R, Raungrattanaamporn O, Bhuripanyo K, Sriratanasathavorn C, Pooranawattanakul S, Punlee K, et al. A randomized clinical trial of the efficacy of radiofrequency catheter ablation and amiodarone in the treatment of symptomatic atrial fibrillation. J Med Assoc Thai. 2003;86(Suppl 1):S8-16.

CHAPTER 50

Atrial Fibrillation Management: Special Situations

INTRODUCTION

As atrial fibrillation (AF) is a common entity and as many of the patients with AF are on anticoagulation therapy, clinicians will face many clinical situations, in which anticoagulants need various modification. The balance between bleeding risk and thrombotic risk lies on a thin edge in those clinical situations.

PERCUTANEOUS CORONARY INTERVENTION

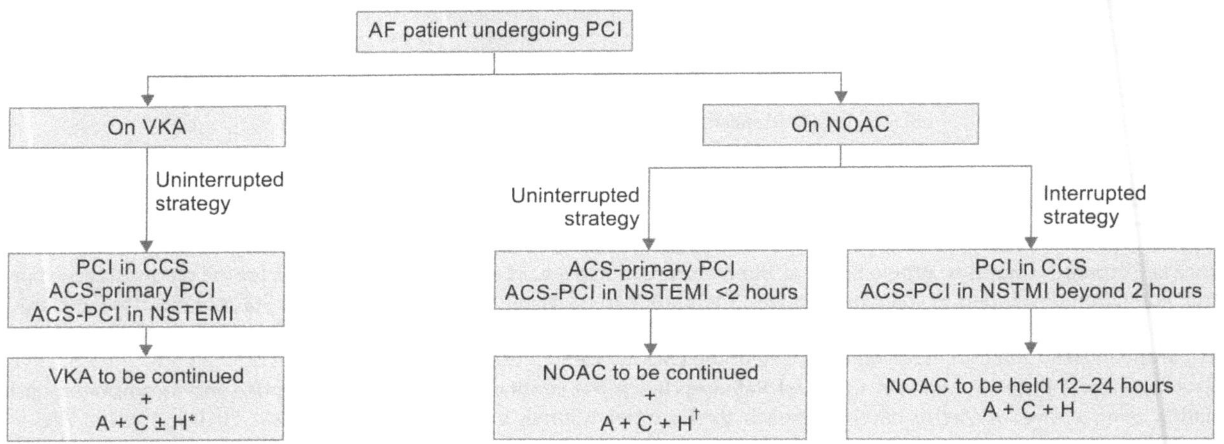

*If INR >2.5: no heparin; If INR <2.5: low-dose heparin/bivalirudin.
†NOAC: A: aspirin; C: clopidogrel; H: heparin; loading dose of clopidogrel in ACS is 600 mg and in CCS is 300 mg.

(ACS: acute coronary syndrome; AF: atrial fibrillation; CCS: chronic coronary syndrome; INR: international normalized ratio; NOAC: non-vitamin-K dependent oral anticoagulant; NSTEMI: non-ST segment elevation myocardial infarction; PCI: percutaneous coronary intervention; VKA: vitamin K antagonist)

Post-percutaneous coronary intervention in patient with atrial fibrillation (AF): Antithrombotic strategy[2]

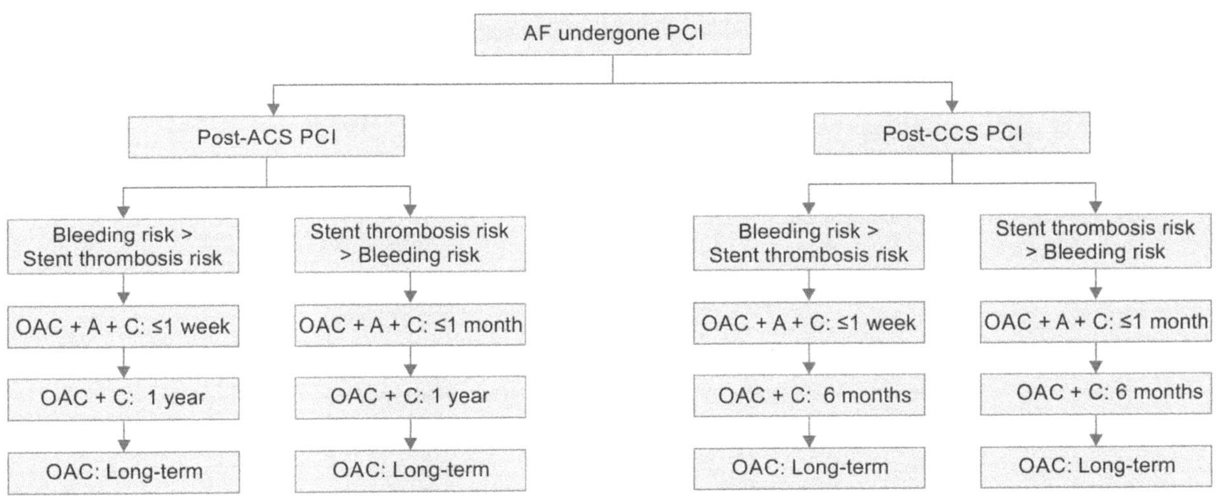

Note: OAC: A: aspirin; C: clopidogrel. When OAC is given in combination with antiplatelets, NOAC is preferred over VKA; amongst P2Y12 inhibitor, clopidogrel is preferred.

(ACS: acute coronary syndrome; AF: atrial fibrillation; CCS: chronic coronary syndrome; OAC: oral anticoagulant; PCI: percutaneous coronary intervention; OAC: oral anticoagulant)

Post-PCI ACS and post-PCI CCS patient with atrial fibrillation: Antithrombotic strategy-2[1]

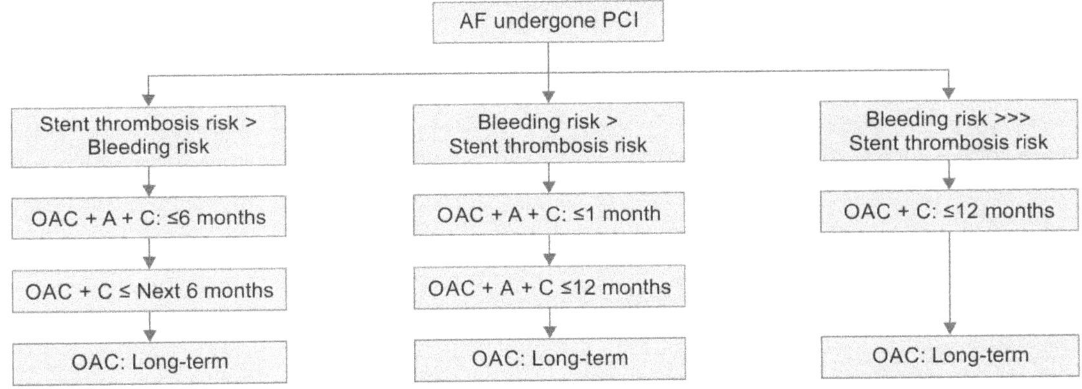

(AF: atrial fibrillation; PCI: percutaneous coronary intervention; OAC: oral anticoagulant)

STROKE

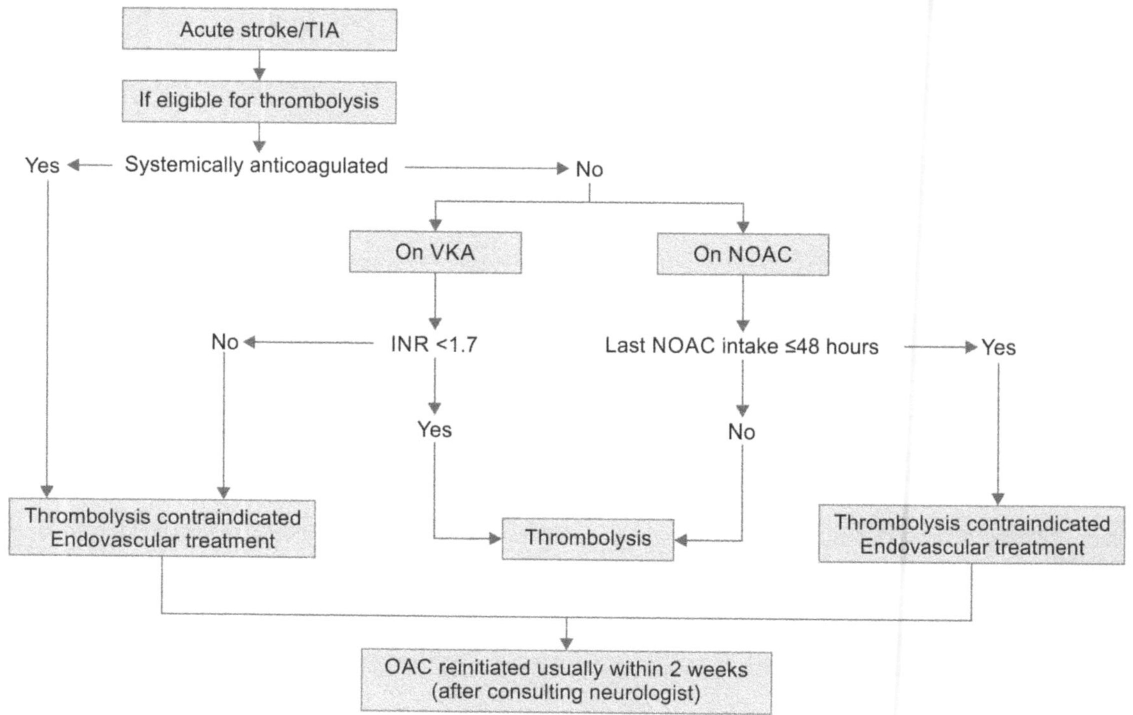

(INR: international normalized ratio; NOAC: non-vitamin-K dependent oral anticoagulant; OAC: oral anticoagulant; TIA: transient ischemic attack; VKA: vitamin K antagonist)

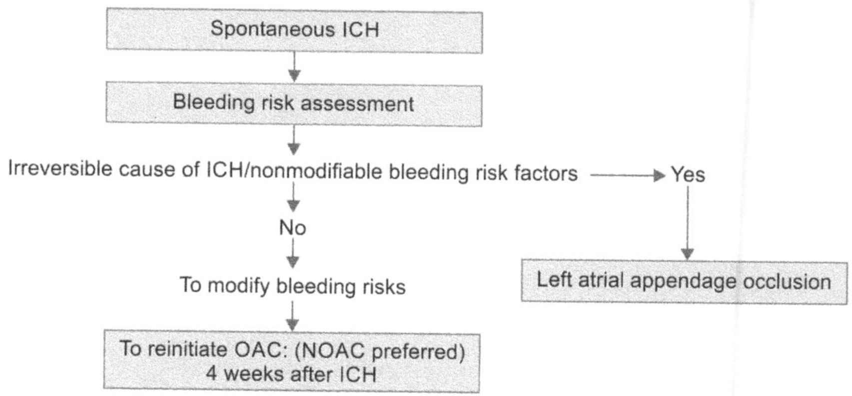

(ICH: intracranial hemorrhage; NOAC: non-vitamin-K dependent oral anticoagulant; OAC: oral anticoagulant)

ACTIVE BLEEDING

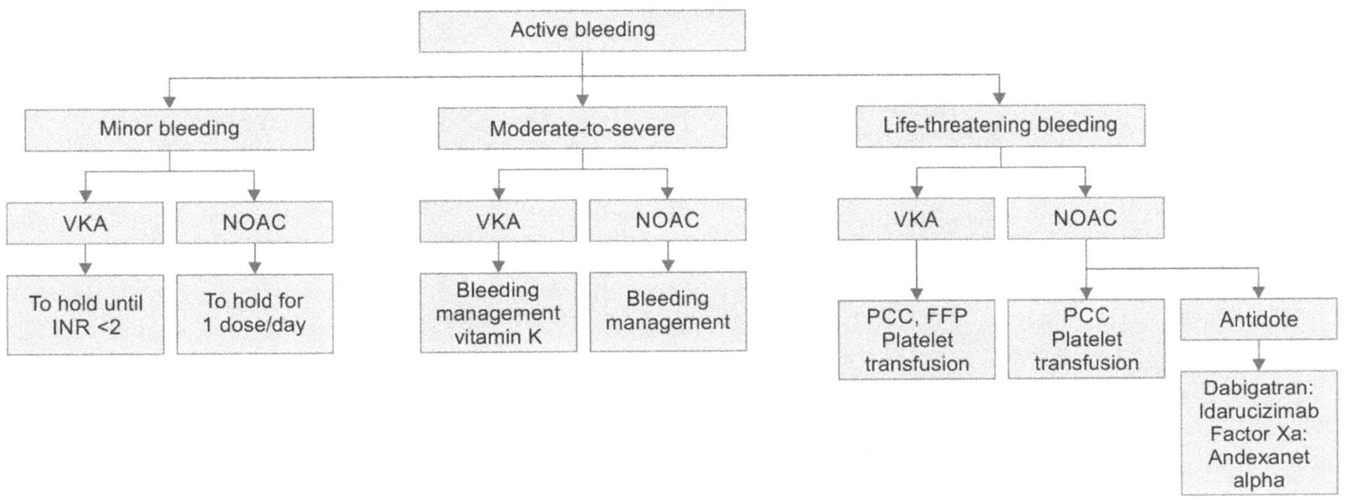

(FFP: fresh frozen plasma; INR: international normalized ratio; NOAC: non-vitamin-K dependent oral anticoagulant; PCC: prothrombin complex concentrate; VKA: vitamin K antagonist)

POSTOPERATIVE ATRIAL FIBRILLATION

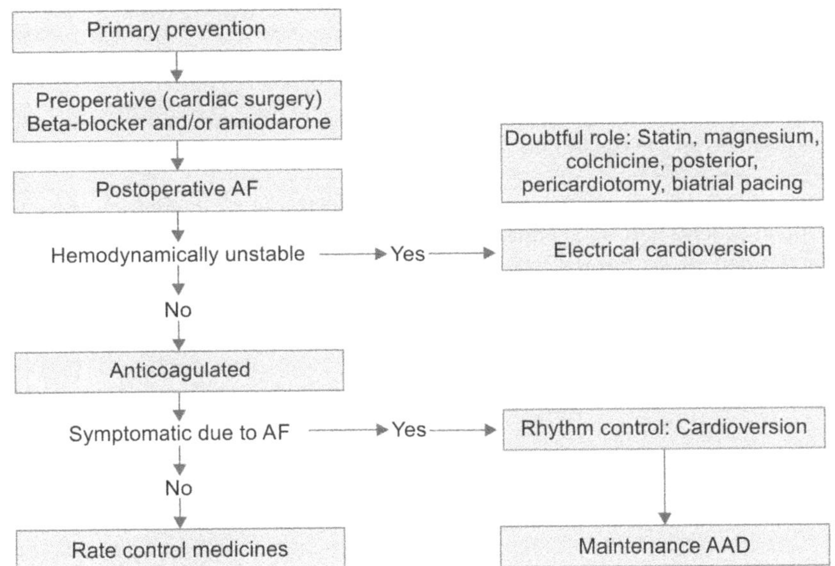

(AAD: antiarrhythmic drugs; AF: atrial fibrillation)

ATRIAL HIGH RATE EPISODE AND SUBCLINICAL ATRIAL FIBRILLATION

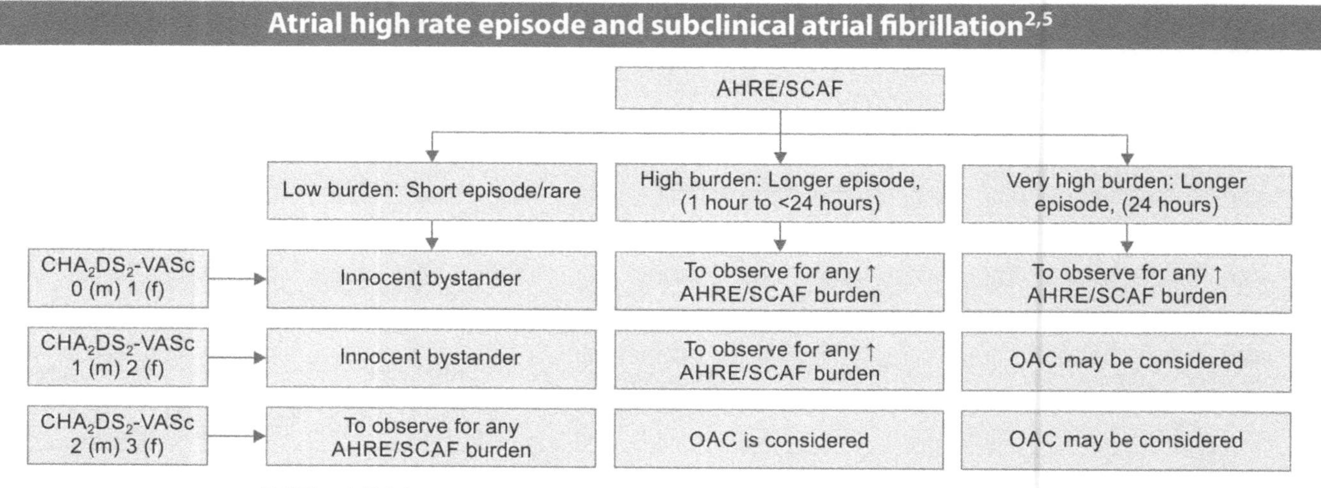

(AHRE: atrial high rate episode; OAC: oral anticoagulant; SCAF: subclinical atrial fibrillation)

REFERENCES

1. Lip GYH, Collet JP, Haude M, Byrne R, Chung EH, Fauchier L, et al; ESC Scientific Document Group. 2018 Joint European consensus document on the management of antithrombotic therapy in atrial fibrillation patients presenting with acute coronary syndrome and/or undergoing percutaneous cardiovascular interventions: a joint consensus document of the European Heart Rhythm Association (EHRA), European Society of Cardiology Working Group on Thrombosis, European Association of Percutaneous Cardiovascular Interventions (EAPCI), and European Association of Acute Cardiac Care (ACCA) endorsed by the Heart Rhythm Society (HRS), Asia-Pacific Heart Rhythm Society (APHRS), Latin America Heart Rhythm Society (LAHRS), and Cardiac Arrhythmia Society of Southern Africa (CASSA). Europace. 2019;21(2):192-3.

2. Hindricks G, Potpara T, Dagres N, Arbelo E, Bax JJ, Blomström-Lundqvist C, et al. 2020 ESC Guidelines for the diagnosis and management of atrial fibrillation developed in collaboration with the European Association for Cardio-Thoracic Surgery (EACTS): The Task Force for the diagnosis and management of atrial fibrillation of the European Society of Cardiology (ESC) Developed with the special contribution of the European Heart Rhythm Association (EHRA) of the ESC. Eur Heart J. 2021;42:373-498.

3. Steffel J, Verhamme P, Potpara TS, Albaladejo P, Antz M, Desteghe L, et al; ESC Scientific Document Group. The 2018 European Heart Rhythm Association Practical Guide on the use of non- vitamin K antagonist oral anticoagulants in patients with atrial fibrillation. Eur Heart J. 2018;39:1330-93.

4. Ruff CT, Giugliano RP, Braunwald E, Hoffman EB, Deenadayalu N, Ezekowitz MD, et al. Comparison of the efficacy and safety of new oral anticoagulants with warfarin in patients with atrial fibrillation: a meta-analysis of randomised trials. Lancet. 2014;383:955-62.

5. Gorenek BC, Bax J, Boriani G, Chen SA, Dagres N, Glotzer TV, et al; ESC Scientific Document Group. Device-detected subclinical atrial tachyarrhythmias: definition, implications and management - an European Heart Rhythm Association (EHRA) consensus document, endorsed by Heart Rhythm Society (HRS), Asia Pacific Heart Rhythm. Society (APHRS) and Sociedad Latinoamericana de Estimulación Cardíaca y Electrofisiología (SOLEACE). Europace. 2017;19:1556-78.

Syncope

CHAPTER 51

Syncope: General Approach

INTRODUCTION

Transient loss of consciousness is defined by the triad of amnesia for the period of unconsciousness, loss of motor control, and unresponsiveness. Syncope is defined as transient loss of consciousness due to cerebral hypoperfusion, characterized by the triad of rapid onset, short duration, and spontaneous complete recovery. Presyncope is defined as prodrome simulating syncope without loss of consciousness. Age wise, the first presentation of syncope has a bimodal presentation between 10 and 30 years of age and above 65 years of age.

There are several etiologies with different mechanisms for syncope. Cessation of cerebral perfusion due to hypotension is the final common pathway for syncope. A cessation for 6–8 seconds can lead to syncope. Systolic pressure of 50–60 mm Hg at the level of heart or 30–40 mm Hg at the level of head leading to cessation of cerebral perfusion even for 6–8 seconds can cause syncope.

A detailed history and clinical examination can differentiate syncope from other causes of transient loss of consciousness in 60% of the cases.[1] History taking is the most important part in diagnosing the etiology for syncope. Eyewitness account is very important. Reflex syncope is the most common cause of syncope in all ages followed by cardiac syncope.

Carotid sinus massage test is recommended in a patient above 40 years of age. Ventricular pause for more than 3 seconds and/or fall of systolic blood pressure of more than 50 mm Hg is defined as carotid sinus hypersensitivity. To define carotid sinus syndrome, there must be syncope during carotid sinus massage associated with ventricular pause, which is usually more than 3 seconds or asymptomatic pause more than 6 seconds. This response is cardioinhibitory response. Only the fall of systolic pressure > 50 mm Hg is vasodepressor response. The complication of carotid sinus massage is stroke or transient ischemic attack (TIA) in 0.24% of cases.[2]

Head-up tilt test (HUTT) is more specific and sensitive for patients presenting with features of vasovagal syncope. However, for other etiologies, the diagnostic role of HUTT is uncertain. In case of unexplained syncope, HUTT is positive only in 30–36% of cases and in 51–60% of cases with history suggestive of reflex syncope.[3] Interestingly, HUTT may be positive even in 45–47% of arrhythmic syncope. HUTT is now taken as a diagnostic tool to detect hypotensive response, which is the mechanism of syncope in reflex syncope, and which may also play a role in cardiac syncope.

Noncardiac syncope with cardioinhibition in the form of asystolic pause >3 seconds or asymptomatic pause >6 seconds during carotid sinus massage or HUTT is an indication of cardiac pacing.

Orthostatic hypotension is defined as the progressive and sustained fall of systolic blood pressure >20 mm Hg, diastolic pressure >10 mm Hg, or systolic pressure falling below 90 mm Hg on active standing from supine posture.

Arrhythmia detected during Holter monitoring without syncope may be found in 15% of cases, which may exclude arrhythmia as a cause of syncope.[4] External loop recorder has a higher yield, nearing 25%. Smartphone used as event recorder is an emerging diagnostic tool with limited applications. Implantable loop recorder (ILR) has a high yield. In unexplained syncope, ILR increases the diagnostic probability three times as compared to conventional diagnostic strategy.[5] Ventricular pause >3 seconds or any supraventricular tachycardia >160 beats/min for more than 32 beats or ventricular tachycardia without symptom has been taken as diagnostic criteria for arrhythmic syncope.[6] Electrophysiology study (EPS) is not very frequently done for evaluation of syncope. Not more than 3% of cases with syncope undergo EPS when syncope is evaluated by a cardiologist.[7] EPS plays an important role in syncope associated with asymptomatic sinus bradycardia, bifascicular block, and suspected tachycardia. In gross sinus bradycardia (heart rate <50 beats/min) or ECG documentation of sinoatrial block, EPS is done to look at sinus node recovery time (SNRT). A corrected SNRT >525 ms or SNRT >1.6 seconds is taken as abnormal response.[8]

Serum level of adenosine has some implication in deciding the etiology of syncope. A low serum level is associated with carotid sinus syncope or atrioventricular (AV) block, whereas a high level is associated with vasovagal syncope. Adenosine challenge test can be done by rapid injection of 20 mg adenosine. Development of complete heart block with asystole >6 seconds in a patient with syncope of unknown origin may add in the decision of cardiac pacing.[9]

Risk stratification is an important task. All the available risk scores have variable fallacies.

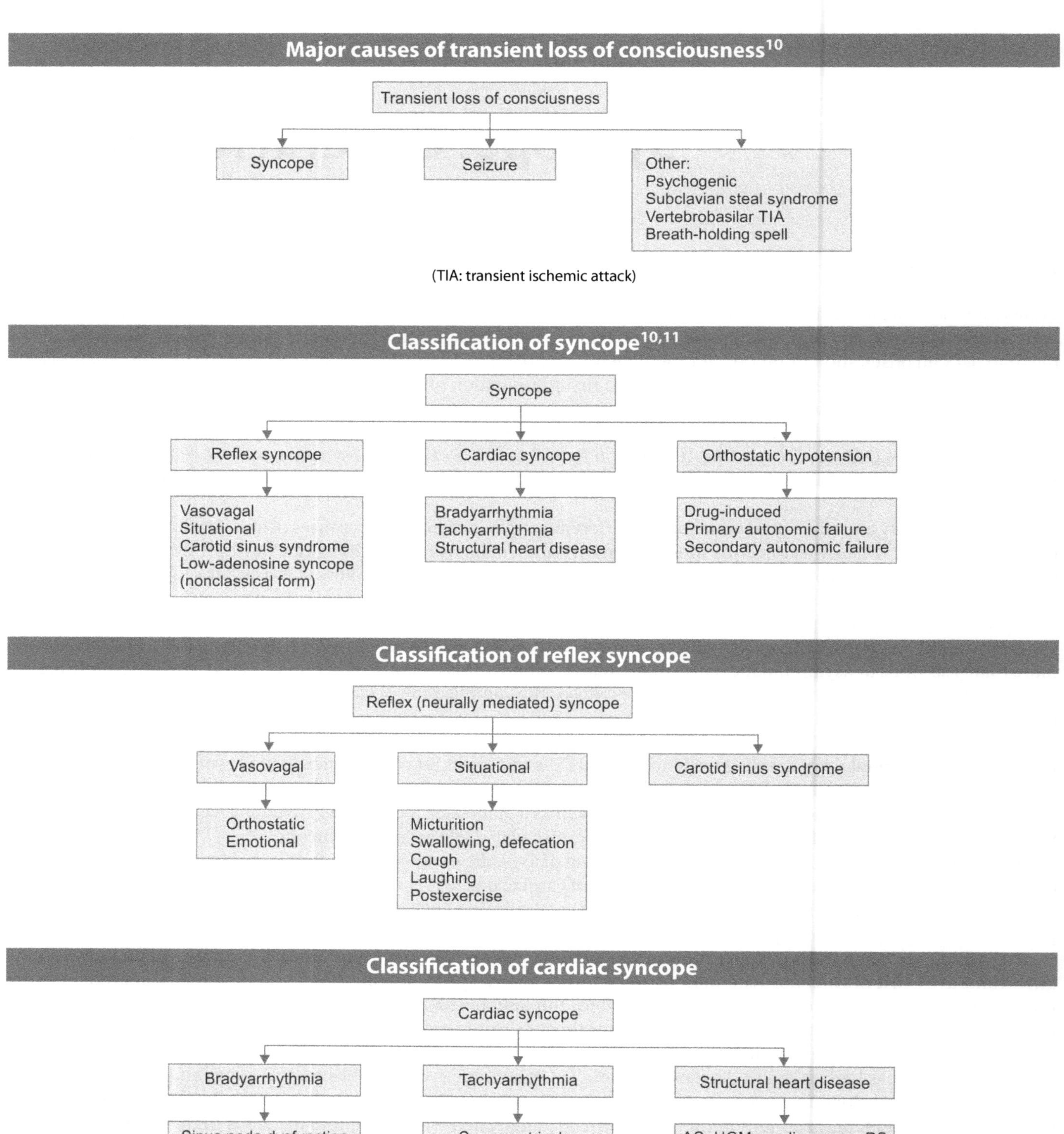

(AS: aortic stenosis; AV: atrioventricular; HCM: hypertrophic cardiomyopathy; PH: pulmonary hypertension; PS: pulmonary stenosis)

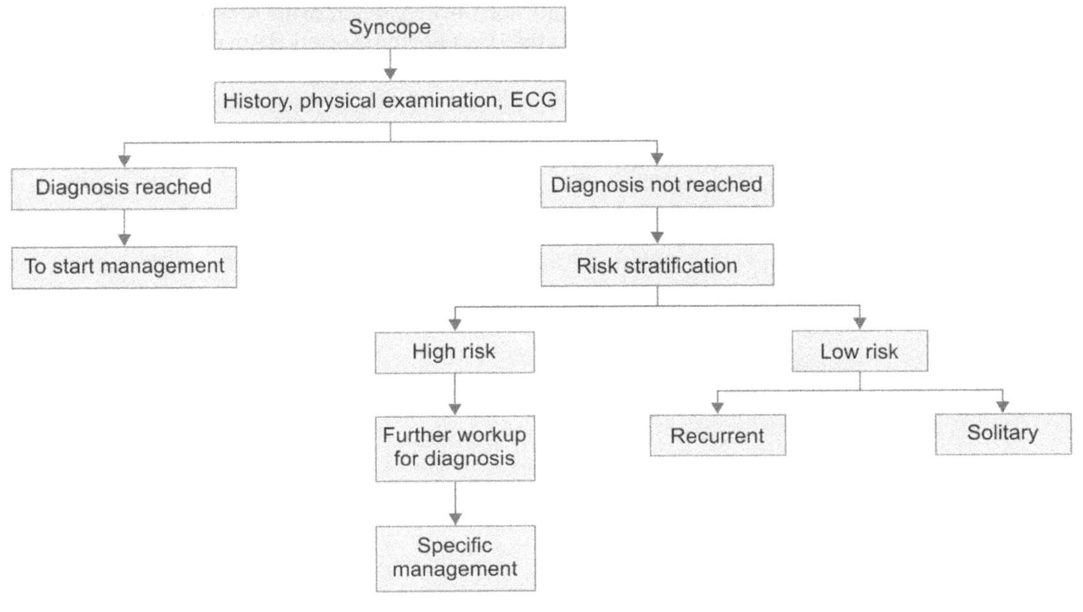

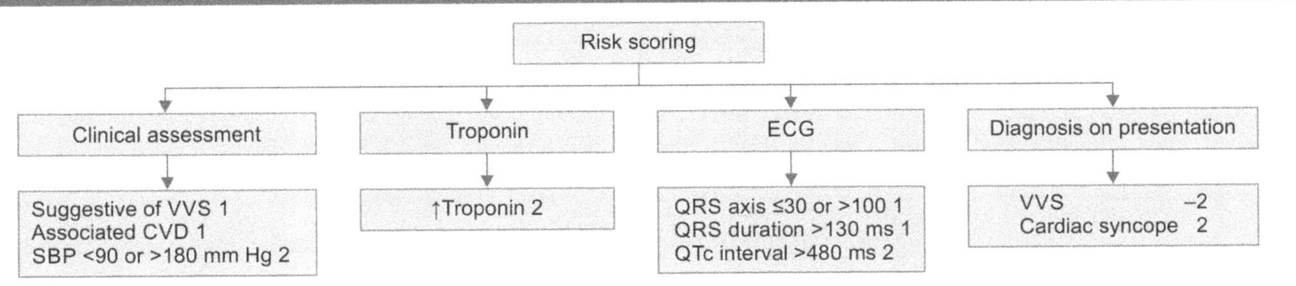

Note: Very low risk: −3 to −2; low risk: −1 to 0; medium risk: 1–3; high risk: 4–5; very high risk: ≥6.

(CVD: cardiovascular disease; ECG: electrocardiogram; SBP: systolic blood pressure; VVS: vasovagal syncope)

REFERENCES

1. van Dijk N, Boer KR, Colman N, Bakker A, Stam J, van Grieken JJ, et al. High diagnostic yield and accuracy of history, physical examination, and ECG in patients with transient loss of consciousness in FAST: the Fainting Assessment study. J Cardiovasc Electrophysiol. 2008;19:48-55.
2. Davies AJ, Kenny RA. Frequency of neurologic complications following carotid sinus massage. Am J Cardiol. 1998;81(10):1256-7.

3. Flevari P, Leftheriotis D, Komborozos C, Fountoulaki K, Dagres N, Theodorakis, G, et al. Recurrent vasovagal syncope: comparison between clomipramine and nitroglycerin as drug challenges during head-up tilt testing. Eur Heart J. 2009;30(18):2249-53.

4. Bass EB, Curtiss EI, Arena VC, Hanusa BH, Cecchetti A, Karpf M, et al. The duration of Holter monitoring in patients with syncope. Is 24 hours enough? Arch Intern Med. 1990;150:1073-8.

5. Farwell DJ, Freemantle N, Sulke N. The clinical impact of implantable loop recorders in patients with syncope. Eur Heart J. 2006;27(3):351-6.

6. Krahn AD, Klein GJ, Yee R, Skanes AC. Detection of asymptomatic arrhythmias in unexplained syncope. Am Heart J. 2004;148:326-32.

7. Brignole M, Menozzi C, Bartoletti A, Giada F, Lagi A, Ungar A, et al. A new management of syncope: prospective systematic guideline-based evaluation of patients referred urgently to general hospitals. Eur Heart J. 2006;27(1):76-82.

8. Dhingra RC. Sinus node dysfunction. Pacing Clin Electrophysiol. 1983;6:1062-9.

9. Deharo JC, Guieu R, Mechulan A, Peyrouse E, Kipson N, Ruf J, et al. Syncope without prodromes in patients with normal heart and normal electrocardiogram: a distinct entity. J Am Coll Cardiol. 2013;62:1075-80.

10. Brignole M, Moya A, de Lange FJ, Deharo JC, Elliot PM, Fanciulli A, et al. 2018 ESC Guidelines for the diagnosis and management of syncope. Eur Heart J. 2018;39:1883-1948.

11. Kusumoto FM, Schoenfeld MH, Barrett C, Edgerton JR, Ellenbogen KA, Gold MR, et al. 2018 ACC/AHA/HRS Guideline on the Evaluation and Management of Patients With Bradycardia and Cardiac Conduction Delay: A Report of the American College of Cardiology/American Heart Association Task Force on Clinical Practice Guidelines and the Heart Rhythm Society. J Am Coll Cardiol. 2019;74:e51-e156.

12. Sutton R, Ricci F, Fedorowski A. Risk stratification of syncope: Current syncope guidelines and beyond. Autonomic neurosci. 2021;238:102929.

CHAPTER 52

Syncope: Management

INTRODUCTION

After a thorough medical examination, recurrence of syncope reduces even without specific management. Recurrence is less than 50% in 1–2 years and in case of recurrence, the syncopal burden is reduced more than 70% as compared to before evaluation is done.[1] Syncope severity is determined by the etiology of syncope. The term "severe syncope" is used when syncope is associated with major morbidity and significant mortality. The severity depends on the severity of underlying disease, rather than the syncope itself. Cardiac syncope is a "severe syncope." Syncope as such causes 1.3 times increased risk of death. Syncope associated with structural heart disease has the highest probability of sudden cardiac death.

Recurrence of syncope is 3% at 1 month and 22% at 2-year follow-up.[2]

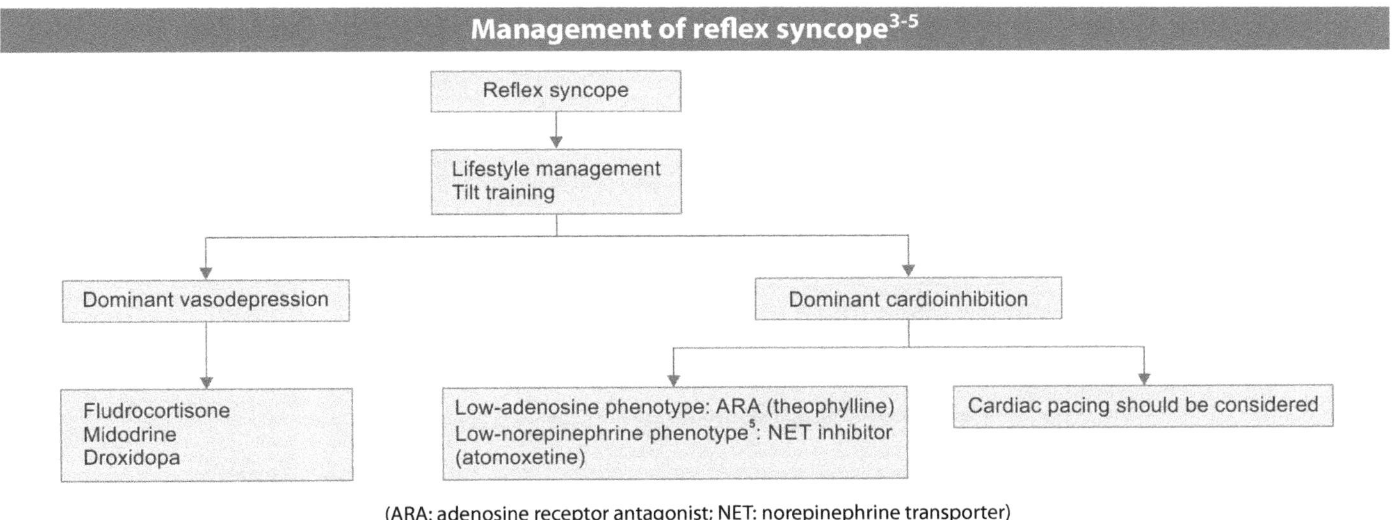

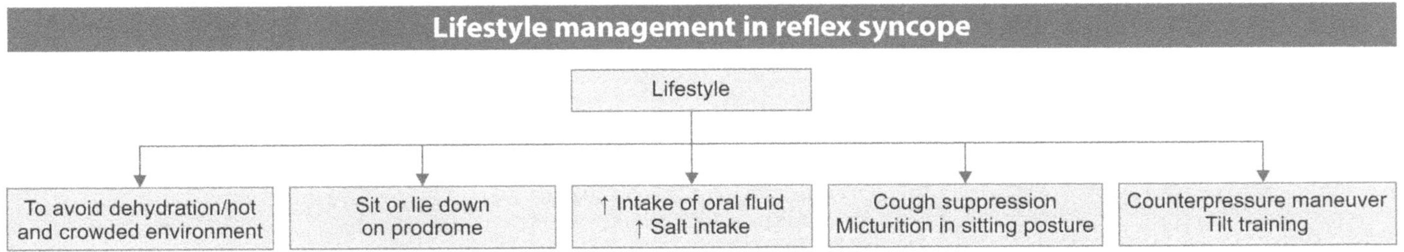

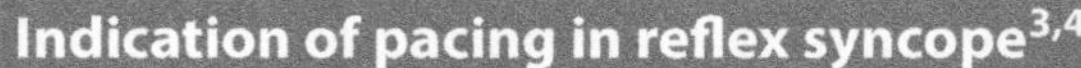

Indication of pacing in reflex syncope[3,4]

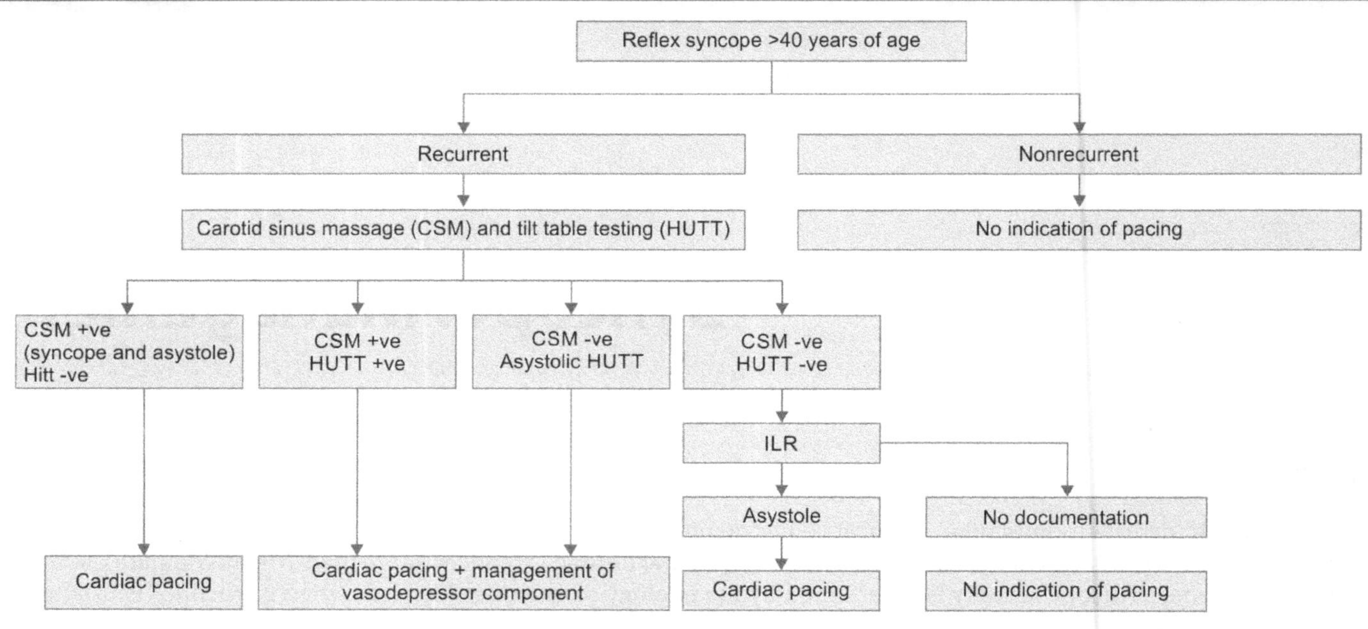

(HUTT: head-up tilt test; ILR: implantable loop recorder)

Management of low-adenosine (nonclassical form) syncope/idiopathic paroxysmal AV block[3,6]

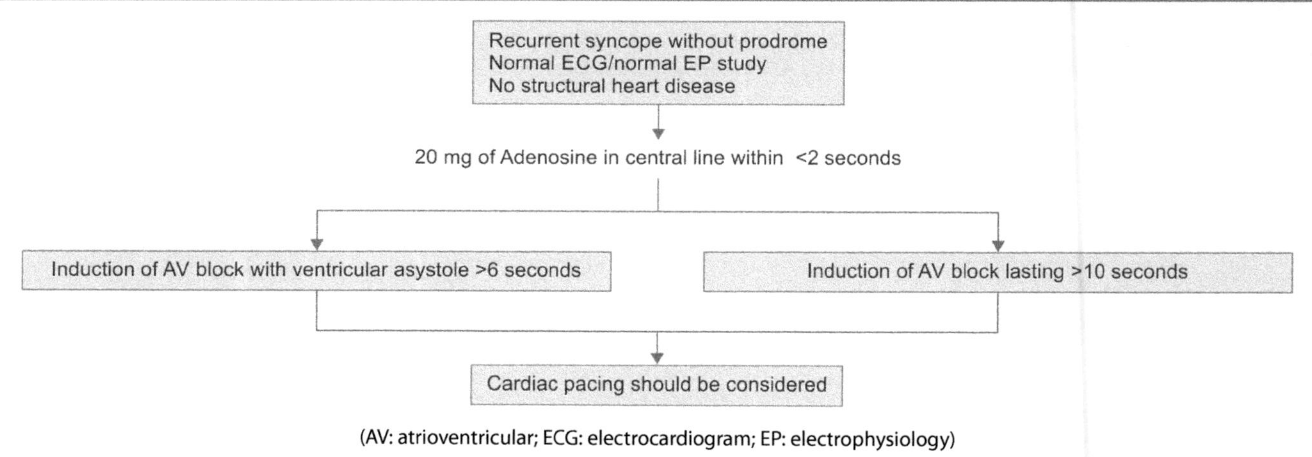

(AV: atrioventricular; ECG: electrocardiogram; EP: electrophysiology)

Outline of management of arrhythmic syncope[3,4]

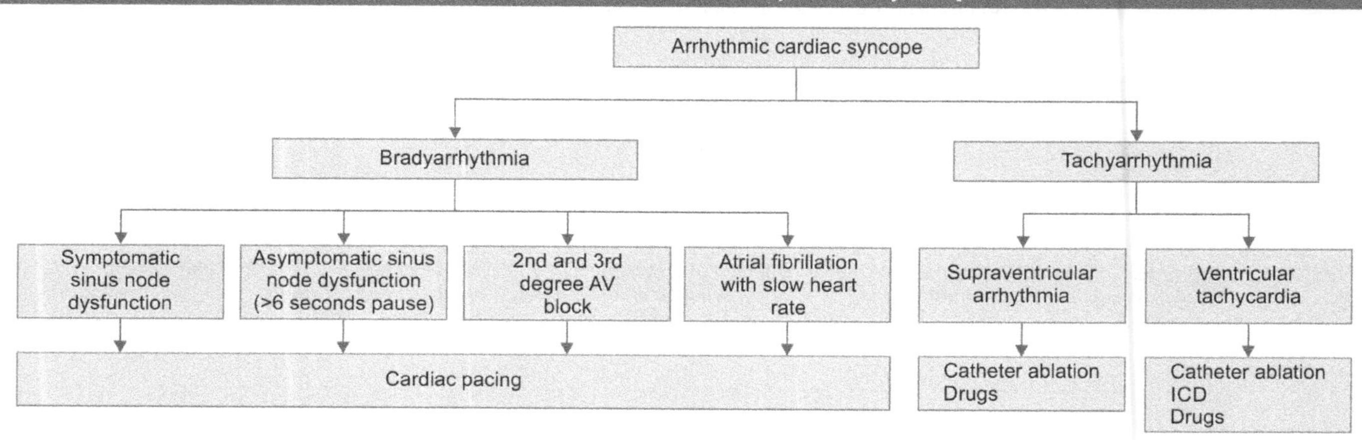

(AV: atrioventricular; ICD: implantable cardioverter defibrillator)

Management of syncope in sick sinus syndrome[7]

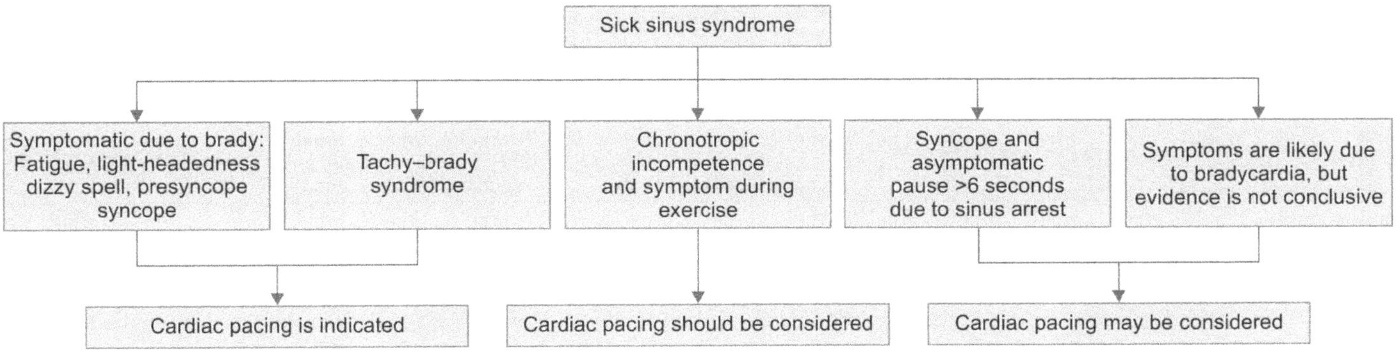

Sick sinus syndrome

Symptomatic due to brady: Fatigue, light-headedness dizzy spell, presyncope syncope

Tachy–brady syndrome

Chronotropic incompetence and symptom during exercise

Syncope and asymptomatic pause >6 seconds due to sinus arrest

Symptoms are likely due to bradycardia, but evidence is not conclusive

Cardiac pacing is indicated

Cardiac pacing should be considered

Cardiac pacing may be considered

Management of syncope in atrioventricular block[7]

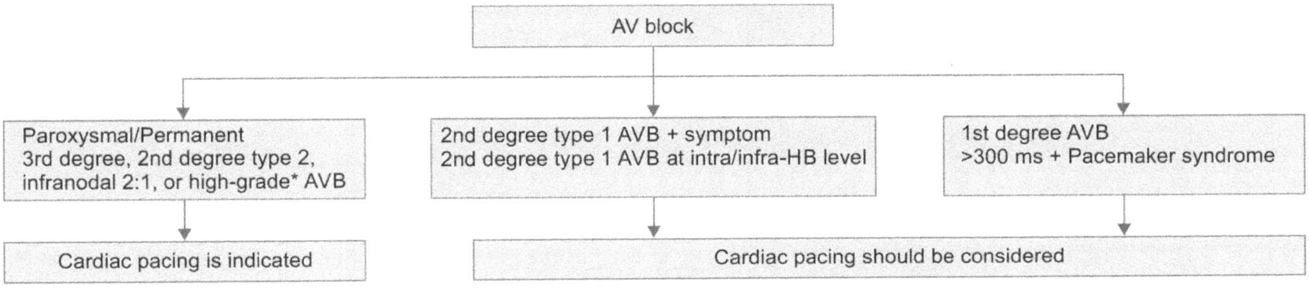

AV block

Paroxysmal/Permanent 3rd degree, 2nd degree type 2, infranodal 2:1, or high-grade* AVB

2nd degree type 1 AVB + symptom 2nd degree type 1 AVB at intra/infra-HB level

1st degree AVB >300 ms + Pacemaker syndrome

Cardiac pacing is indicated

Cardiac pacing should be considered

*High grade AV block: where P:QRS ratio is 3:1 or higher.
(AVB: atrioventricular block; HB: His bundle)

Management of syncope with bifascicular block[7]

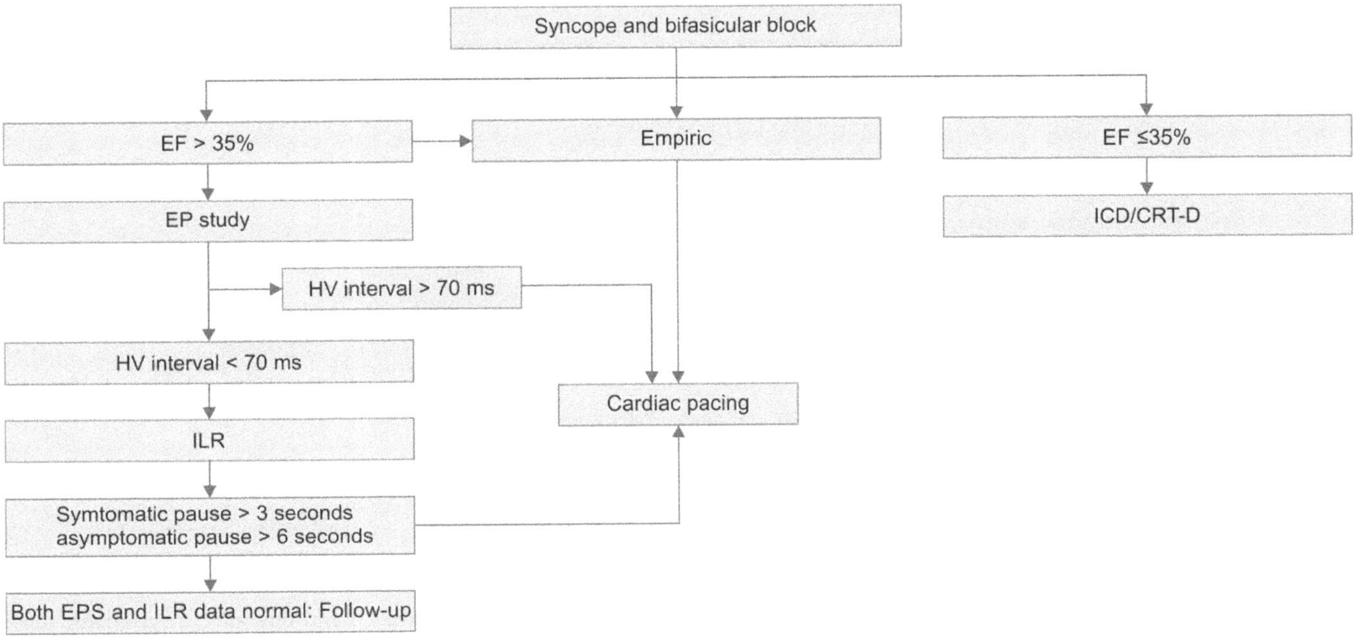

Syncope and bifasicular block

EF > 35%

Empiric

EF ≤35%

EP study

ICD/CRT-D

HV interval > 70 ms

HV interval < 70 ms

Cardiac pacing

ILR

Symtomatic pause > 3 seconds asymptomatic pause > 6 seconds

Both EPS and ILR data normal: Follow-up

(CRT-D: cardiac resynchronization therapy with defibrillator; EF: ejection fraction; EP: electrophysiologic; EPS: electrophysiology study; ICD: implantable defibrillator; ILR: implantable loop recorder)

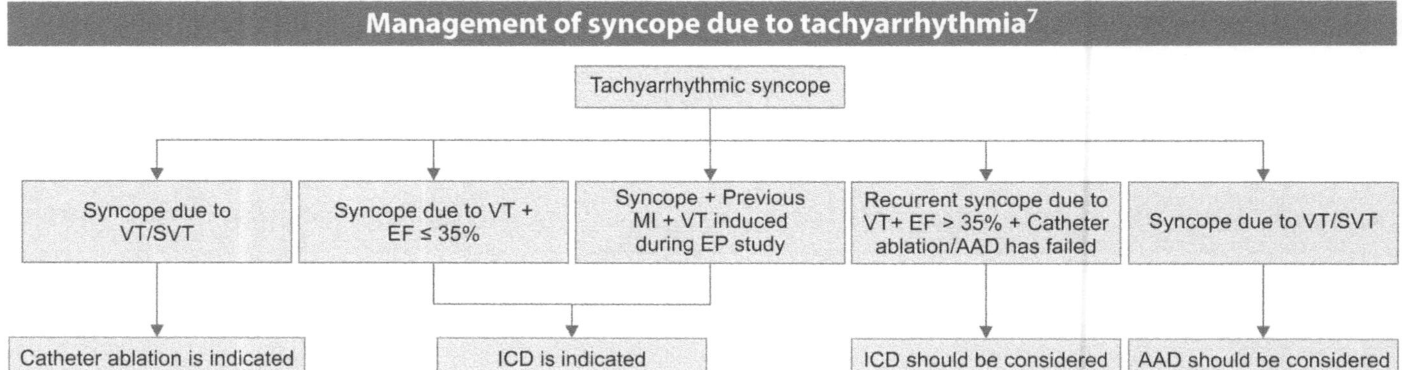

(AAD: antiarrhythmic drug; EF: ejection fraction; EP: electrophysiologic; ICD: implantable defibrillator; MI: myocardial infarction; SVT: supraventricular tachycardia; VT: ventricular tachycardia)

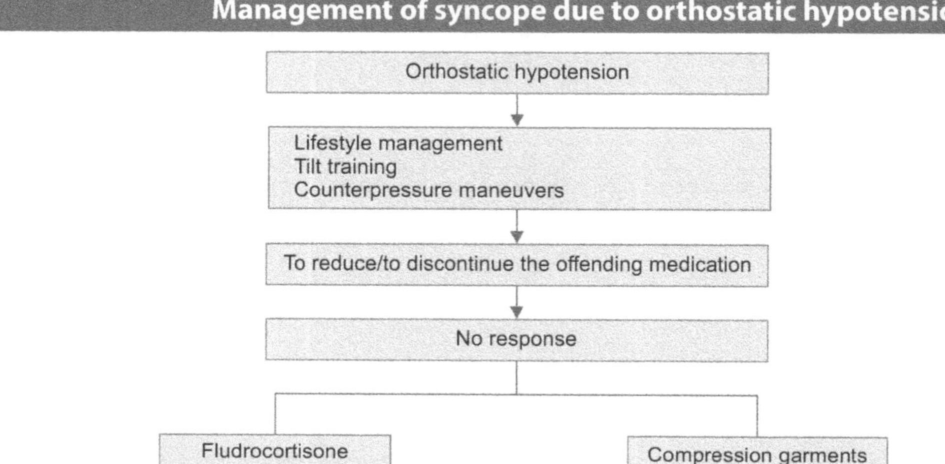

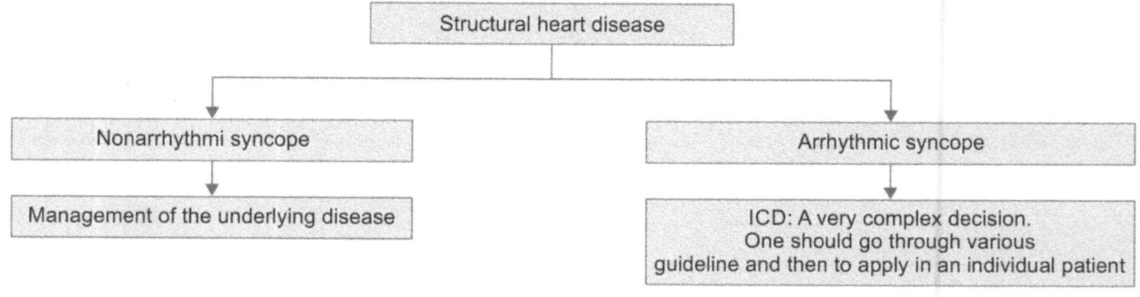

(ICD: implantable defibrillator)

REFERENCES

1. Sud S, Massel D, Klein GJ, Leong-Sit P, Yee R, Skanes AC, et al. The expectation effect and cardiac pacing for refractory vasovagal syncope. Am J Med. 2007;120:54-62.
2. Solbiati M, Casazza G, Dipaola F, Rusconi AM, Cernuschi G, Barbic F, et al. Syncope recurrence and mortality: a systematic review. Europace. 2015;17:300-8.
3. Brignole M, Moya A, de Lange FJ, Deharo JC, Elliot PM, Fanciulli A, et al. 2018 ESC Guidelines for the diagnosis and management of syncope. Eur Heart J. 2018;39:1883.

4. Kusumoto FM, Schoenfeld MH, Barrett C, Edgerton JR, Ellenbogen KA, Gold MR, et al. 2018 ACC/AHA/HRS Guideline on the Evaluation and Management of Patients With Bradycardia and Cardiac Conduction Delay: A Report of the American College of Cardiology/American Heart Association Task Force on Clinical Practice Guidelines and the Heart Rhythm Society. J Am Coll Cardiol. 2019;74:e51-e156.
5. Sheldon RS, Lei L, Guzman JC, Kus T, Ayala-Paredes FA, Angihan J, et al. A proof of principle study of atomoxetine for the prevention of vasovagal syncope: the prevention of syncope trial VI. Europace. 2019;21(11):1733-41.
6. Brignole M, Deharo JC, De Roy L, Menozzi C, Blommaert D, Dabiri L, et al. Syncope due to idiopathic paroxysmal atrioventricular block: long-term follow-up of a distinct form of atrioventricular block. J Am Coll Cardiol. 2011;58:167-73.
7. Glikson M, Nielsen JC, Konborg MB, Michowitz Y, Auricchio A, Barbash IM, et al. 2021 ESC Guidelines on cardiac pacing and cardiac resynchronization therapy. Eur Heart J. 2021;42(35):3427-520.

Primary Electrical Abnormality

CHAPTER 53

Primary Electrical Abnormality: Cardiac Channelopathy

INTRODUCTION

Ventricular arrhythmias are the major underlying rhythm, leading to sudden cardiac death (SCD). Coronary artery disease is the most common disease leading to SCD in patients over the age of 40 years, whereas primary electrical abnormality and inherited cardiomyopathy are prevailing in younger patients. Primary electrical abnormality, also known as cardiac channelopathies, may contribute up to 30% of all SCD in younger patients.[1] The common pathophysiology of this group of channelopathies is the mutations in genes encoding cardiac ion channels or their regulatory proteins. Mutations modify the cardiac action potentials and cellular calcium handling which lead to electrical instability and life-threatening ventricular arrhythmia.

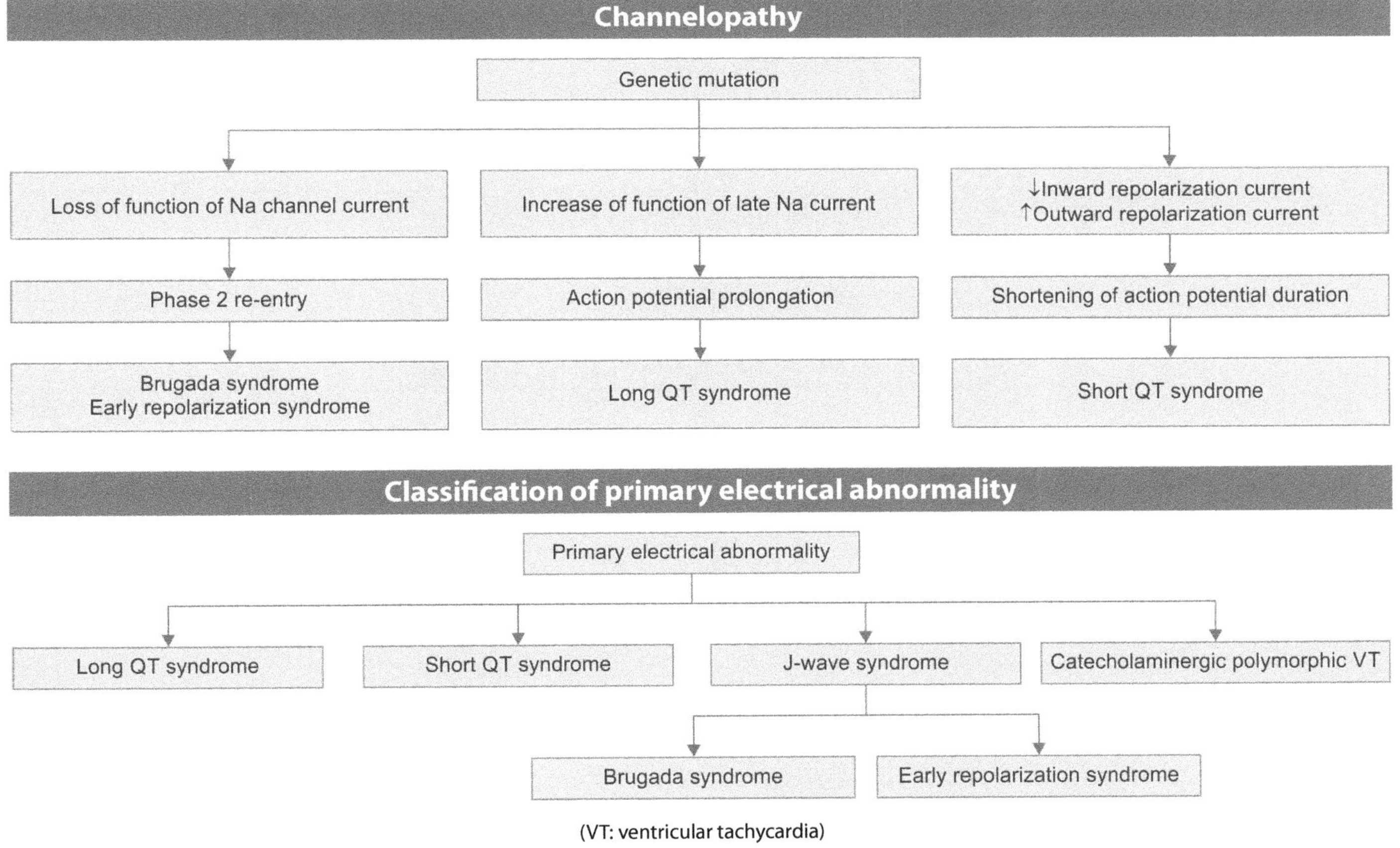

REFERENCE

1. Puranik R, Chow CK, Duflou JA, Kilborn MJ, McGuire MA. Sudden death in the young. Heart Rhythm. 2005;2:1277-82.

CHAPTER 54

Primary Electrical Abnormality: Congenital Long QT Syndrome

INTRODUCTION

Congenital long QT syndrome (LQTS) is an inherited electrical disorder with an abnormally prolonged QT interval on the electrocardiogram (ECG) in absence of structural heart disease and external precipitating factors. Initially, LQTS was described in two types, Jervell and Lange–Nielsen syndrome (associated with deafness: autosomal recessive LQTS 1) and Romano–Ward syndrome (without deafness: autosomal recessive LQTS 1). Subsequently, according to underlying genetic defects, different subtypes have been described.[1]

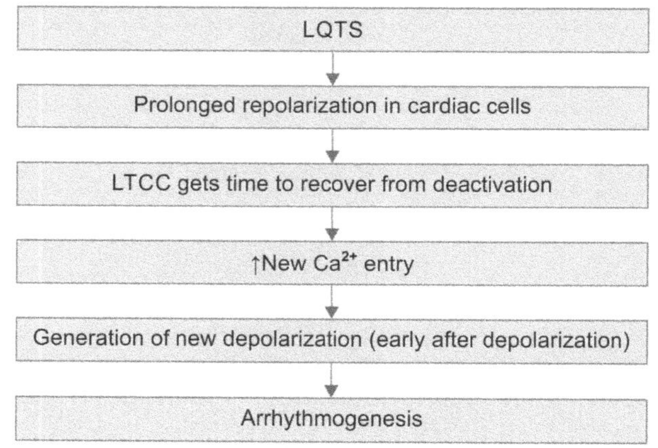

(LTTC: L-type voltage-dependent calcium channel; LQTS: long QT syndrome)

Different genetic types of congenital LQTS

LQTS

Major genes
- LQT1: *KCNQ1* (40–55%)
- LQT2: *KCNH2* (30–45%)
- LQT3: *SCN5A* (5–10%)

Syndrome
- RWS/JLNS
- RWS
- RWS

Minor genes
- LQT4: *ANKB* (<1%)
- LQT5: *KCNE1* (<1%)
- LQT6: *KCNE2* (<1%)
- LQT7: *KCNJ2* (<1%)
- LQT8: *CACNA1C* (<1%)

Syndrome
- RWS
- JLNS
- RWS
- AS
- TS

(AS: Anderson syndrome; JLNS: Jervell and Lange–Nielsen syndrome; LQTS: long QT syndrome; RWS: Romano–Ward syndrome; TS: Timothy syndrome)

T-wave in ECG and different precipitating factors in LQTS

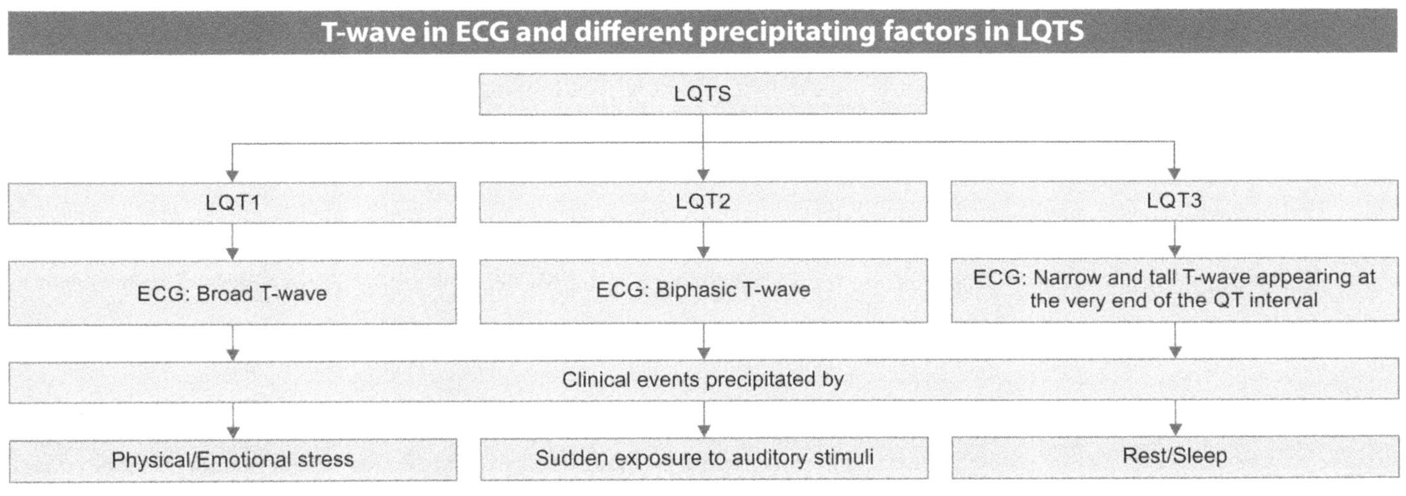

(ECG: electrocardiogram; LQTS: long QT syndrome)

Schwartz score for LQTS[2]

LQTS

ECG

QTc interval:
≥480 ms 3
460–479 ms 2
450–459 ms 1
≥480 ms during
2nd–4th minute of
recovery from exercise
testing 1

TDP 2

T-wave alternans 1

Notched T-wave in three leads 1

Resting heart rate below 2nd percentile for age 0.5

Clinical history

Syncope
With stress 2
Without stress 1
Congenital deafness 0.5

Family history

Relative with LQTS 1
Unexplained sudden cardiac death in immediate relative <30 years of age 0.5

Note: Probability of LQTS: Total score ≤1 (low); 2–3 (intermediate); ≥3.5 (high).
(ECG: electrocardiogram; LQTS: long QT syndrome; TDP: torsades de pointes)

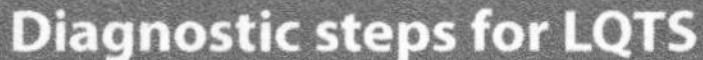

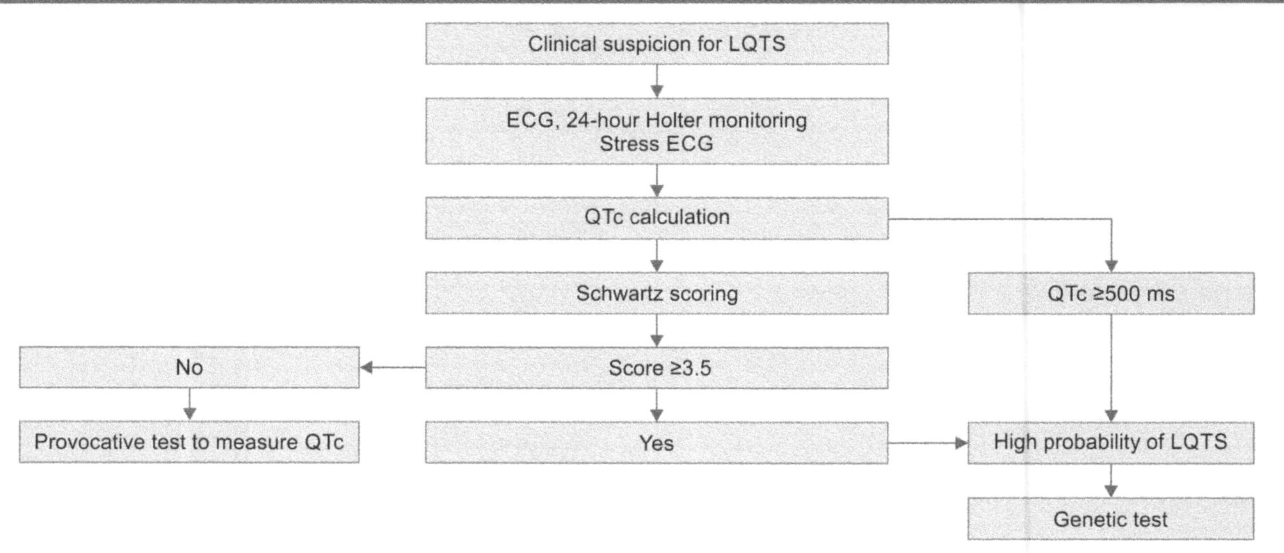

(ECG: electrocardiogram; LQTS: long QT syndrome)

Risk stratification in LQTS

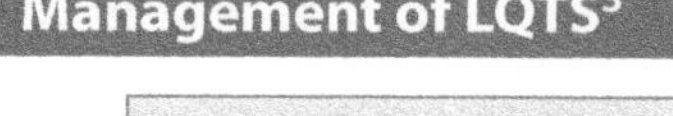

(JLNS: Jervell and Lange–Nielsen syndrome; LQTS: long QT syndrome)

Management of LQTS[3]

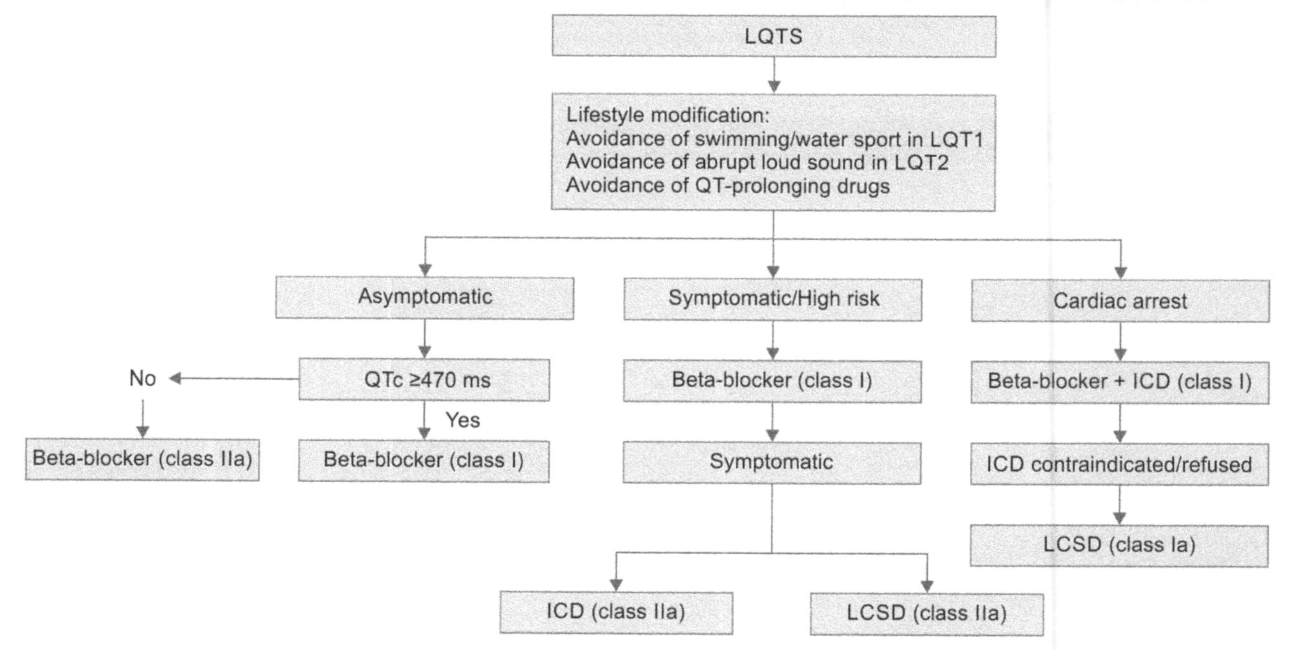

(ICD: implantable cardioverter-defibrillator; LCSD: left cardiac sympathetic denervation; LQTS: long QT syndrome)

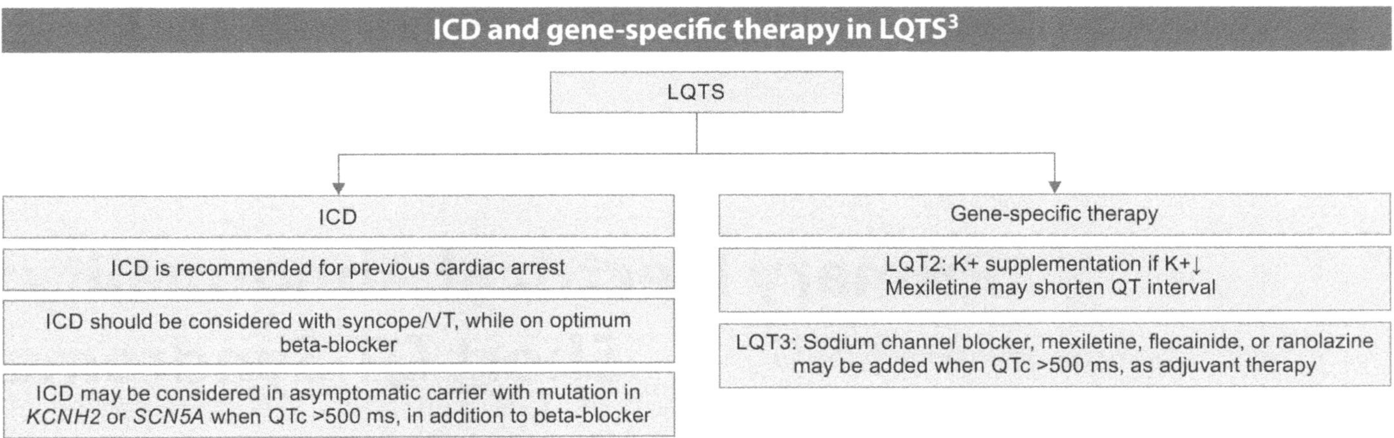

(ICD: implantable cardioverter-defibrillator; LQTS: long QT syndrome)

REFERENCES

1. Schwartz PJ, Ackerman MJ. The long QT syndrome: a transatlantic clinical approach to diagnosis and therapy. Eur Heart J. 2013;34(40): 3109-16.
2. Priori SG, Blomström-Lundqvist C, Mazzanti A, Blom N, Borggrefe M, Camm J, et al. 2015 ESC Guidelines for the management of patients with ventricular arrhythmias and the prevention of sudden cardiac Death. The Task Force for the Management of Patients with Ventricular Arrhythmias and the Prevention of Sudden Cardiac Death of the European Society of Cardiology. G Ital Cardiol (Rome). 2016;17(2):108-70.
3. Wilde AA, Amin AS, Postem PG. Diagnosis, management and therapeutic strategies for congenital long QT syndrome. Heart 2022;108: 332-8.

CHAPTER 55

Primary Electrical Abnormality: Short QT Syndrome

INTRODUCTION

Short QT syndrome (SQTS) is an inherited disorder, belonging to channelopathy characterized by short QT interval on ECG and presenting as fatal arrhythmia. Short QT interval in ECG is due to accelerated cardiac repolarization and shorter refractory period. A reduction in inward repolarization current or enhancement of outward repolarization will set in early repolarization, leading to shortening of action potential duration and thereof QT shortening. It predisposes to re-entry phenomenon and ventricular tachycardia (VT) and atrial fibrillation (AF). SQTS may remain asymptomatic in 40% of cases. Infants are vulnerable with this syndrome with 4% rate of cardiac arrest.[1] The first year of life and age period between 20 and 40 years of life are the periods when two peaks of sudden cardiac death (SCD) occur. AF is one of the most common presentations in SQTS. Thus, when a young patient presents with lone AF, vigilant assessment should be done for associated SQTS.

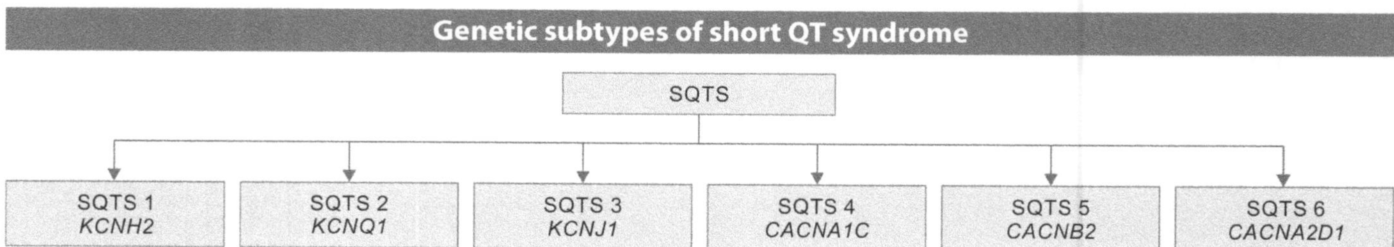

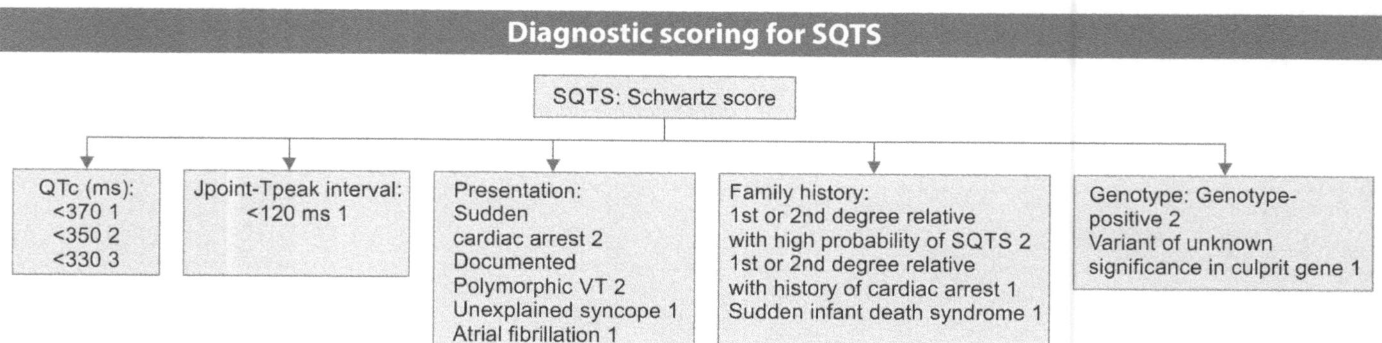

Note: Low probability of SQTS: Total score ≤2; intermediate probability: total score: 3; high probability: total score ≥4.
(SQTS: short QT syndrome; VT: ventricular tachycardia)

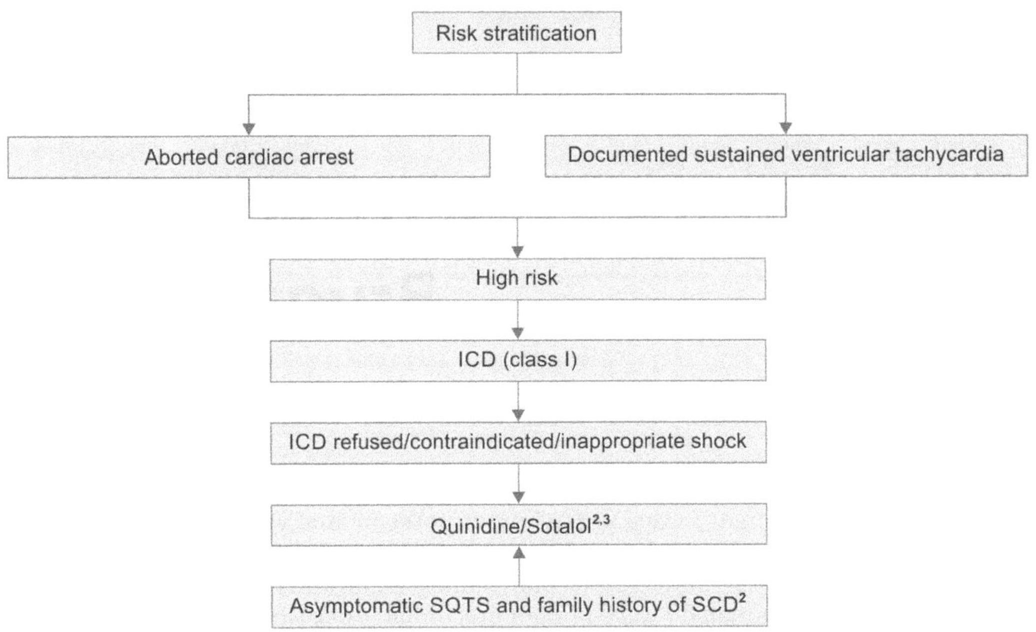

(ICD: implantable cardioverter-defibrillator; SCD: sudden cardiac death; SQTS: short QT syndrome)

REFERENCES

1. Mazzanti A, Kanthan A, Monteforte N, Memmi M, Bloise R, Novelli V, et al. Novel insight into the natural history of short QT syndrome. J Am Coll Cardiol. 2014;63:1300-8.
2. Priori SG, Blomström-Lundqvist C, Mazzanti A, Blom N, Borggrefe M, Camm J, et al. 2015 ESC Guidelines for the management of patients with ventricular arrhythmias and the prevention of sudden cardiac Death. The Task Force for the Management of Patients with Ventricular Arrhythmias and the Prevention of Sudden Cardiac Death of the European Society of Cardiology. G Ital Cardiol (Rome). 2016;17(2):108-70.
3. Giustetto C, Schimpf R, Mazzanti A, Scrocco C, Maury P, Anttonen O, et al. Long-term follow- up of patients with short QT syndrome. J Am Coll Cardiol. 2011;58:587-95.

CHAPTER 56

Primary Electrical Abnormality: Brugada Syndrome

J-WAVE SYNDROME

Association of accentuated and prominent J wave in ECG predisposes to fatal ventricular arrhythmia and is known as J-wave syndrome, which includes Brugada syndrome (BrS) and early repolarization syndrome (ERS). J wave has been described in three segments, the start, peak, and terminal part, namely Jo, Jp, and Jt.[1] The anterior right ventricular outflow tract is involved in BrS, leading to accentuated J wave in right precordial leads, whereas ERS affects the inferior surface of the left ventricle, expressed in the lateral or inferolateral leads.

BRUGADA SYNDROME

Brugada syndrome is a channelopathy/arrhythmogenic cardiomyopathy characterized by typical ECG change in right precordial leads and a predisposition to ventricular arrhythmia and sudden cardiac death (SCD). There is an imbalance between outward and inward current in early phase 1 of repolarization, leading to phase-2 re-entry and ventricular reentrant arrhythmia. Prevalence of BrS ranges from 1 in 5,000 to 1 in 2,000. BrS is responsible for 4–12% of all SCD. It is 10 times more prevalent in men than women. Testosterone has been ascribed for this significant male dominance. Typical symptoms are syncope, seizure, or nocturnal agonal breathing, occurring typically during rest or sleep, induced by vagal dominance or bradycardia. Symptoms have also been described during febrile illness. Atrial fibrillation (AF) may occur in 30% of cases. Genetically, BrS is an autosomal dominant disorder, tmajority located at *SCN5A*. BrS has been included in the entity of arrhythmogenic cardiomyopathy,[2] because of microanatomical changes that have been detected in endomyocardial biopsy in patients with BrS. The changes include increased collagen, fibrosis, and reduced gap junction expression, suggestive of pan-myocardial inflammation, which may be responsible for arrhythmic susceptibility.

Different types of Brugada syndrome[3,4]

BrS

- **Type 1 "Coved"**
  - J-point amplitude or ST-segment elevation ≥2 mm in ≥1 of leads V_1–V_3, followed by an R wave and a concave or straight ST segment which crosses the baseline, followed by negative and symmetric T-wave

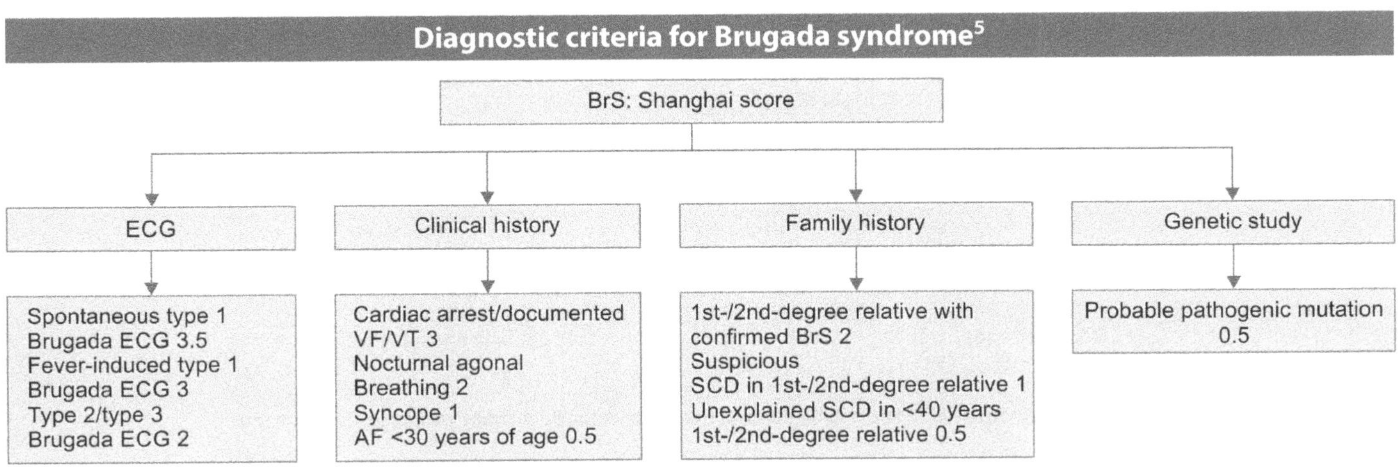

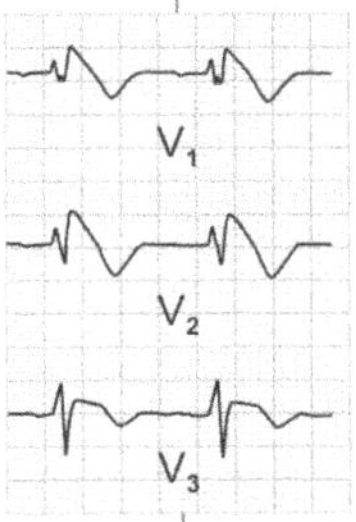

- **Type 2 Saddle-back**
  - J-point elevation ≥2 mm in ≥1 of leads V_1–V_3, followed by a slow downward convex ST segment slope which remains ≥1 mm elevated above the baseline, followed by positive or biphasic T-wave in V_2 and variable morphology in V_1

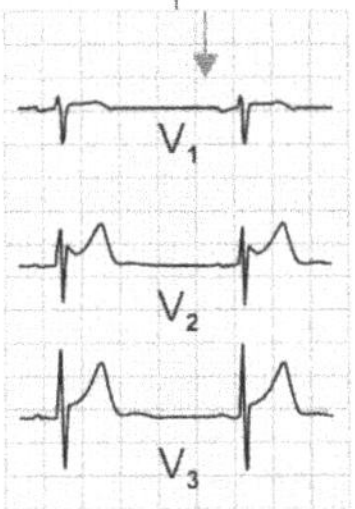

- **Type 3**
  - Saddleback or coved appearance with ST-segment elevation <1 mm

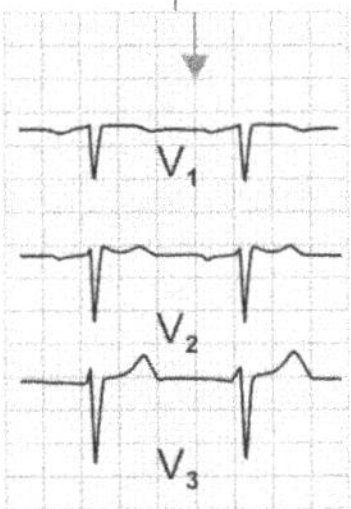

Drugs used to unmask Brugada ECG

- Ajmaline
- Flecainide
- Procainamide
- Pilsicainide

(BrS: Brugada syndrome; ECG: electrocardiogram)

Diagnostic criteria for Brugada syndrome[5]

BrS: Shanghai score

- **ECG**
  - Spontaneous type 1 Brugada ECG 3.5
  - Fever-induced type 1 Brugada ECG 3
  - Type 2/type 3 Brugada ECG 2
- **Clinical history**
  - Cardiac arrest/documented VF/VT 3
  - Nocturnal agonal Breathing 2
  - Syncope 1
  - AF <30 years of age 0.5
- **Family history**
  - 1st-/2nd-degree relative with confirmed BrS 2
  - Suspicious SCD in 1st-/2nd-degree relative 1
  - Unexplained SCD in <40 years 1st-/2nd-degree relative 0.5
- **Genetic study**
  - Probable pathogenic mutation 0.5

Note: ≥3.5 points: Probable/definite BrS; 2–3 points: possible BrS; <2 points: non-diagnostic.

(AF: atrial fibrillation; BrS: Brugada syndrome; ECG: electrocardiogram; SCD: sudden cardiac death; VF: ventricular fibrillation; VT: ventricular tachycardia)

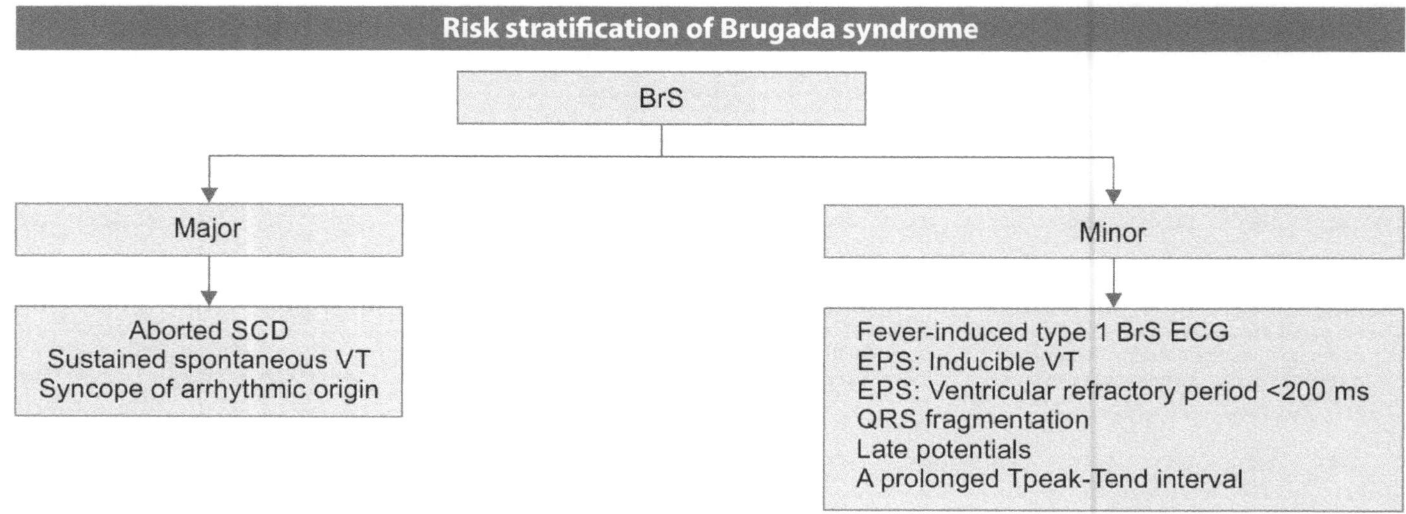

(BrS: Brugada syndrome; ECG: electrocardiogram; EPS: electrophysiologic study; SCD: sudden cardiac death; VT: ventricular tachycardia)

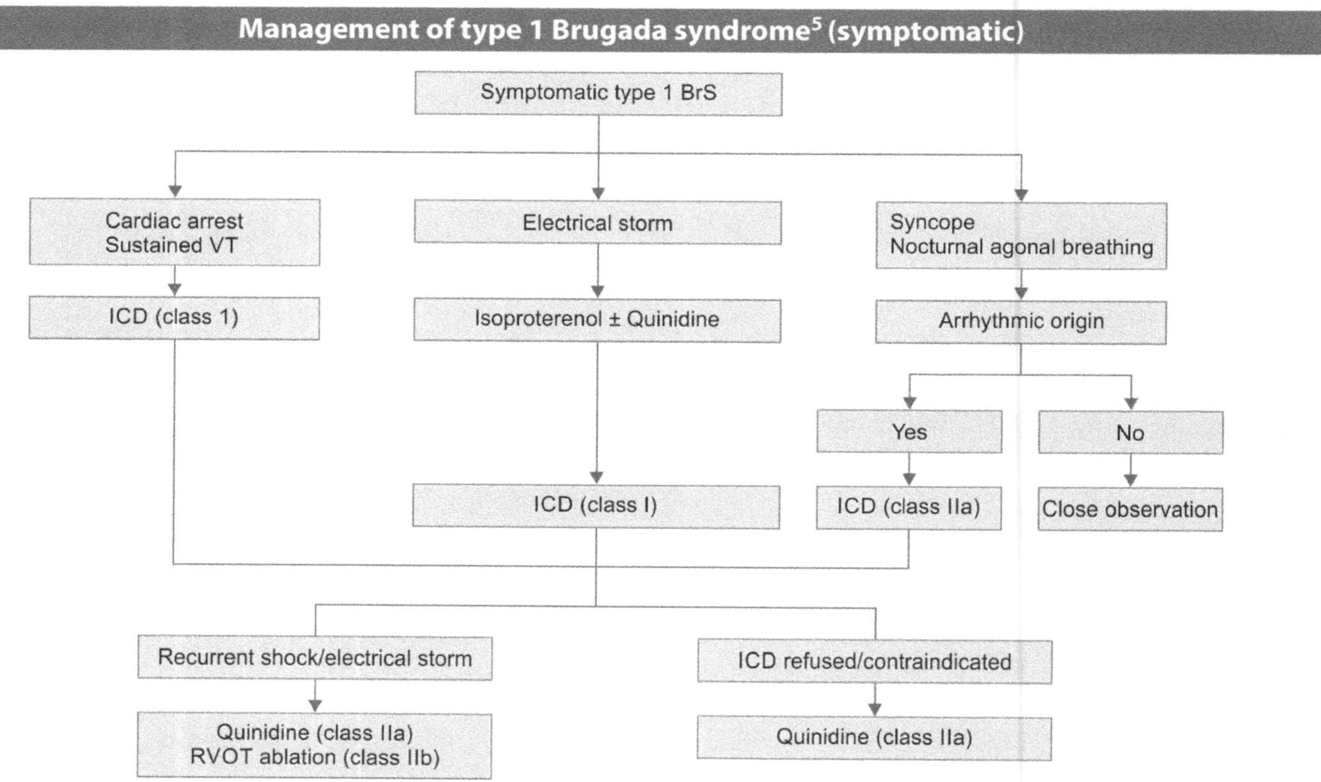

(BrS: Brugada syndrome; ICD: implantable cardioverter-defibrillator; RVOT: right ventricular outflow tract)

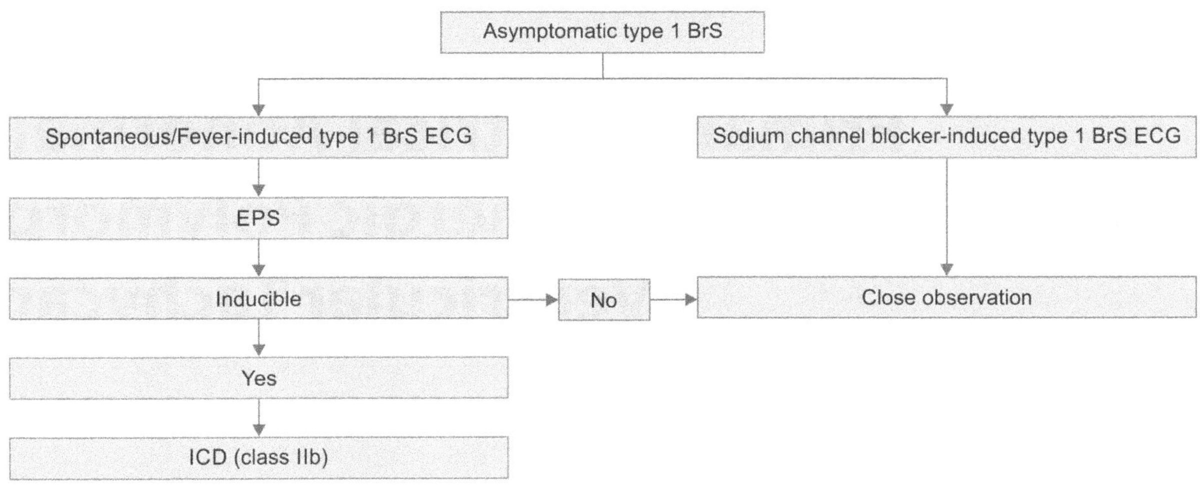

(BrS: Brugada syndrome; ECG: electrocardiogram; EPS: electrophysiological study)

REFERENCES

1. Macfarlane P, Antzelevitch C, Haissaguerre M, Huikuri HV, Potse M, Rosso R, et al. The early repolarization pattern: consensus paper. J Am Coll Cardiol. 2015;66:470-7.
2. Towbin JA, McKenna WJ, Abrams DJ, Ackerman MJ, Calkins H, Darrieux FCC, et al. 2019 HRS expert consensus statement on evaluation, risk stratification, and management of arrhythmogenic cardiomyopathy. Heart Rhythm. 2019;16:e373-e407.
3. Brugada J. Management of patients with a Brugada ECG pattern. E-journal of cardiology practice 2009;7:1-15.
4. Brugada J, Campuzano O, Arbelo E, Sarquella-Brugada G, Brugada R, et al. Present status of Brugada syndrome. J Am Coll Cardiol. 2018;72:1046-59.
5. Antzelevitch C, Yan G-X, Ackerman MJ, Borggrefe M, Corrado D, Guo J, et al. J-wave syndromes expert consensus conference report: emerging concepts and gaps in knowledge. Europace. 2017;19:665-94.

CHAPTER 57

Primary Electrical Abnormality: Catecholaminergic Polymorphic Ventricular Tachycardia

INTRODUCTION

Catecholaminergic polymorphic ventricular tachycardia (CPVT) is a channelopathy, characterized by bidirectional and polymorphic ventricular tachycardia (VT), commonly presenting in the first to second decade of life. It is an uncommon primary electrical abnormality with a prevalence estimated to be 1:10,000 in Europe. The mortality of CPVT is very high, amounting as high as 31% by the age of 30 years.[1] The disease is inherited as an autosomal dominant form. The mutation occurs in the gene *CPVT1* modulating the cardiac ryanodine receptor 2 (*RYR2*), which are calcium release channels present in the sarcoplasmic reticulum. There is also an autosomal recessive form of inheritance due to mutation in *CPVT2* gene. Syncope is associated with seizure, precipitated by physical or emotional stress. Family history of syncope or sudden cardiac death (SCD) induced by physical stress is found in 30% of the patients. Beta-blocker without intrinsic sympathetic activity is the anchoring medicine in management. Nadolol is the preferred agent.

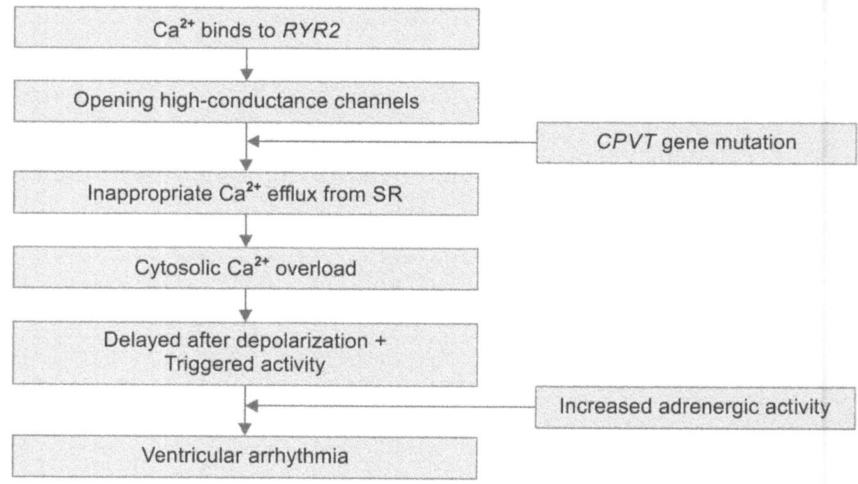

(CPVT: catecholaminergic polymorphic ventricular tachycardia; RYR2: ryanodine receptor 2)

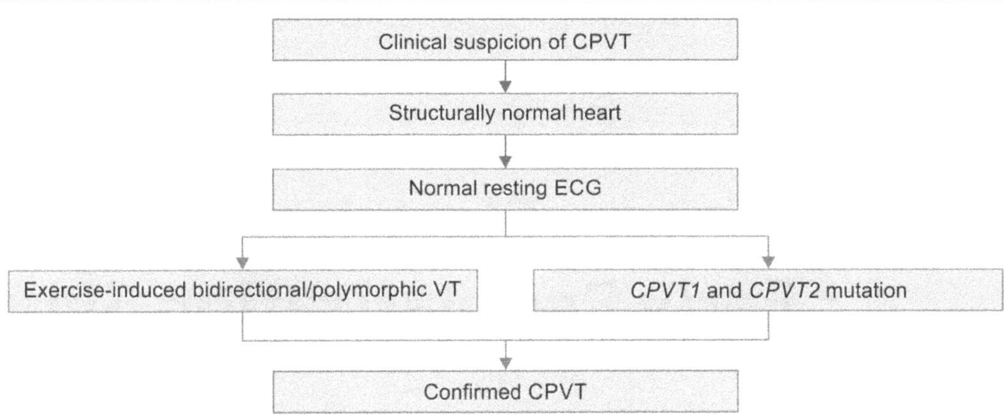

(CPVT: catecholaminergic polymorphic ventricular tachycardia; ECG: electrocardiogram; VT: ventricular tachycardia)

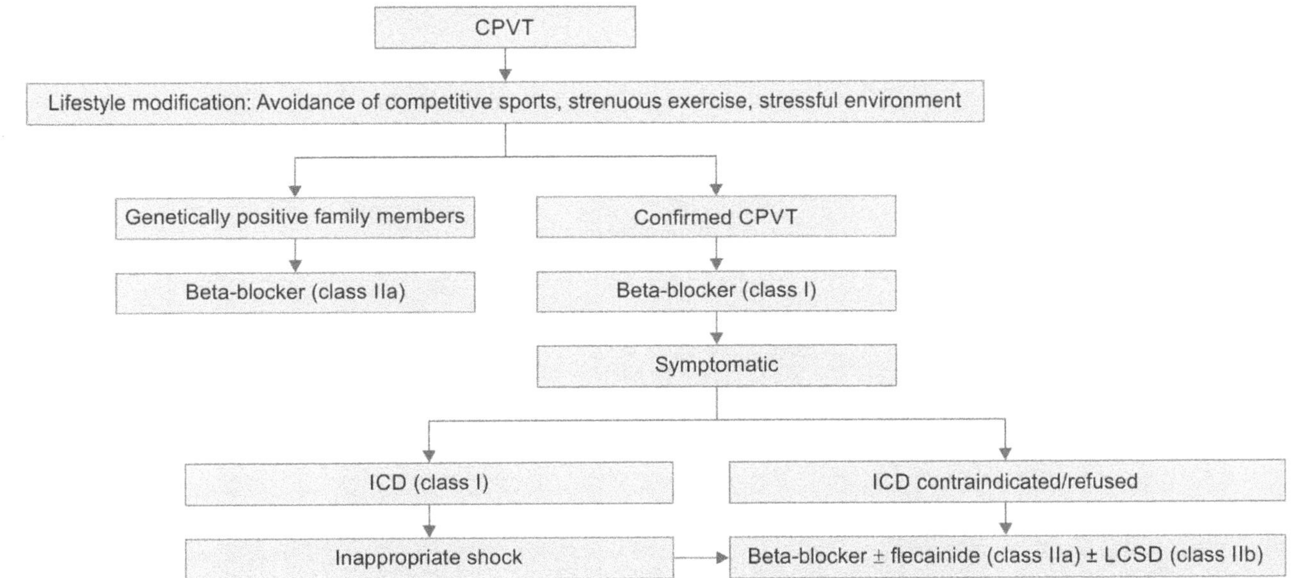

(CPVT: catecholaminergic polymorphic ventricular tachycardia; ICD: implantable cardioverter-defibrillator; LCSD: left cardiac sympathetic denervation)

REFERENCES

1. Reid DS, Tynan M, Braidwood L, Fitzgerald GR. Bidirectional tachycardia in a child. A study using His bundle electrography. Br Heart J. 1975;37:339-44.
2. Priori SG, Blomström-Lundqvist C, Mazzanti A, Blom N, Borggrefe M, Camm J, et al. 2015 ESC Guidelines for the management of patients with ventricular arrhythmias and the prevention of sudden cardiac death: The Task Force for the Management of Patients with Ventricular Arrhythmias and the Prevention of Sudden Cardiac Death of the European Society of Cardiology (ESC). Endorsed by: Association for European Paediatric and Congenital Cardiology (AEPC). Eur Heart J. 2015;36:2793-867.

CHAPTER 58

Primary Electrical Abnormality: Early Repolarization Syndrome

INTRODUCTION

Early repolarization syndrome (ERS) is characterized by feature of early repolarization (ER) in inferior and/or lateral leads in electrocardiogram (ECG) and a predisposition for malignant ventricular arrhythmia and sudden cardiac death (SCD). ER is commonly found in healthy individuals, more commonly in blacks and athletes. Certain situations, like hypothermia and ischemia, also induce ER.

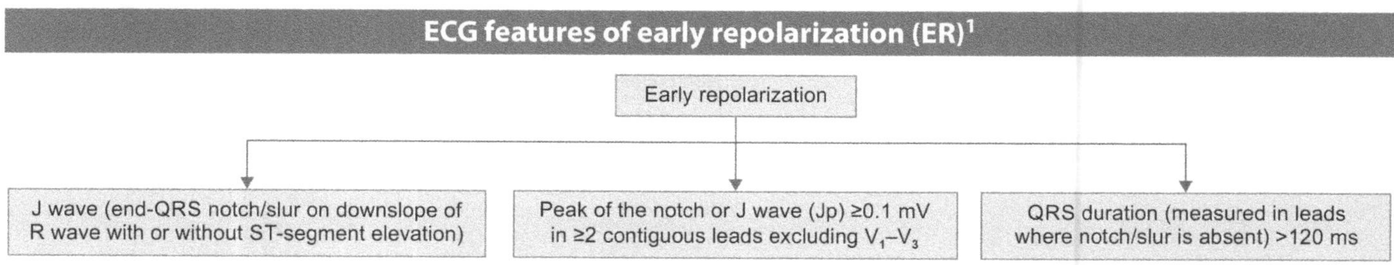

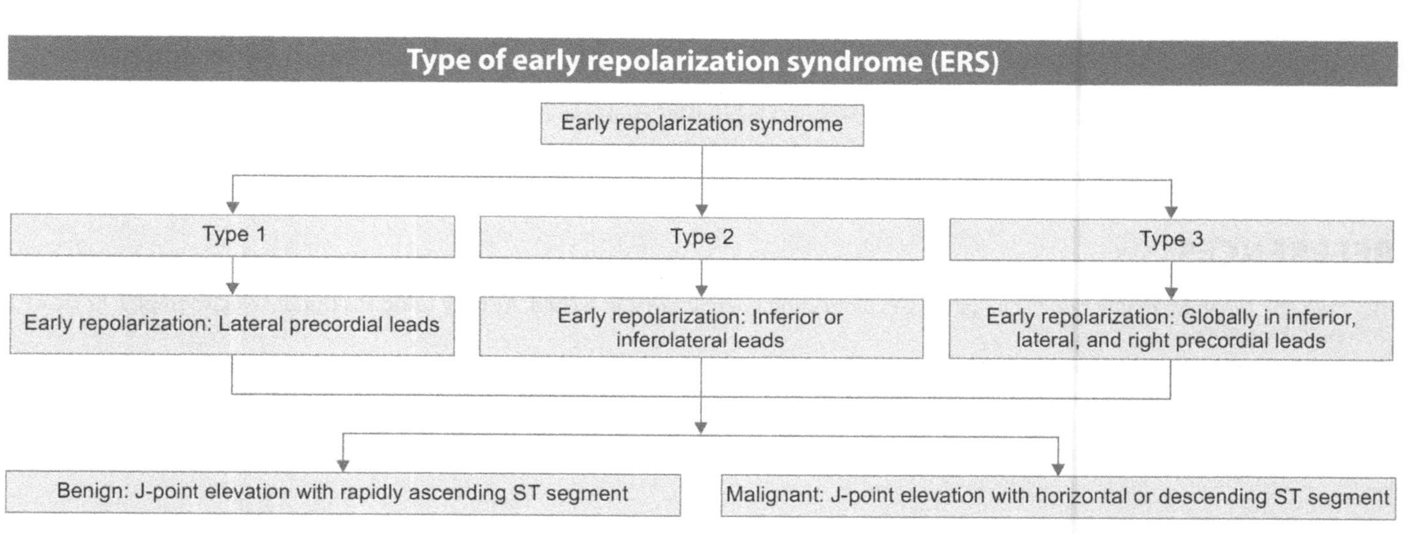

Diagnostic score for early repolarization syndrome (ERS)[1,2]

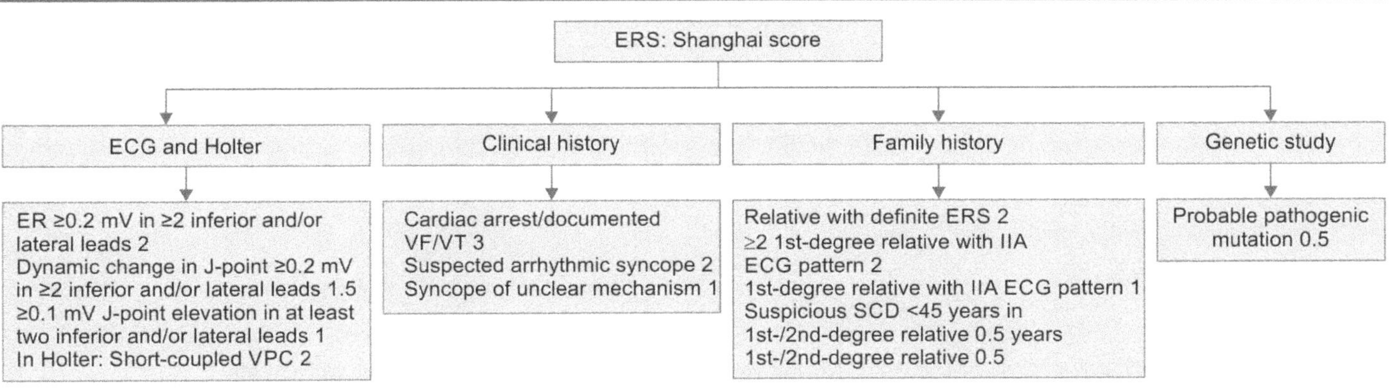

Note: ≥5 points: Probable/Definite ERS; 3–4.5 points: possible ERS; <3 points: nondiagnostic.
(ERS: early repolarization syndrome; VF: ventricular fibrillation; VPC: ventricular premature complex; VT: ventricular tachycardia)

Risk stratification for early repolarization syndrome (ERS)

(ERS: early repolarization syndrome; SCD: sudden cardiac death)

Management of early repolarization syndrome (ERS)[1] (symptomatic)

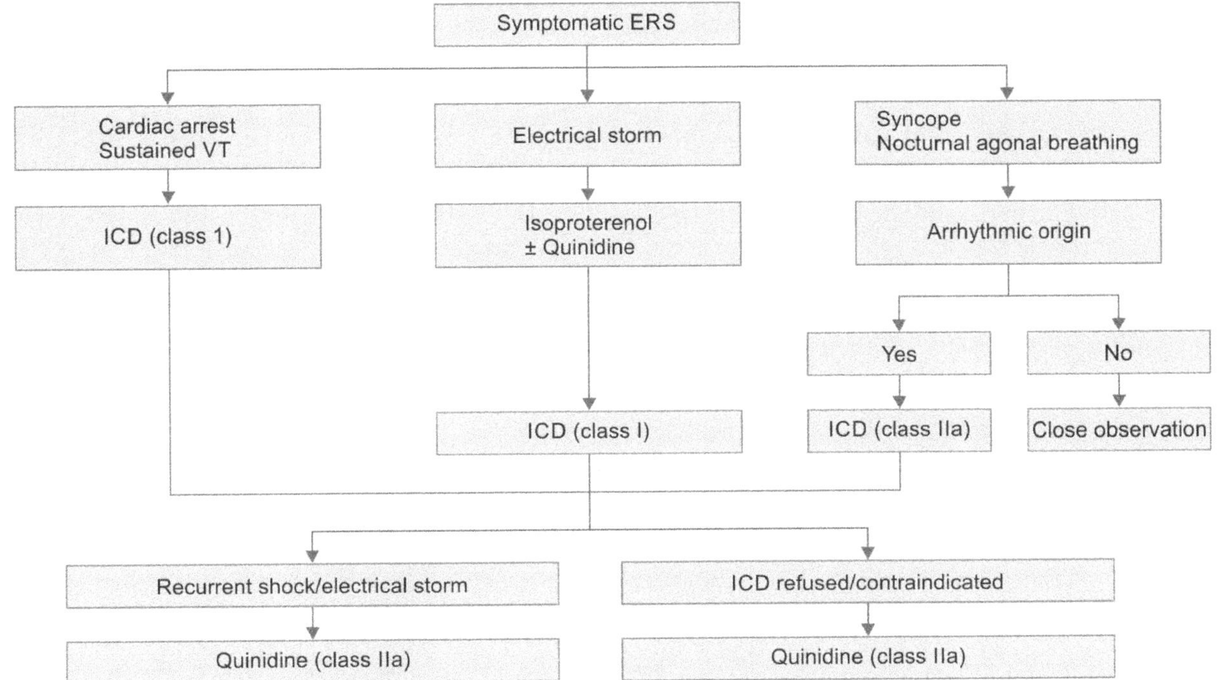

(ERS: early repolarization syndrome; ICD: implantable cardioverter-defibrillator; VT: ventricular tachycardia)

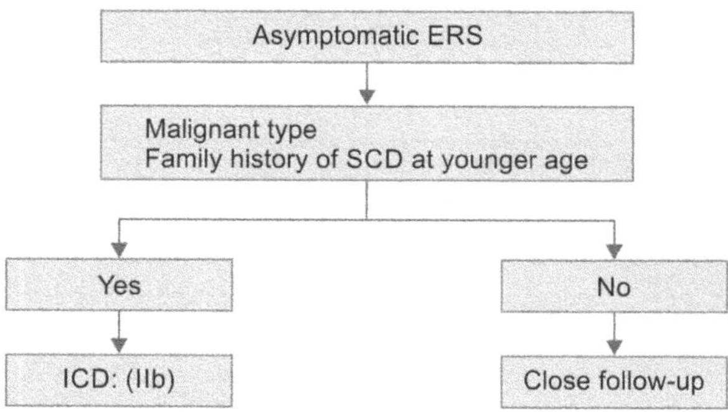

(ERS: early repolarization syndrome; ICD: implantable cardioverter-defibrillator; SCD: sudden cardiac death)

REFERENCES

1. Antzelevitch C, Yan G-X, Ackerman MJ, Borggrefe M, Corrado D, Guo J, et al. J-wave syndromes expert consensus conference report: emerging concepts and gaps in knowledge. Europace. 2017;19:665-94.
2. Patton KK, Ellinor PT, Ezekowitz M, Kowey P, Lubitz SA, Perez M, et al. Electrocardiographic early repolarization: a scientific statement from the American Heart Association. Circulation. 2016;133:1520-9.

Sudden Cardiac Death

CHAPTER 59

Sudden Cardiac Death: General Approach

INTRODUCTION

Sudden cardiac death (SCD) is defined in witnessed case as an unforeseen and unexpected death either within 1 hour of symptoms or in unwitnessed case, within 24 hours of last being seen alive.[1] The incidence is very high, amounting to 5 million cases of SCD per year globally with an annual incidence of 50–100 per 100,000 in western country. However, there is a significant decline in the incidence of SCD over the last few decades. There is a lower rate in Asian countries. The incidence of SCD increases with age with a bimodal peak presentation between 1 and 5 years of age and between 75 and 80 years of age. SCD patients are becoming older, majority of whom are male. Out-of-hospital cardiac arrest (OHCA) is common with a distinct circadian variation with peak incidence occurring in the morning hours.

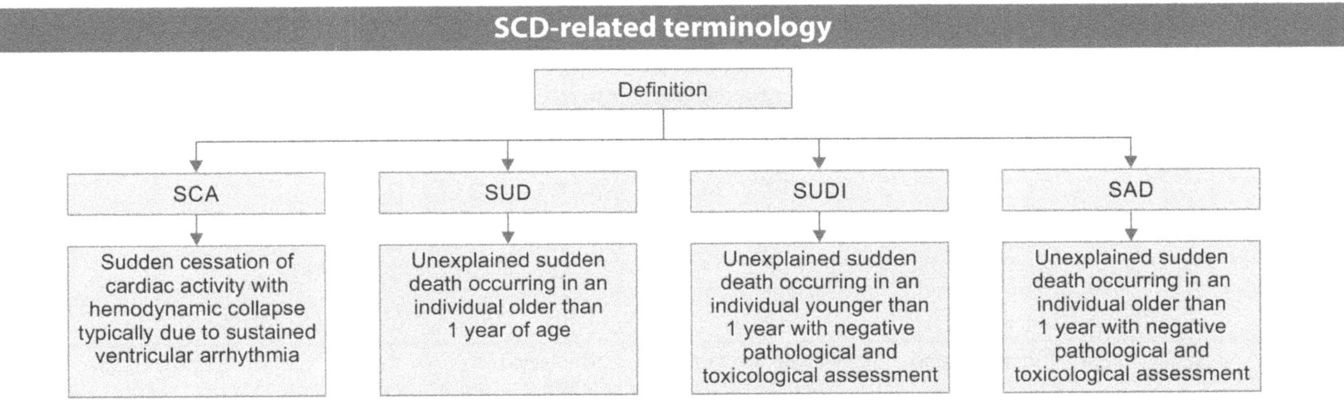

(SAD: sudden arrhythmic death; SCA: sudden cardiac arrest; SUD: sudden unexplained death; SUDI: sudden unexplained death in infant)

Three-staged events in SCD

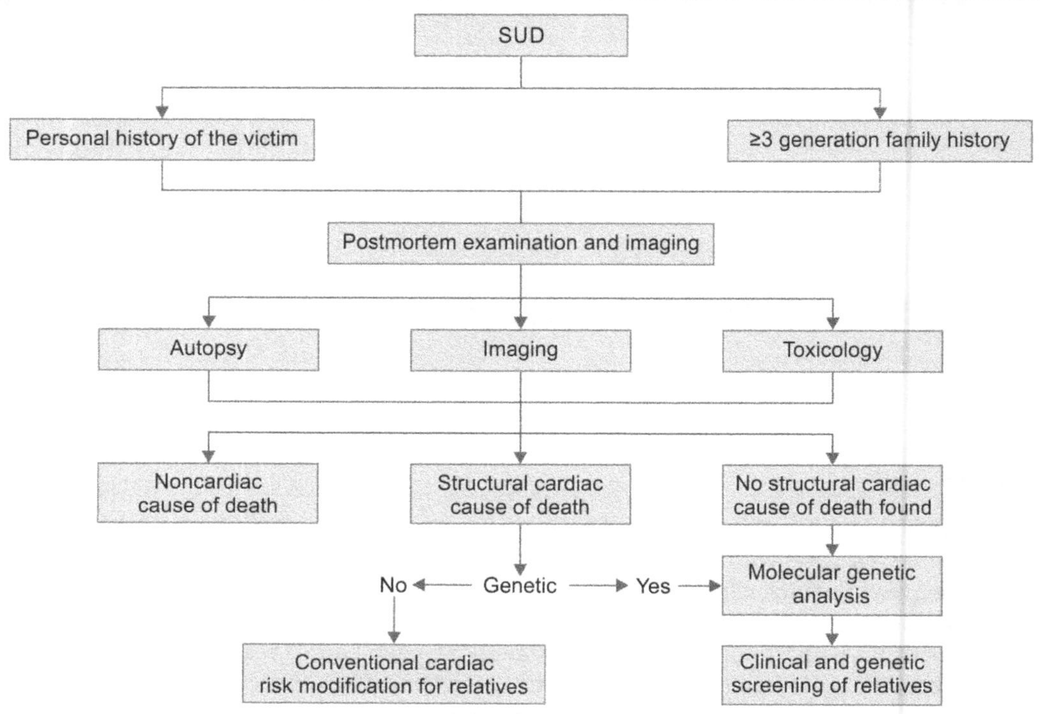

(SCD: sudden cardiac death)

Cardiac condition leading to SCD[2]

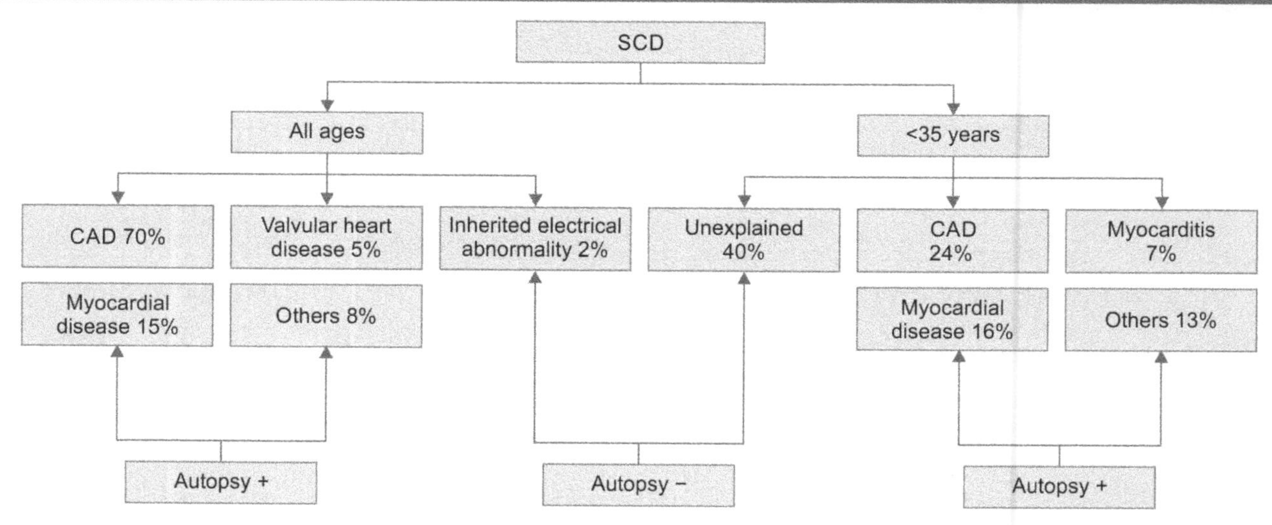

(CAD: coronary artery disease; SCD: sudden cardiac death)

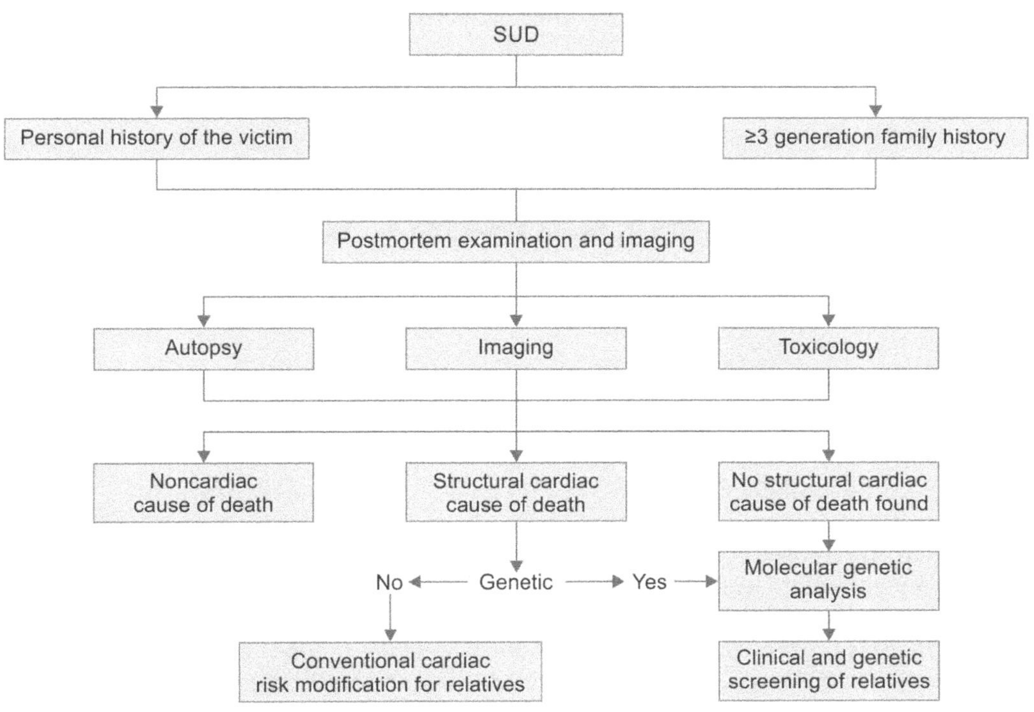

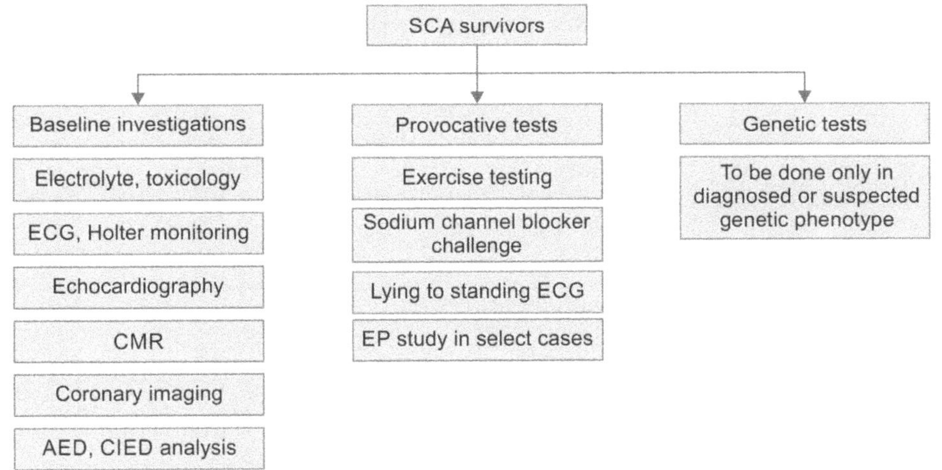

REFERENCES

1. Isbister J, Semsarian C. Sudden cardiac death: an update. Intern Med J. 2019;49:826-33.
2. Wong CX, Brown A, Lau DH, Chugh SS, Albert CM, Kalman JM, et al. Epidemiology of sudden cardiac death: global and regional perspectives. Heart Lung Circ. 2019;28:6-14.
3. Basso C, Aguilera B, Banner J, Cohle S, d'Amati G, de Gouveia RH, et al. Guidelines for autopsy investigation of sudden cardiac death: 2017 update from the Association for European Cardiovascular Pathology. Virchows Arch. 2017;471:691-705.
4. Stiles MK, Wilde AA, Abrams DJ, Ackerman MJ, Albert CM, Behr ER, et al. 2020 APHRS/HRS Expert Consensus Statement on the Investigation of Decedents with Sudden Unexplained Death and Patients with Sudden Cardiac Arrest, and of Their Families. J Arrhythmia. 2021;18:e1-e50.

CHAPTER 60

Sudden Cardiac Death in General Population

INTRODUCTION

Sudden cardiac death (SCD) is the eventuality of sudden cardiac arrest (SCA). In general population, SCD is a major worldwide health problem. The mortality of SCA is nearing 90%. The risk for SCD is highest in patients with ischemic heart disease or lower left ventricular ejection fraction. However, the risk is lower in general population. The lifetime risk for SCD is 10% in middle-aged men and 3% in middle-aged women, who do not have any known cardiac disease. In around 50% of total SCD cases, there is no known heart disease at the time of the indexed event, though majority of those cases have undiagnosed ischemic heart disease. The annual incidence is quite high, ranging from 30 to 100 cases per 100,000 person-years.[1] In 50% cases, SCA is due to noncardiac cause. When etiology can be established, ischemic heart disease is responsible for 80% of all cases of SCD. However, in population younger than 35 years, arrhythmic cause is responsible in 20–30% of cases.[2]

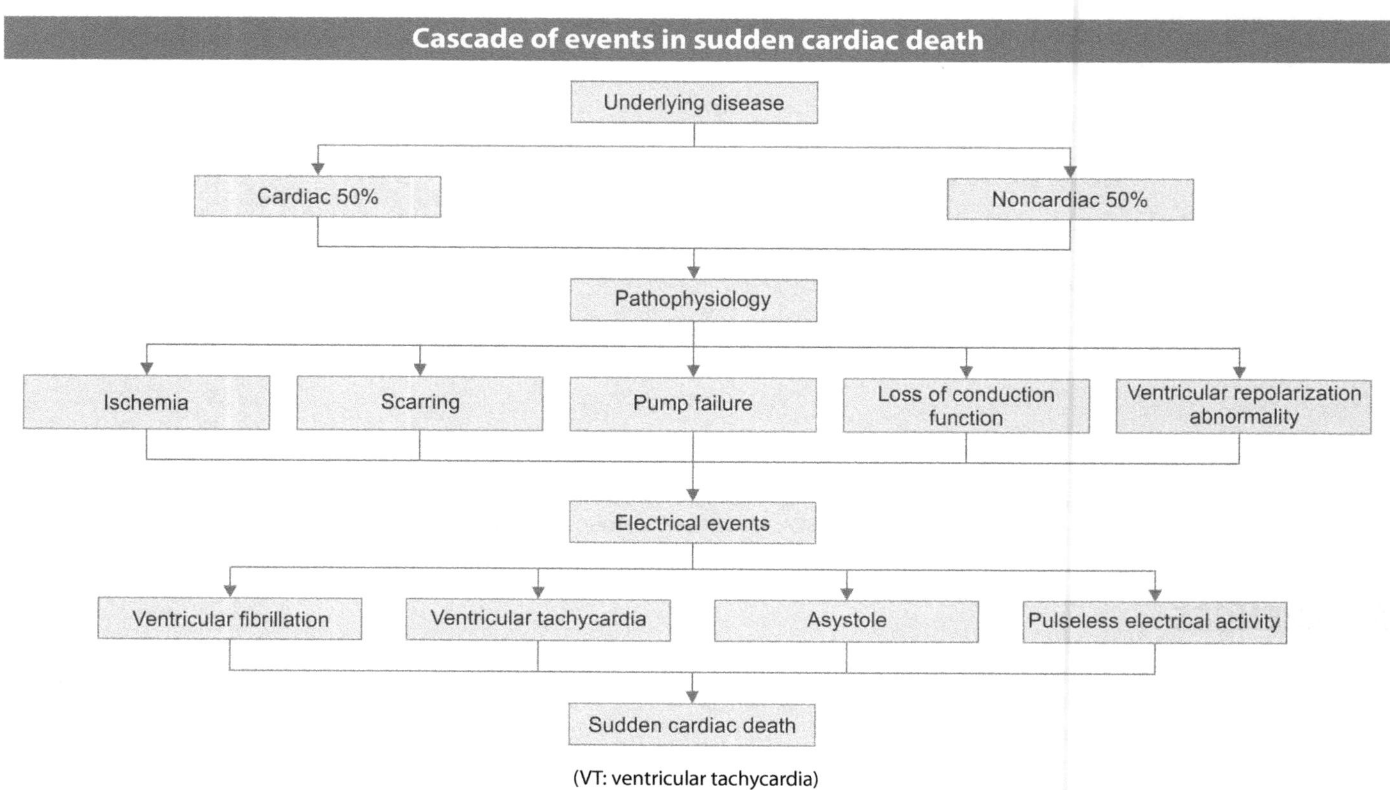

(VT: ventricular tachycardia)

High-risk factors for SCD in general population[3]

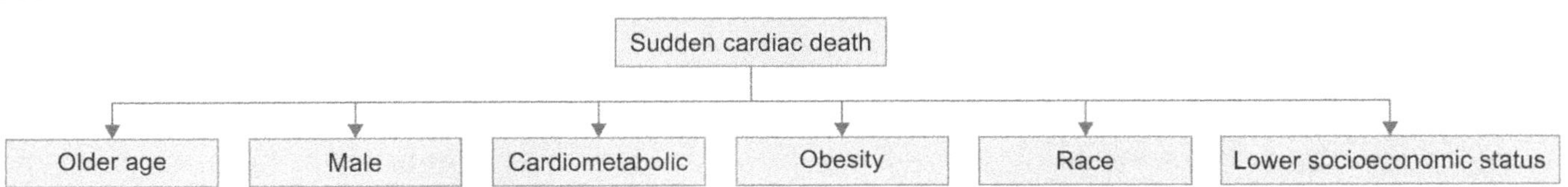

Risk markers for SCD in general population[3]

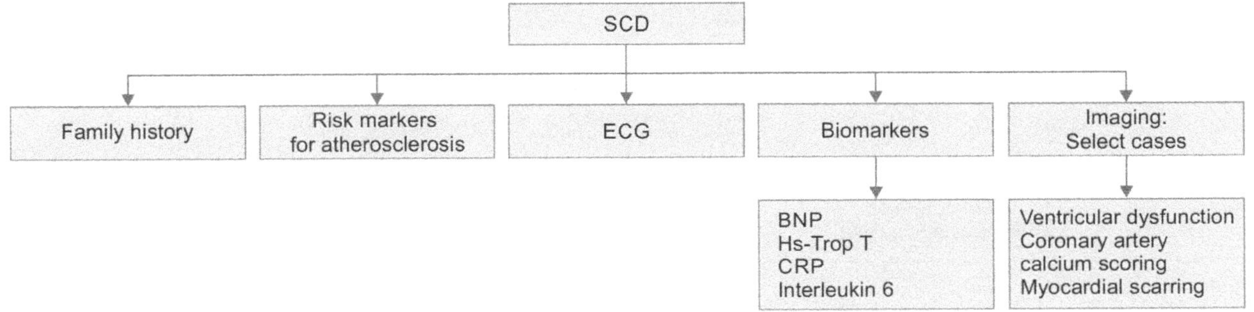

(BNP: B-type natriuretic peptide; CRP: C-reactive protein; ECG: electrocardiogram; Hs-Trop T: high-sensitivity cardiac troponin test; SCD: sudden cardiac death)

ECG risk markers for SCD

(ECG: electrocardiogram; LVH: left ventricular hypertrophy; SCD: sudden cardiac death)

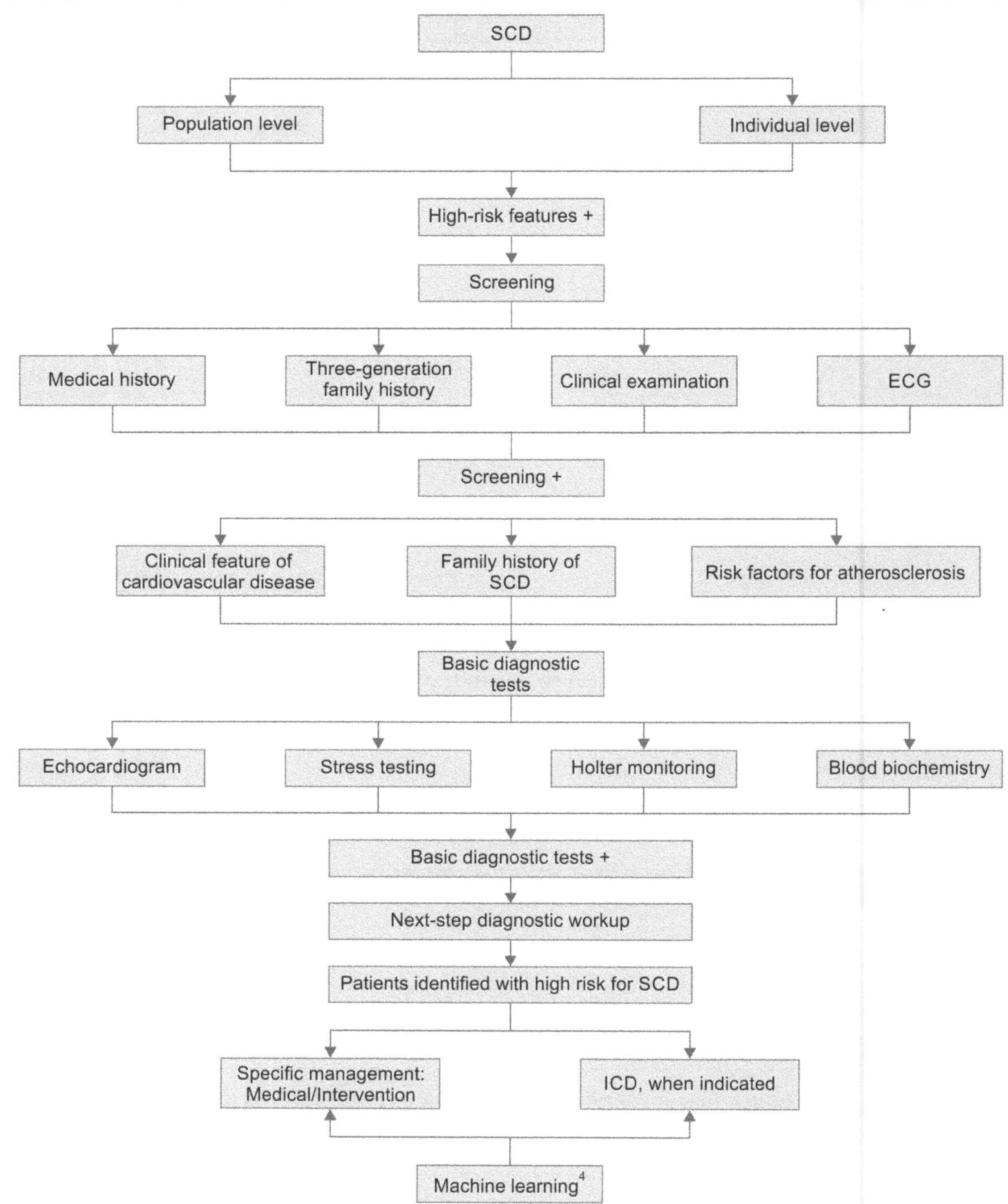

(ICD: implantable cardioverter- defibrillator; ECG: electrocardiogram; SCD: sudden cardiac death)

REFERENCES

1. Narayan SM, Wang PJ, Daubert JP. New concepts in sudden cardiac arrest to address an intractable epidemic: JACC state-of-the-art review. J Am Coll Cardiol. 2019;73:70-88.

2. Jayaraman R, Reinier K, Nair S, Aro AL, Uy-Evanado A, Rusinaru C, et al. Risk factors of sudden cardiac death in the young: multiple-year community-wide assessment. Circulation. 2018;137:1561-70.

3. Ha ACT, Doumouras BS, Wang CN, Tranmer J, Lee DS, et al. Prediction of Sudden Cardiac Arrest in the General Population: Review of Traditional and Emerging Risk Factors. Can J Cardiol. 2022;38:465-78.

4. Andaur Navarro CL, Damen JAA, Takada T, Nijman SW, Dhiman P, Ma J, et al. Risk of bias in studies on prediction models developed using supervised machine learning techniques: systematic review. BMJ 2021;375:n2281.

CHAPTER 61

Sudden Cardiac Death in Dilated Cardiomyopathy

INTRODUCTION

Dilated cardiomyopathy (DCM) accounts for a good proportion of sudden cardiac death (SCD) with an annual incidence of 2–3%, out of which 40–50% cases occur out of hospital. Implantable cardioverter-defibrillator (ICD) is the most important measure to prevent SCD and left ventricular ejection fraction (LVEF) is the most important determinant for risk of SCD. However, most of the trials have failed to show any significant reduction in all-cause mortality with ICD therapy in patients with DCM and LVEF <35%.[1] Moreover, most patients with SCD in community have near-normal LVEF and patients with severely depressed left ventricular function constitute a smaller part of total SCD cases.

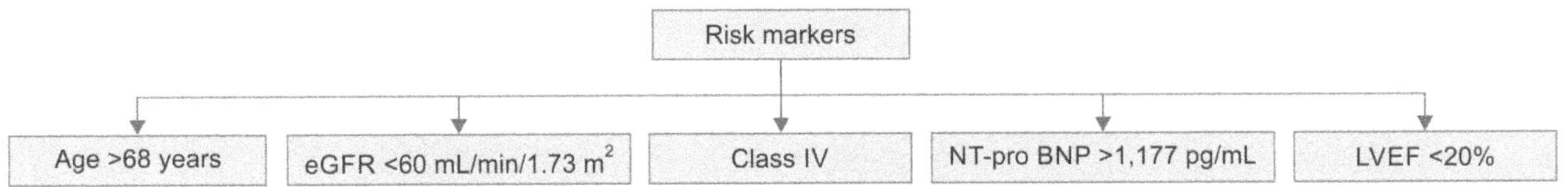

(eGFR: estimated glomerular filtration rate; LVEF: left ventricular ejection fraction; NT-pro BNP: N-terminal pro B-type natriuretic peptide)

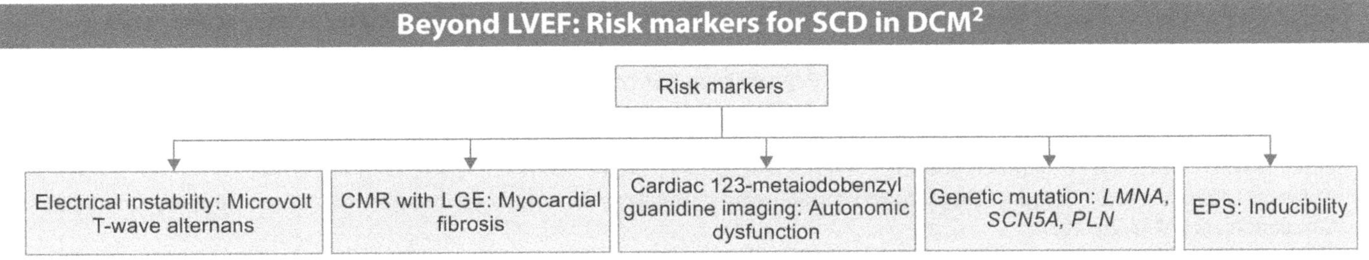

(CMR: cardiovascular magnetic resonance; EPS: electrophysiological study; LGE: late gadolinium enhancement; LMNA: lamin A/C; PLN: phospholamban; SCN5A: sodium channel type 5)

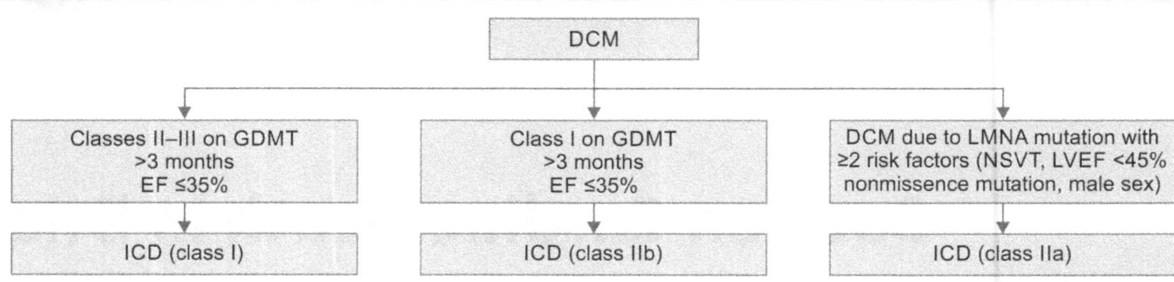

(DCM: dilated cardiomyopathy; EF: ejection fraction; GDMT: guideline-directed medical therapy; ICD: implantable cardioverter-defibrillator; LMNA: lamin A/C; LVEF: left ventricular ejection fraction; NSVT: non-sustained ventricular tachycardia)

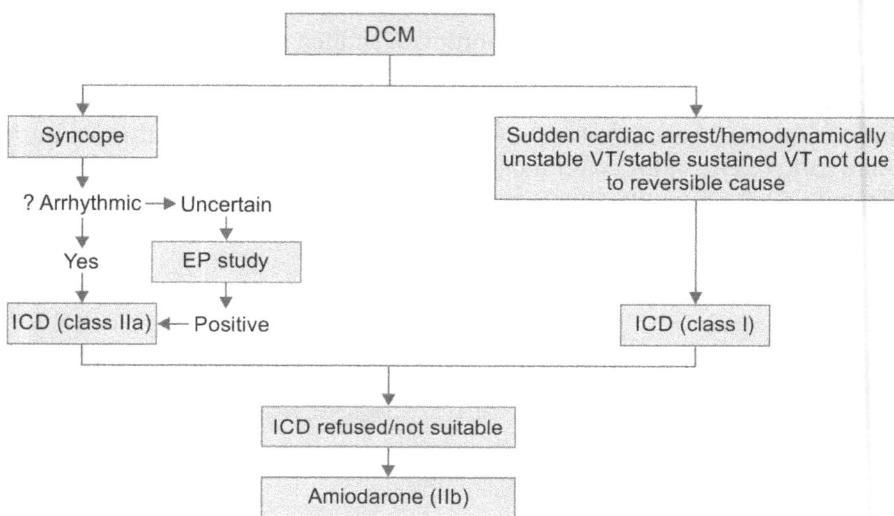

(DCM: dilated cardiomyopathy; EP: electrophysiological; ICD: implantable cardioverter-defibrillator; VT: ventricular tachycardia)

REFERENCES

1. Køber L, Thune JJ, Nielsen JC, Haarbo J, Videbæk L, Korup E, et al; DANISH Investigators. Defibrillator implantation in patients with nonischemic systolicheart failure. N Engl J Med. 2016;375:1221-30.

2. Halliday BP, Cleland JGF, Goldberger JJ, Prasad SK. Personalizing Risk Stratification for Sudden Death in Dilated Cardiomyopathy The Past, Present, and Future Circulation 2017;136:215-31.

3. Priori SG, Blomstrom-Lundqvist C, Mazzanti A, Blom N, Borggrefe M, Camm J, et al. 2015 ESC guidelines for the management of patients with ventricular arrhythmias and the prevention of sudden cardiac death. Europace. 2015;17:1601-87.

4. Golwala H, Bajaj NS, Arora G, Arora P. Implantable cardioverter- defibrillator for nonischemic cardiomyopathy: an updated meta-analysis. Circulation. 2017;135:201203.

5. Al-Khatib SM, Stevenson WG, Ackerman MJ, et al. 2017 AHA/ACC/HRS guideline for management of patients with ventricular arrhythmias and the prevention of sudden cardiac death: a report of the American College of Cardiology/American Heart Association Task Force on Clinical Practice Guidelines and the Heart Rhythm Society. Circulation. 2018;138:e272-e391.

CHAPTER 62

Sudden Cardiac Death in Ischemic Cardiomyopathy

INTRODUCTION

A standardized definition of ischemic cardiomyopathy (ICM) is left ventricular dysfunction in the presence of severe coronary artery disease, including at least one of the following criteria: (1) prior revascularization or acute myocardial infarction, (2) 75% luminal stenosis in the left main stem of left anterior descending artery, and (3) two or more coronary arteries with >75% luminal stenosis.[1]

Pathophysiology of ischemic cardiomyopathy (ICM)[2]

Pathophysiology

Acute ischemia	Recurrent ischemic episode	Prolonged sustained ischemia
Preserved resting myocardial flow ↓Coronary flow reserve	↓Resting myocardial flow ↓Coronary flow reserve	↓↓Resting myocardial flow ↓↓Coronary flow reserve
Preserved contractile reserve and metabolic capacity	Downregulated contractile reserve and metabolic capacity	Myocardial necrosis ↓↓Metabolic capacity
Myocardial stunning	Myocardial hibernation	Myocardial scarring
Inflammation	Coronary microvascular dysfunction	Remodeling

Ischemic cardiomyopathy

Risk factors for SCD in ischemic cardiomyopathy (ICM)

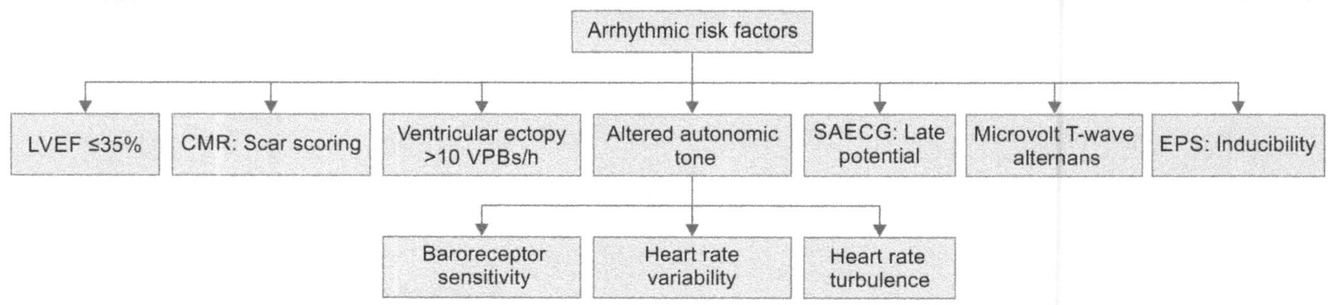

(CMR: cardiac magnetic resonance; EPS: electrophysiological study; LVEF: left ventricular ejection fraction; SAECG: signal-averaged echocardiogram; VPBs: ventricular premature beats)

Primary prevention of SCD in ischemic cardiomyopathy

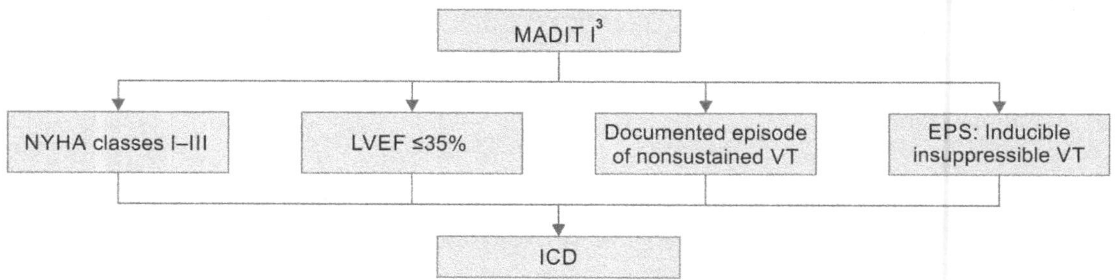

(EPS: electrophysiological study; ICD: implantable cardioverter-defibrillator; LVEF: left ventricular ejection fraction; MADIT: multicenter automatic defibrillator implantation trial; NYHA: New York Heart Association; VT: ventricular tachycardia)

Primary prevention of SCD in ischemic cardiomyopathy

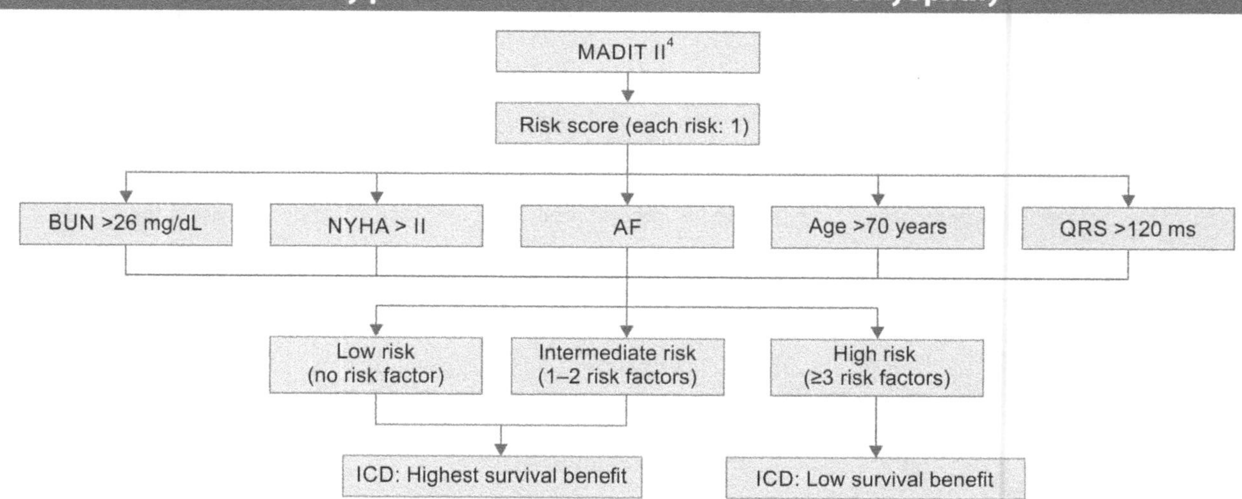

(AF: atrial fibrillation; BUN: blood urea nitrogen; ICD: implantable cardioverter-defibrillator; MADIT: multicenter automatic defibrillator implantation trial; NYHA: New York Heart Association)

Primary prevention of SCD in ischemic cardiomyopathy

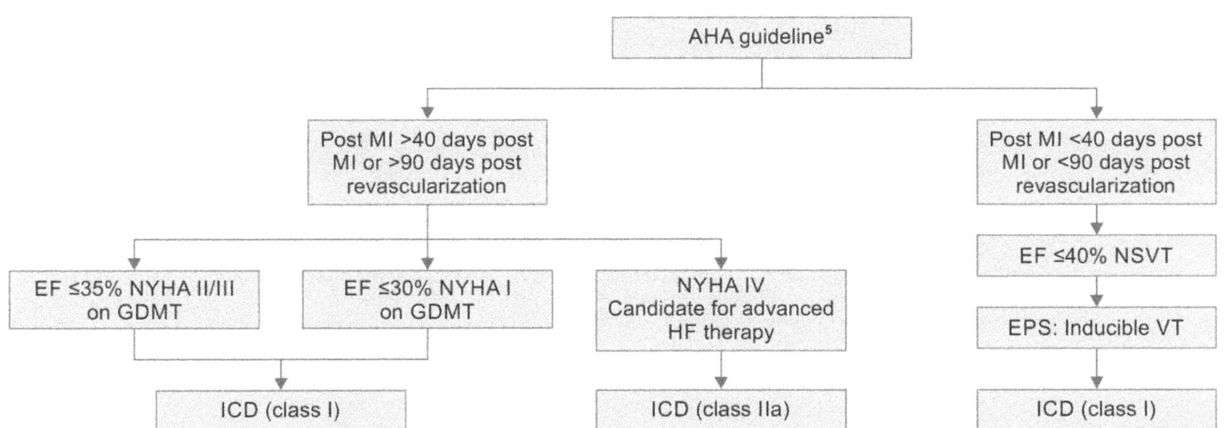

(AHA: American Heart Association; EF: ejection fraction; EPS: electrophysiological study; GDMT: guideline-directed medical therapy; HF: heart failure; ICD: implantable cardioverter-defibrillator; MI: myocardial infarction; NSVT: non-sustained ventricular tachycardia; NYHA: New York Heart Association; VT: ventricular tachycardia)

Secondary prevention of SCD in ischemic cardiomyopathy

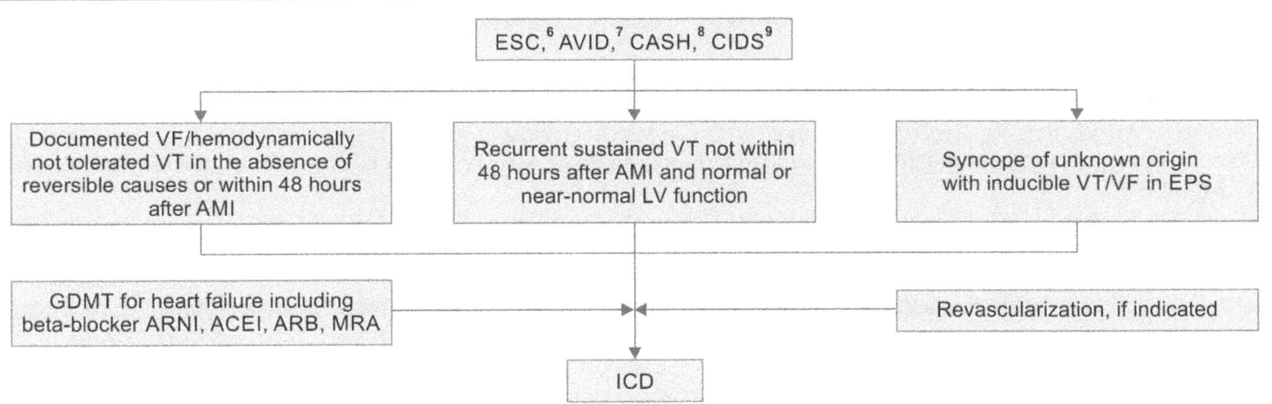

(ACEI: angiotensin-converting enzyme inhibitor; ARB: angiotensin-receptor blocker; AMI: acute myocardial infarction; ARNI: angiotensin receptor-neprilysin inhibitor; AVID: antiarrhythmics versus implantable defibrillators; CASH: cardiac arrest study Hamburg; CIDS: Canadian implantable defibrillator study; EPS: electrophysiological study; ESC: European Society of Cardiology; GDMT: guideline directed medical therapy; ICD: implantable cardioverter-defibrillator; LV: left ventricular; MRA; mineralocorticoid receptor antagonist; VF: ventricular fibrillation; VT: ventricular tachycardia)

Secondary prevention of SCD in ischemic heart disease

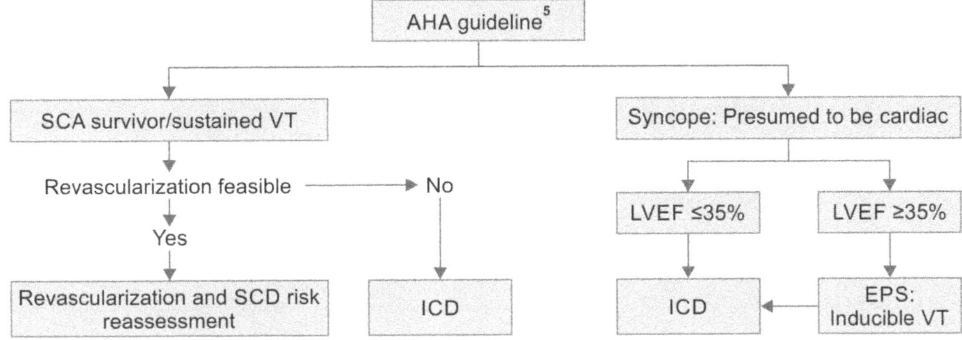

(AHA: American Heart Association; EPS: electrophysiological study; ICD: implantable cardioverter-defibrillator; LVEF: left ventricular ejection fraction; SCA: sudden cardiac arrest; SCD: sudden cardiac death; VT: ventricular tachycardia)

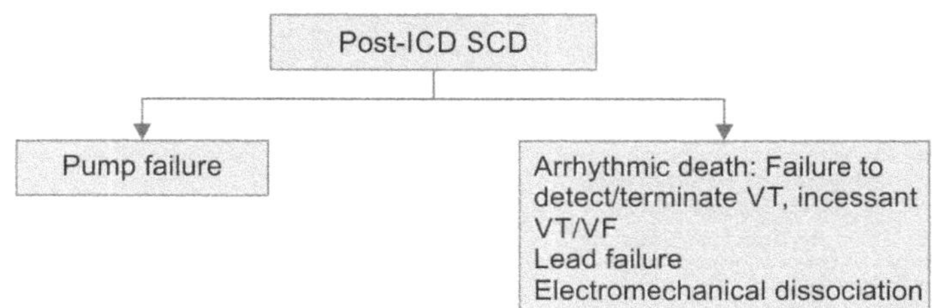

(ICD: implantable cardioverter defibrillator; SCD: sudden cardiac death; VF: ventricular fibrillation; VT: ventricular tachycardia)

REFERENCES

1. Felker GM, Shaw LK, O'Connor CM. A standardized definition of ischemic cardiomyopathy for use in clinical research. J Am Coll Cardiol. 2002;39:210-8.

2. Caba-Pogorevic I, Muk B, Rustamova Y, Kalogeropoulos A, Tzeis S, Vardaset P. Ischaemic cardiomyopathy. Pathophysiological insights, diagnostic management and the roles of revascularisation and device treatment. Gaps and dilemmas in the era of advanced technology. Eur J Heart Fail. 2020;22:789-99.

3. Moss AJ, Hall WJ, Cannom DS, Daubert JP, Higgins SL, Klein H, et al. Improved survival with an implanted defibrillator in patients with coronary disease at high risk for ventricular arrhythmias. Multicenter Automatic Defibrillator Implantation Trial Investigators. N Engl J Med. 1996;335:1933-40.

4. Goldenberg I, Vyas AK, Hall WJ, Moss AJ, Wang H, He H, et al. Risk stratification for primary implantation of a cardioverter- defibrillator in patients with ischemic left ventricular dysfunction. J Am Coll Cardiol. 2008;51:288-96.

5. Heidenreich PA, Bozkurt B, Aguilar D, Allen LA, Byun JJ, Colvin MM, et al. 2022 AHA/ACC/HFSA Guideline for the Management of Heart Failure: A Report of the American College of Cardiology/American Heart Association Joint Committee on Clinical Practice Guidelines 2022;145:e1-e138.

6. Al-Khatib SM, Stevenson WG, Ackerman MJ, Bryant WJ, Callans DJ, Curtis AB, et al. 2017 AHA/ACC/HRS guideline for management of patients with ventricular arrhythmias and the prevention of sudden cardiac death: a report of the American College of Cardiology/American Heart Association Task Force on Clinical Practice Guidelines and the Heart Rhythm Society. Circulation. 2018;138:e272-e391.

7. The Antiarrhythmics Versus Implantable Defibrillators (AVID) Investigators. A comparison of antiarrhythmic drug therapy with implantable defibrillators in patients resuscitated from near-fatal ventricular arrhythmias. N Engl J Med. 1997;337:1576-83.

8. Kuck KH, Cappato R, Siebels J, Ruppel R. Randomized comparison of antiarrhythmic drug therapy with implantable defibrillators in patients resuscitated from cardiac arrest: the Cardiac Arrest Study Hamburg (CASH). Circulation. 2000;102:748-54.

9. Connolly SJ, Gent M, Robers RS, Dorian P, Roy D, Sheldon RS, et al. Canadian Implantable Defibrillator Study (CIDS): a randomized trial of the implantable defibrillator against amiodarone. Circulation. 2000;101:1297-302.

Sudden Cardiac Death in Hypertrophic Cardiomyopathy

INTRODUCTION

Hypertrophic cardiomyopathy (HCM) is an autosomal dominant genetic cardiomyopathy, due to sarcomeric protein gene mutation with a prevalence in general population of 1:200 to 1:500. The most feared consequence of the disease is sudden cardiac death (SCD), particularly in young population. The annual incidence of SCD in adult population is 1%, whereas in children the incidence is between 1 and 7.2%.[1] SCD risk extends in mid-40s, but is infrequent in patients older than 60 years. Race or gender does not affect the incidence of SCD.

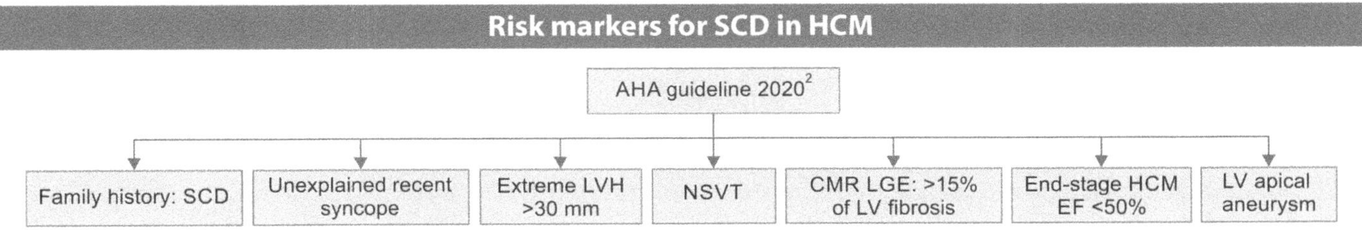

(AHA: American Heart Association; CMR: cardiovascular magnetic resonance; EF: ejection fraction; LGE: late gadolinium enhancement; LV: left ventricular; LVH: left ventricular hypertrophy; NSVT: nonsustained ventricular tachycardia; SCD: sudden cardiac death)

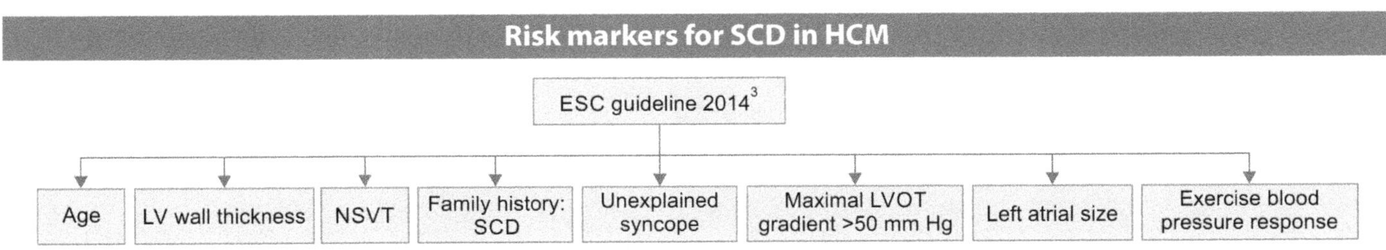

Note: The HCM Risk-SCD formula is as follows:

$$\text{Probability}_{\text{SCD at 5 years}} = 1 - 0.998^{\exp(\text{Prognostic index})}$$

Where Prognostic index = [0.15939858 × maximal wall thickness (mm)] − [0.00294271 × maximal wall thickness^2 (mm^2)] + [0.0259082 × left atrial diameter (mm)] + [0.00446131 × maximal (rest/Valsalva) LVOT gradient (mm Hg)] + [0.4583082 × family history SCD] + [0.82639195 × NSVT] + [0.71650361 × unexplained syncope] − [0.01799934 × age at clinical evaluation (years)].

(ESC: European Society of Cardiology; LV: left ventricular; LVOT: left ventricular outflow tract; NSVT: nonsustained ventricular tachycardia; SCD: sudden cardiac death)

Risk markers for SCD beyond guideline[4]

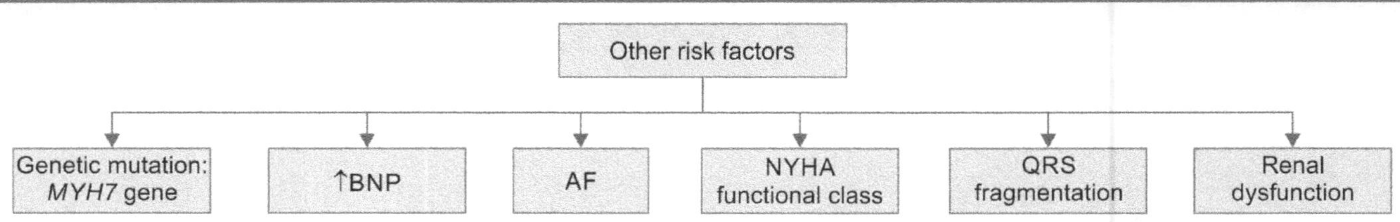

(AF; atrial fibrillation; BNP; B-type natriuretic peptide; NYHA: New York Heart Association)

Mechanism of arrhythmogenicity in HCM[5]

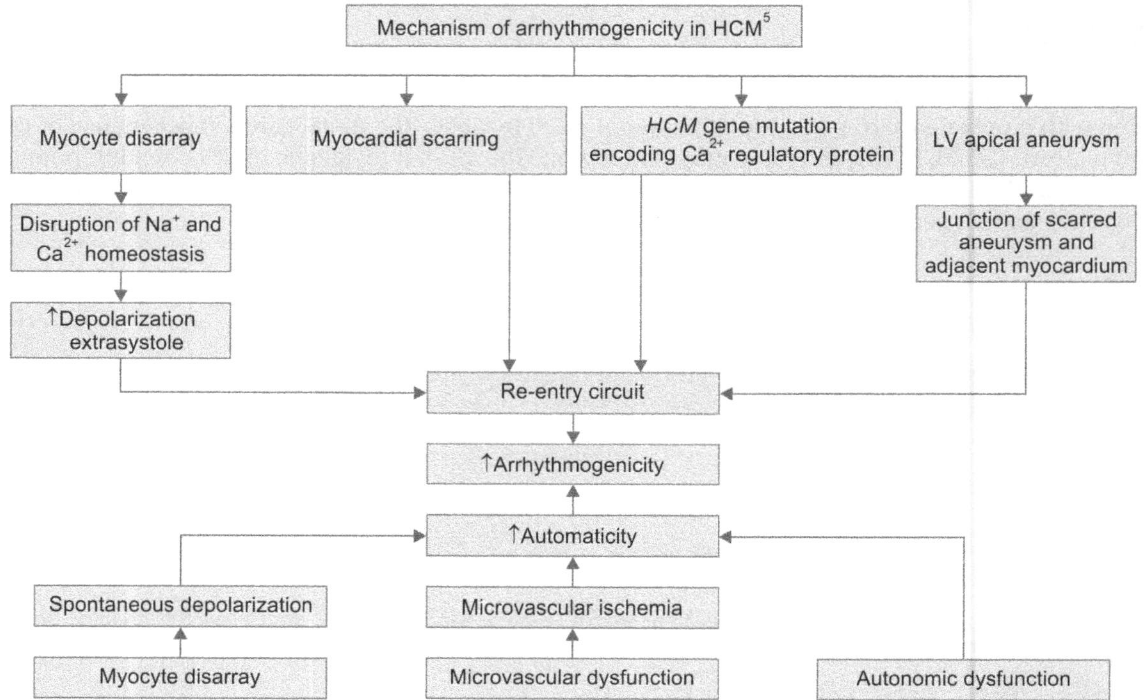

(HCM: hypertrophic cardiomyopathy; LV: left ventricular)

Prevention of SCD in HCM: AHA guideline[2]

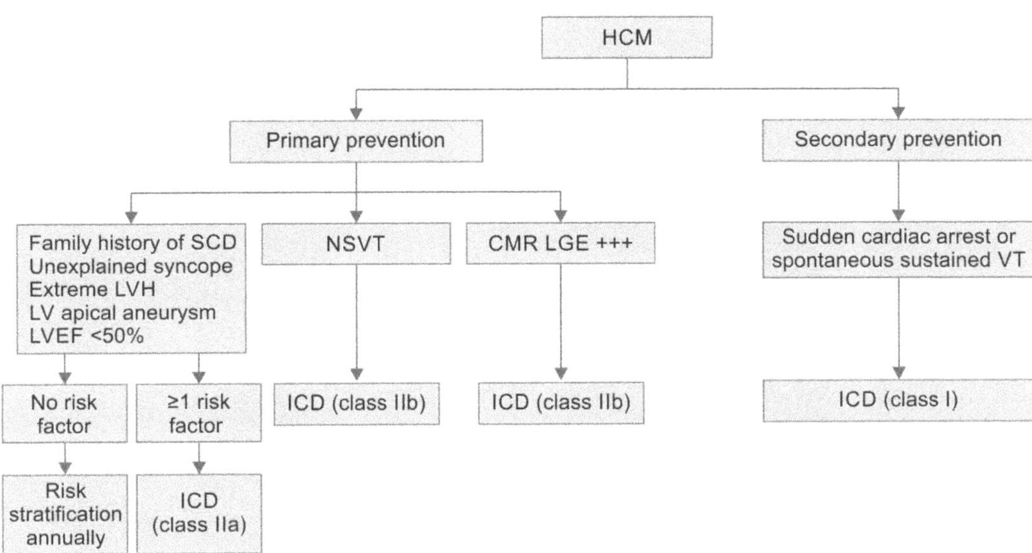

(AHA: American Heart Association; CMR: cardiovascular magnetic resonance; HCM: hypertrophic cardiomyopathy; ICD: implantable cardioverter-defibrillator; LGE: late gadolinium enhancement; LV: left ventricular; LVEF: left ventricular ejection fraction; LVH: left ventricular hypertrophy; NSVT: nonsustained ventricular tachycardia; VT: ventricular tachycardia)

Prevention of SCD in children with HCM: AHA guideline[2]

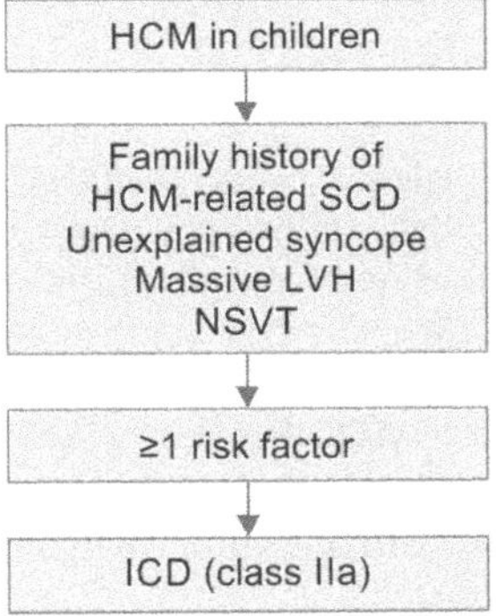

(AHA: American Heart Association; HCM: hypertrophic cardiomyopathy; ICD: implantable cardioverter-defibrillator; LVH: left ventricular hypertrophy; NSVT: nonsustained ventricular tachycardia; SCD: sudden cardiac death)

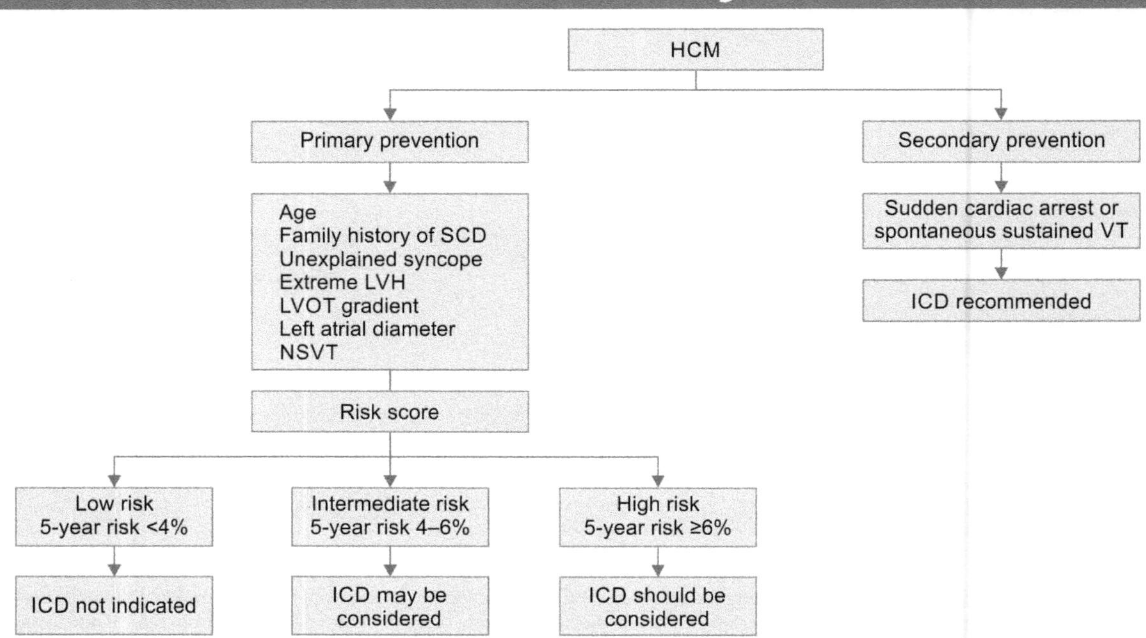

(HCM: hypertrophic cardiomyopathy; ICD: implantable cardioverter-defibrillator; LVH: left ventricular hypertrophy; LVOT: left ventricular outflow tract; NSVT: nonsustained ventricular tachycardia; SCD: sudden cardiac death; VT: ventricular tachycardia)

REFERENCES

1. Ostman-Smith I, Wettrell G, Keeton B, Holmgren D, Ergander U, Gould S, et al. Age- and gender-specific mortality rates in childhood hypertrophic cardiomyopathy. Eur Heart J. 2008;29:1160-7.

2. Ommen SR, Mital S, Burke MA, Day SM, Deswal A, Elliott P, et al. 2020AHA/ACC Guideline for the and Diagnosis and Treatment of Patients With Hypertrophic Cardiomyopathy: executive summary: a report of the American College of Cardiology/American Heart Association Joint Committee on Clinical Practice Guidelines. Circulation. 2020;142:e533-e557.

3. Elliott PM, Anastasakis A, Borger MA, Borggrefe M, Cecchi F, Charron P, et al; Authors/Task Force members. 2014 ESC Guidelines on diagnosis and management of hypertrophic cardiomyopathy: the Task Force for the Diagnosis and Management of Hypertrophic Cardiomyopathy of the European Society of Cardiology (ESC). Eur Heart J. 2014;35:2733-79.

4. Hong Y, Su WW, Li X. Risk factors for sudden cardiac death in Hypertrophic Cardiomyopathy. Curr Opin Cardiol. 2022;37:15-21.

5. Maron BJ, Rowin EJ, Maron MS. Paradigm of sudden death prevention in hypertrophic cardiomyopathy. Circ Res. 2019;125(4):370-8.

Cardio-Oncology

CHAPTER 64

Cardio-Oncology: General Approach

INTRODUCTION

Cardio-Oncology is an emerging field in cardiology, which deals with cardiovascular disease in patients with cancer. Cardio-Oncology paradigm is the prevention, diagnosis, and treatment of cardiotoxicity resulting from radiotherapy and chemotherapy. In the recent past, remarkable progress has been made in oncology science that has translated to immense improvement in long-term survival.[1] At the same time, remarkable advance in cardiovascular disease management has led to considerable improvement in mortality in patients with cardiac disease. These trends have resulted in a considerable population with coexisting cancer and cardiovascular disease. The most common cardiotoxicity is myocardial dysfunction.

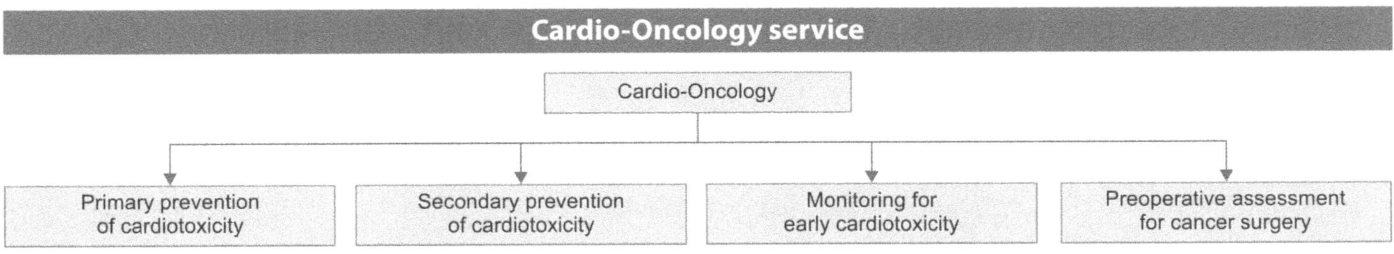

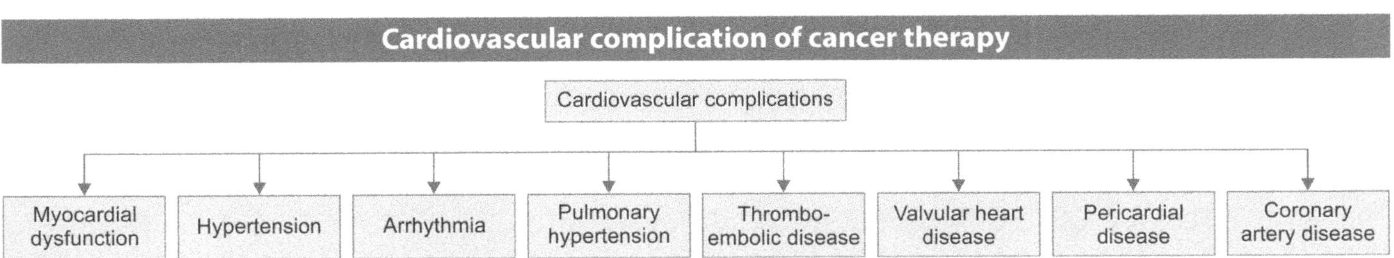

Parameters for higher risk of cardiotoxicity[2]

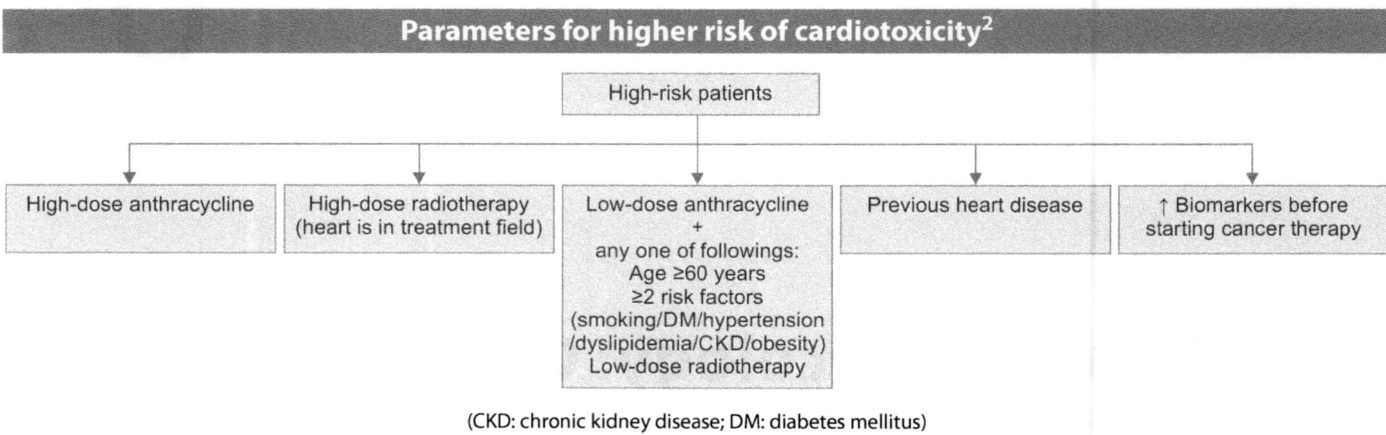

(CKD: chronic kidney disease; DM: diabetes mellitus)

Mechanism and staging of myocardial dysfunction in cancer therapy

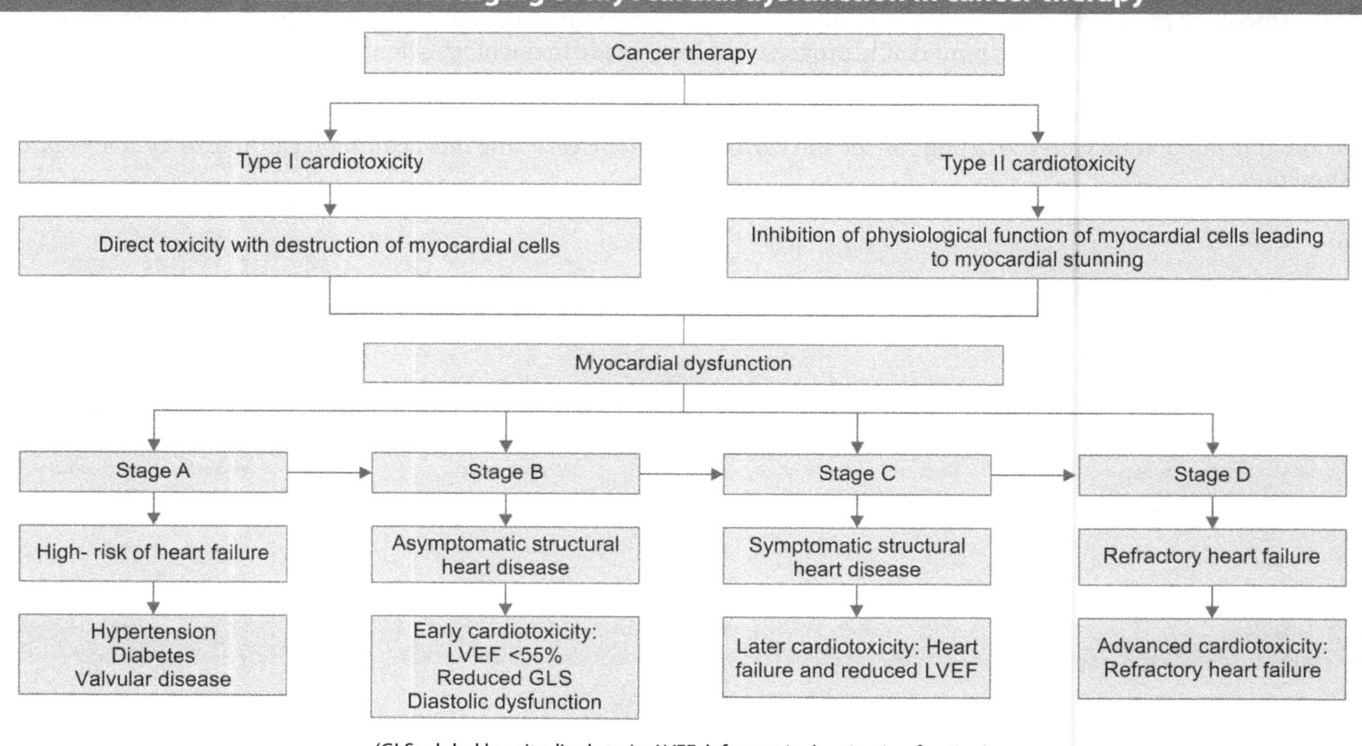

(GLS: global longitudinal strain; LVEF: left ventricular ejection fraction)

Cardio-Oncological evaluation[3]

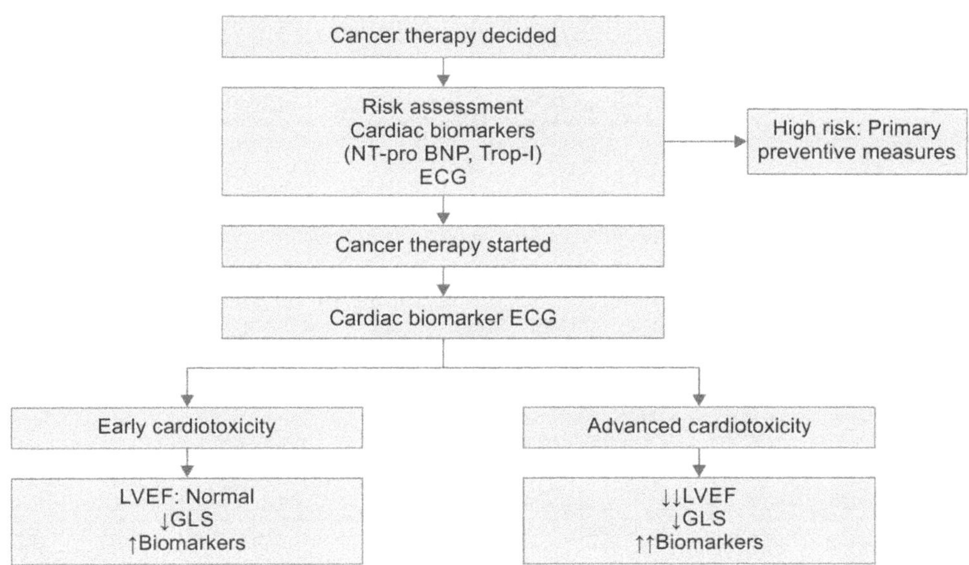

(ECG: electrocardiogram; GLS: global longitudinal strain; LVEF: left ventricular ejection fraction; NT-pro BNP: N-terminal pro-brain natriuretic peptide; Trop-I: troponin-I)

Management of early myocardial toxicity[4,5]

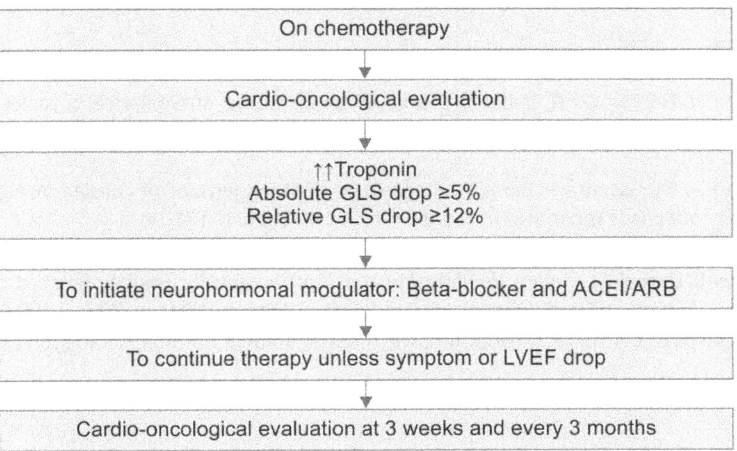

(ACEI: angiotensin-converting enzyme inhibitor; ARB: angiotensin-receptor blocker; GLS: global longitudinal strain; LVEF: left ventricular ejection fraction)

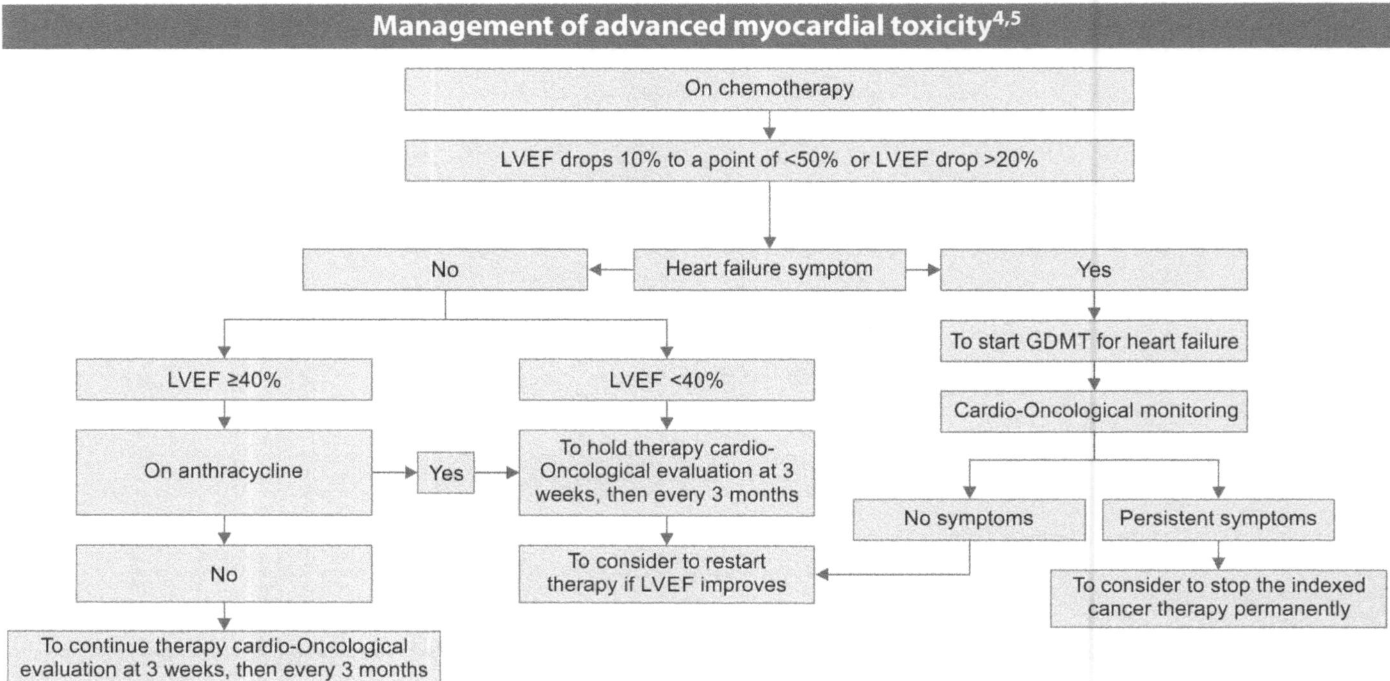

(GDMT: guideline-directed medical therapy; LVEF: left ventricular ejection fraction)

REFERENCES

1. Allemani C, Weir HK, Carreira H, Harewood R, Spika D, Wang XS, et al. Global surveillance of cancer survival 1995–2009: analysis of individual data for 25,676,887 patients from 279 population-based registries in 67 countries (CONCORD-2). Lancet. 2015;385: 977-1010.
2. Curigliano G, Lenihan D, Fradley M, Ganatra S, Barac A, Blaes A, et al. Management of cardiac disease in cancer patients throughout oncological treatment: ESMO consensus recommendations. Ann Oncol. 2020;31:171-90.
3. Cubbon RM, Lyon AR. Cardio-oncology: concepts and practice. Ind Heart J. 2016;68:S77-85.
4. Alexandre J, Cautela J, Ederhy S, Damaj GL, Salem JE, Barlesi F, et al. Cardiovascular Toxicity Related to Cancer Treatment: A Pragmatic Approach to the American and European Cardio-Oncology Guidelines J Am Heart Assoc. 2020;9:e08403.
5. Koutsoukis A, Ntalianis A, Repasos E, Kastritis E, Dimopoulos MA, Paraskevaidis I. Cardio-oncology: A Focus on Cardiotoxicity Eur Cardiol. 2018;13:64-9.

CHAPTER 65

Cardio-Oncology: Chemotherapy

INTRODUCTION

Anthracycline is one of the oldest chemotherapeutic agents. Anthracycline-induced cardiotoxicity was first reported in the early 1970s.[1] Over the last two decades, newer molecules for cancer therapy have been developed, most of which block the growth and spread cancer by interfering with specific molecules. This is called targeted therapy which is associated with various cardiovascular complications, the most common of which is heart failure and left ventricular dysfunction and myocarditis. Different terminologies have been used to describe the cardiovascular side effects, like cardiotoxicity, cardiotoxic cardiomyopathy, or cancer therapy-related cardiac dysfunction (CTRCD). Doxorubicin, trastuzumab, and sunitinib are associated with cardiotoxicity in 3–26, 2–28, and 2.7–11% of treated cases, respectively.[2]

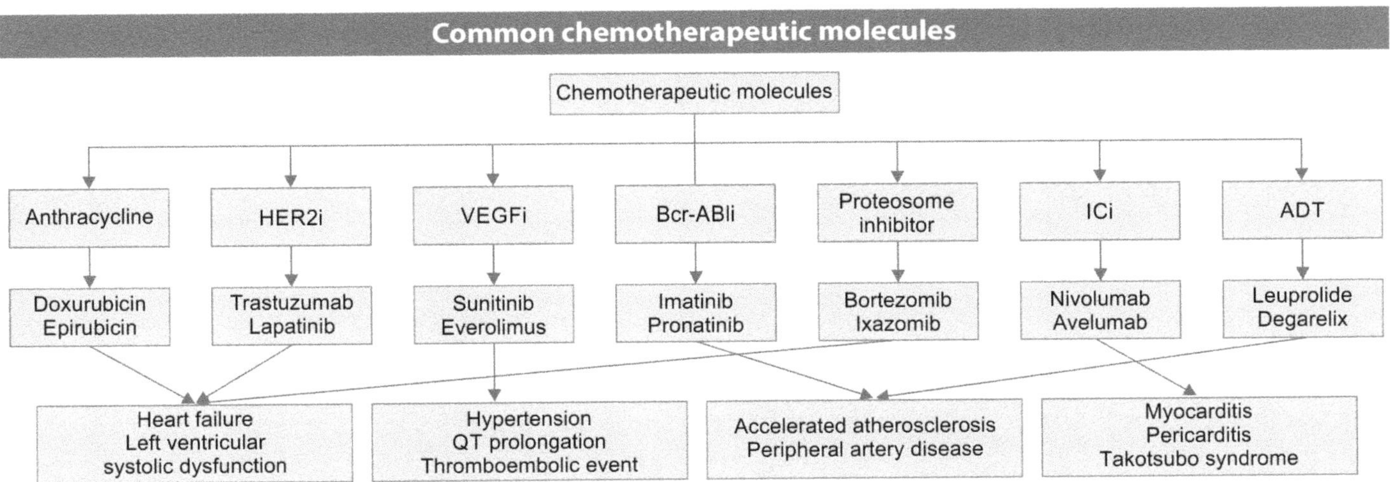

(ADT: androgen deprivation therapy; Bcr-ABIi: Bcr-ABI kinase inhibitor; HER2i: human epidermal growth factor 2 inhibitor; ICi: immune check point inhibitor; VEGFi: vascular endothelial growth factor inhibitor)

Management protocol for anthracycline-induced cardiotoxicity[3,4]

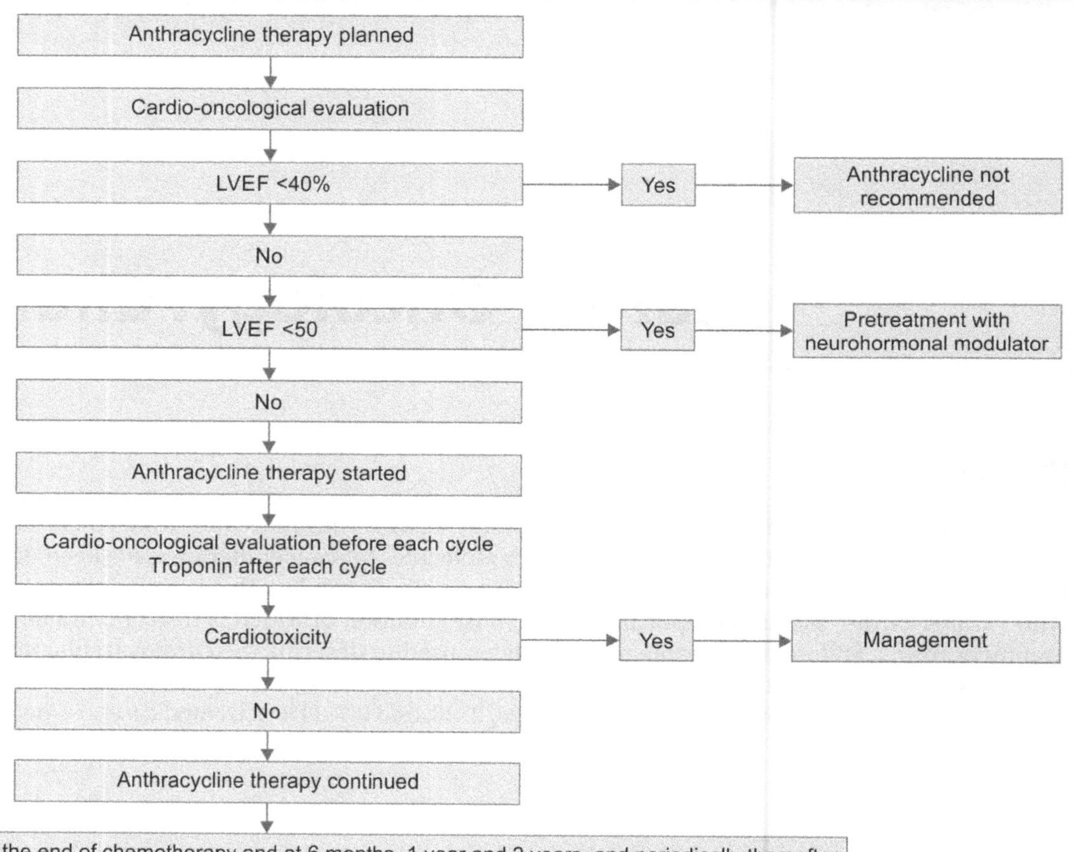

(LVEF: left ventricular ejection fraction)

Management protocol for HER2i-induced cardiotoxicity[3,4]

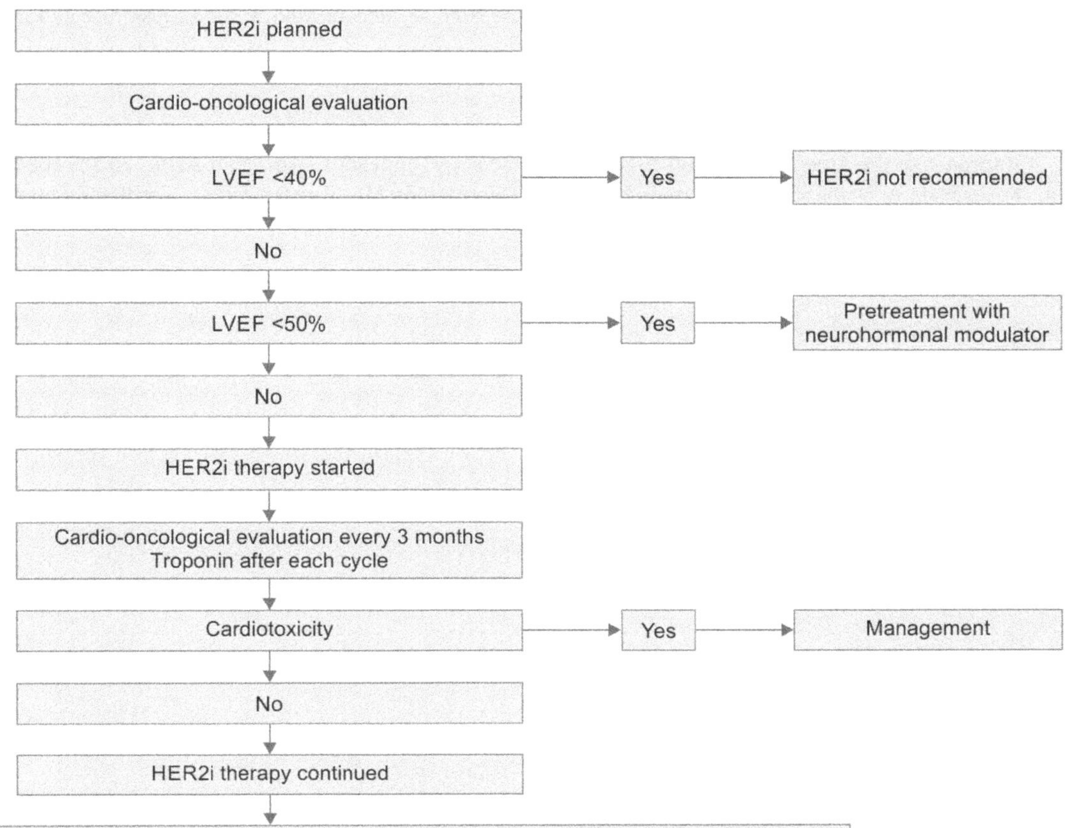

(HER2i: human epidermal growth factor 2 inhibitor; LVEF: left ventricular ejection fraction)

Management protocol for immune checkpoint inhibitor therapy[3,4]

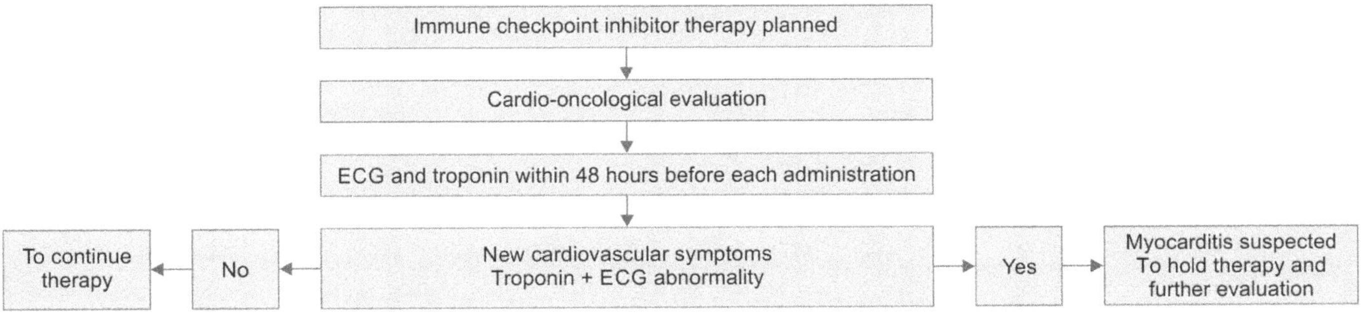

REFERENCES

1. Von Hoff DD, Layard MW, Basa P, Davis HL Jr, Von Hoff AL, Rozencweig M, et al. Risk factors for doxorubicin-induced congestive heart failure. Ann Intern Med. 1979;91:710-7.
2. Yeh ET, Bickford CL. Cardiovascular complications of cancer therapy: incidence, pathogenesis, diagnosis, and management. J Am Coll Cardiol. 2009;53:2231-47.
3. Alexandre J, Cautela J, Ederhy S, Damaj GL, Salem JE, Barlesi F, et al. Cardiovascular Toxicity Related to Cancer Treatment: A Pragmatic Approach to the American and European Cardio-Oncology Guidelines J Am Heart Assoc. 2020;9:e08403.
4. Koutsoukis A, Ntalianis A, Repasos E, Kastritis E, Dimopoulos MA, Paraskevaidis I. Cardio-oncology: A Focus on Cardiotoxicity. Eur Cardiol. 2018;13:64-9.

CHAPTER 66

Cardio-Oncology: Radiation Therapy

INTRODUCTION

Radiation therapy (RT) is used in more than 50% of cancer patients. In fact, RT has changed the prognosis and survival of the cancer patients. At the same time, RT has led to significant adverse effects, including adverse cardiovascular effects, which add to significant morbidity and mortality in cancer survivors.[1] The effect is dose related, and a cumulative dose of 0.5 Gy increases the cardiovascular risk. Even a dose <2 Gy may increase the rate of ischemic heart disease significantly.[2] Cardiovascular complications take long time to develop after RT. The first sign of cardiac toxicity appears 10–15 years after RT.

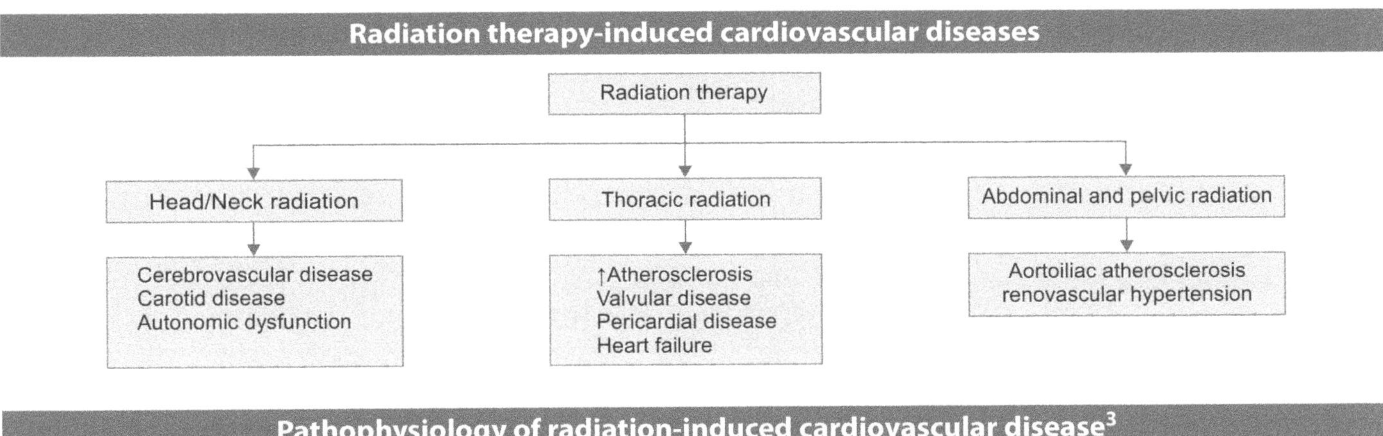

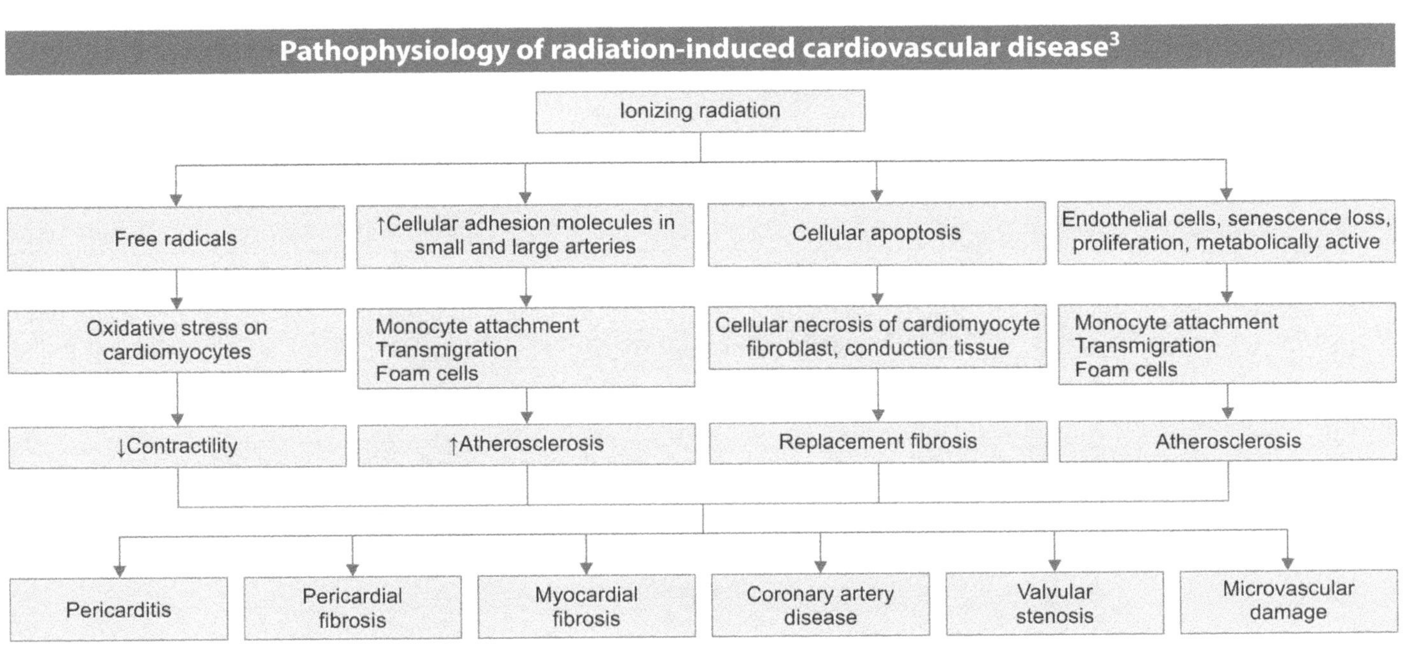

Prevention of cardiovascular disease on radiation therapy

Before RT

- Optimum screening of CV risk factors and CV disease
- To look for available CT-chest image for coronary artery/aortic calcium load to assess coronary artery disease
- To maximally reduce radiation dose to CV structure without compromising cancer treatment
- Deep inspiratory breath holding during RT through cardiac structure

(CT: computed tomography; CV: cardiovascular; RT: radiation therapy)

Prevention of cardiovascular disease on radiation therapy

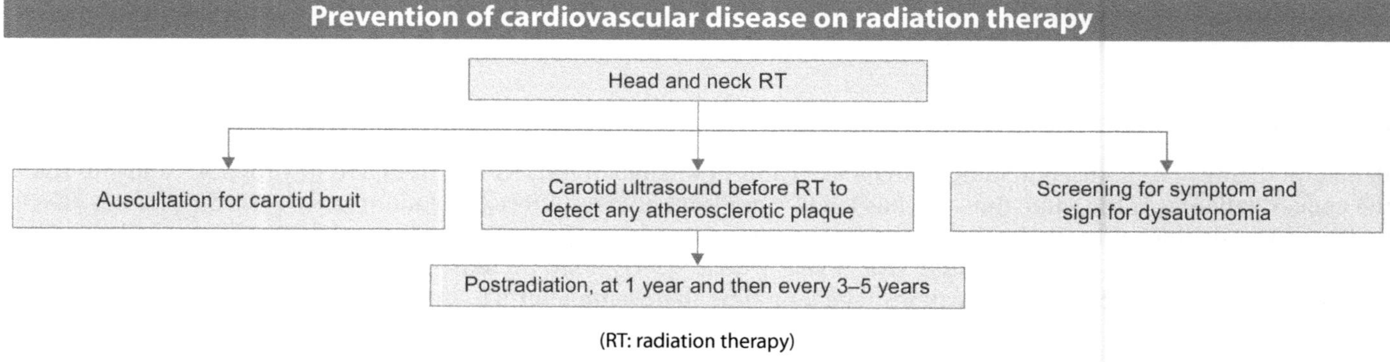

(RT: radiation therapy)

Prevention of cardiovascular disease on radiation therapy

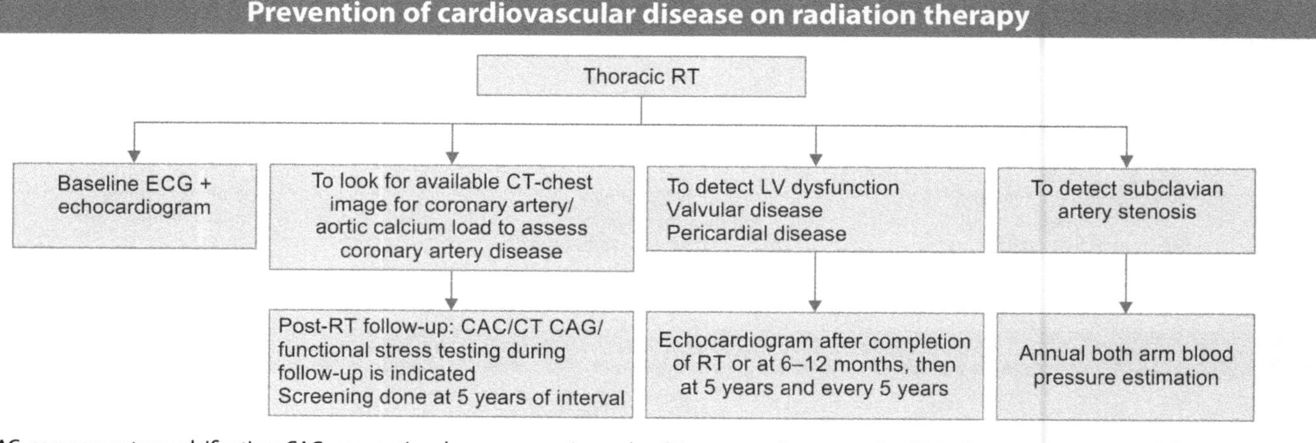

(CAC: coronary artery calcification; CAG: conventional coronary angiography; CT: computed tomography; ECG: electrocardiogram; LV: left ventricular; RT: radiation therapy)

Prevention of cardiovascular disease on radiation therapy

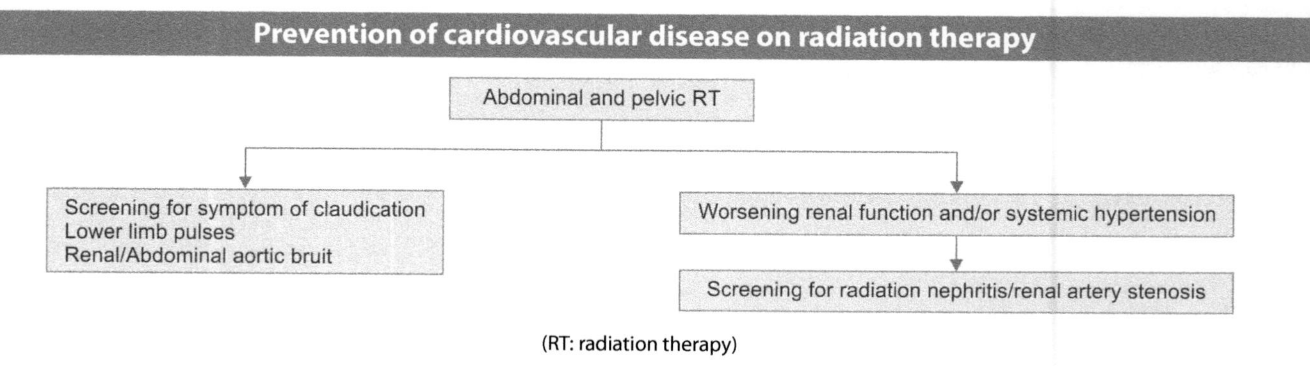

(RT: radiation therapy)

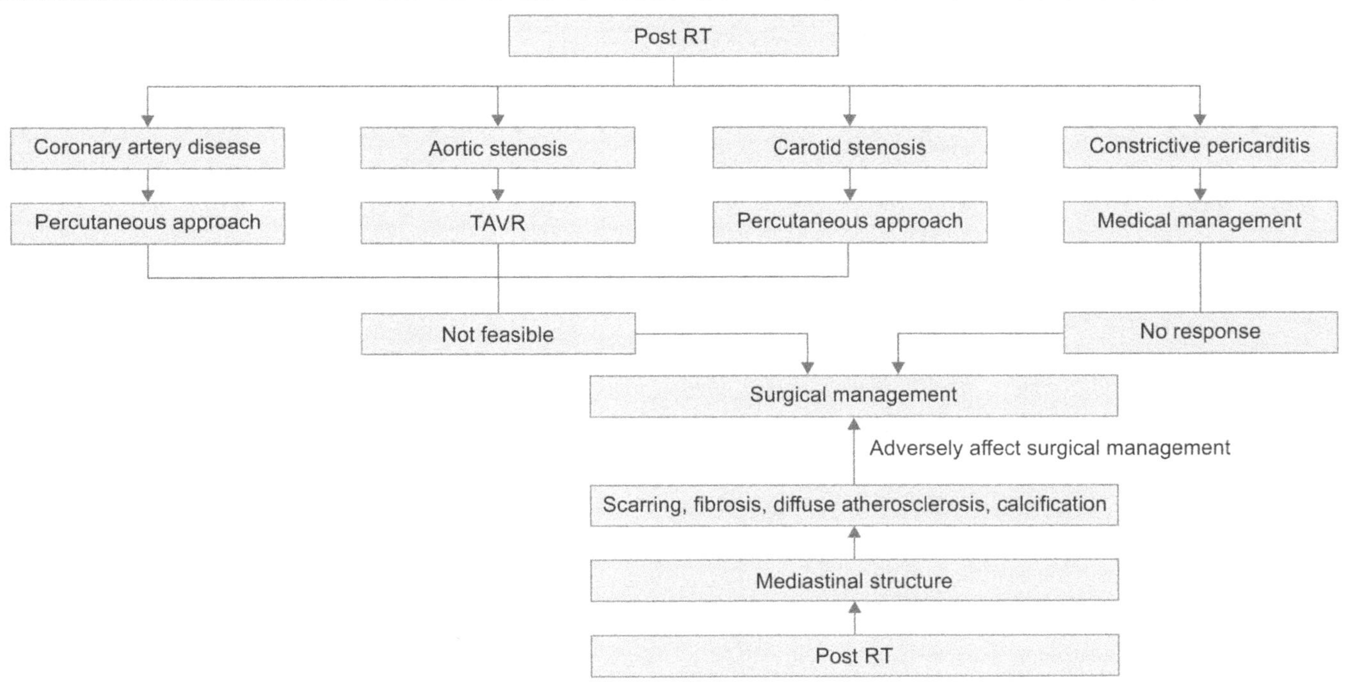

(RT: radiation therapy; TAVR: transcatheter aortic valve replacement)

REFERENCES

1. Atkins KM, Rawal B, Chaunzwa TL, Lamba N, Bitterman DS, Williams CL, et al. Cardiac radiation dose, cardiac disease, and mortality in patients with lung cancer. J Am Coll Cardiol. 2019;73:2976-87.
2. Darby SC, Ewertz M, McGale P, Bennet AM, Blom-Goldman U, Brønnum D, et al. Risk of ischemic heart disease in women after radiotherapy for breast cancer. N Engl J Med. 2013;368:987-98.
3. Tapio S. Pathology and biology of radiation-induced cardiac disease. J Radiat Res. 2016;57:439-48.
4. Mitchell JD, Cehic DA, Morgia M, Bergom C, Toohey J, Guerrero PA, et al. Cardiovascular Manifestations From Therapeutic Radiation: A Multidisciplinary Expert Consensus Statement From the International Cardio-Oncology Society. JACC: Oncology. 2021;3:360-38.

Geriatric Cardiology

CHAPTER 67

Degenerative Cardiovascular Disease

INTRODUCTION

Aging is a major risk factor for cardiovascular disease.[1] Up to 65% of older persons more than 70 years of age die due to heart disease. The cardiovascular system is affected by the aging process of degeneration at the organismal, cellular, and molecular levels, leading to degenerative cardiovascular disease (DCD) of the elderly.

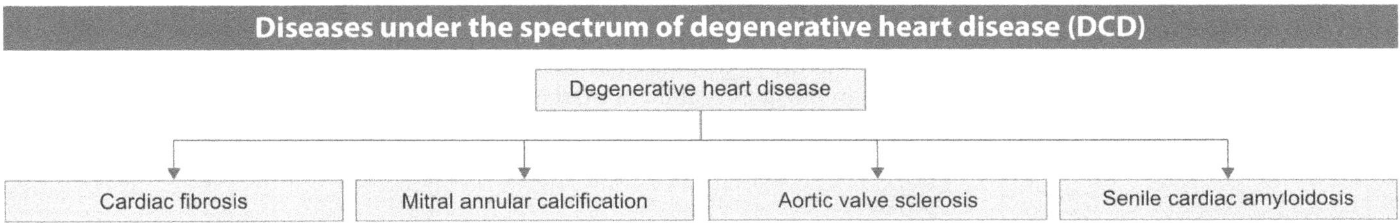

CARDIAC FIBROSIS

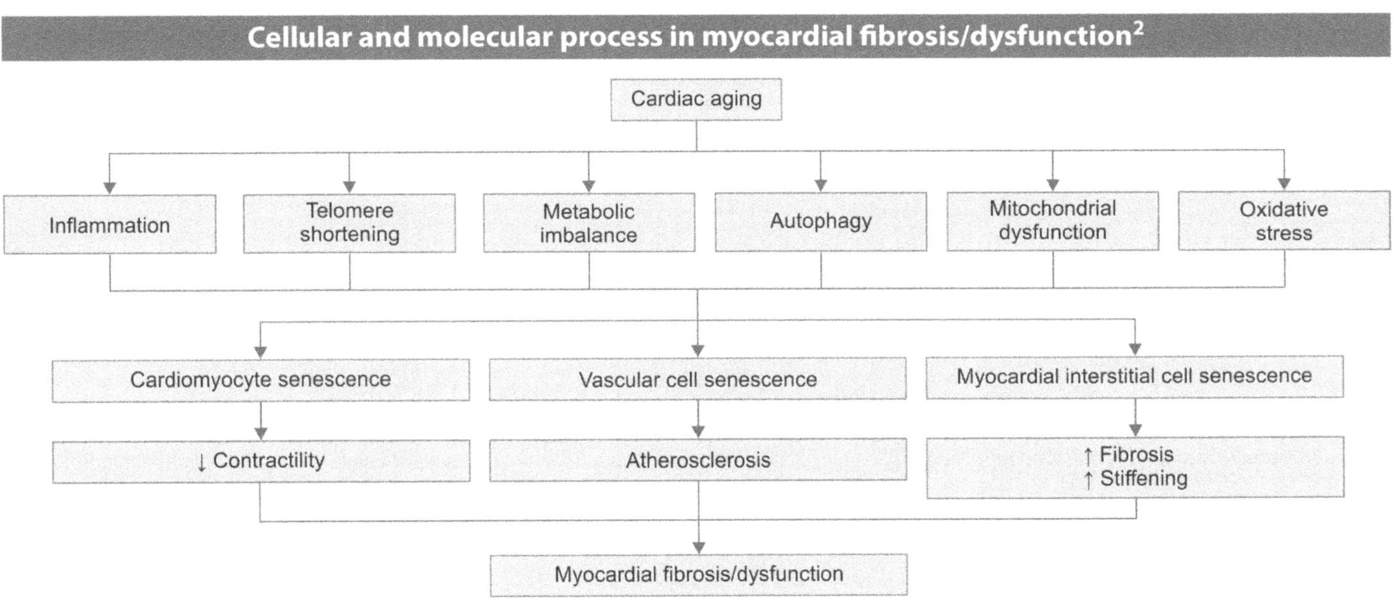

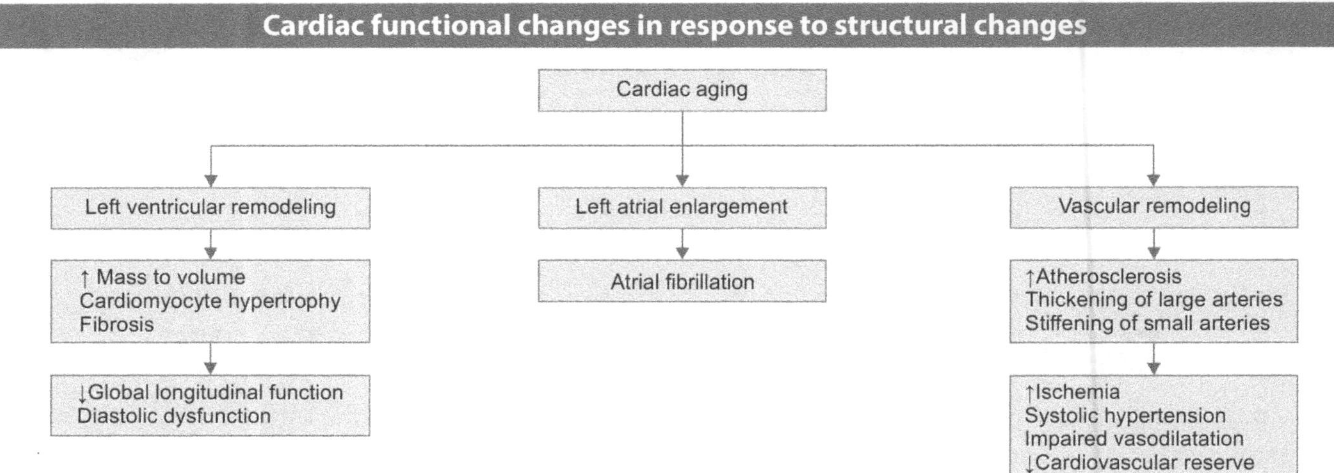

MITRAL ANNULAR CALCIFICATION

Mitral annular calcification (MAC) is defined as a DCD involving fibrous supporting structure of the mitral valve.[3] There is accumulation of calcium along the annulus, predominantly along the posterior annulus. In severe cases, calcification extends to the anterior aspect and even aortic annulus. Like calcific aortic stenosis, MAC is now considered not only as a passive degeneration but also as active process of injury, lipid deposition, inflammation, and bone formation. Its prevalence increases with age, amounting to 10% of the population and 40% in the septuagenarians. MAC is more common in women. The clinical significance of MAC lies in the facts that it is a marker of adverse events and mortality and it may be associated with mitral valve dysfunction. For every 1 mm increase in MAC, there is a 10% increased risk for cardiovascular disease, mortality, and all-cause mortality.[4]

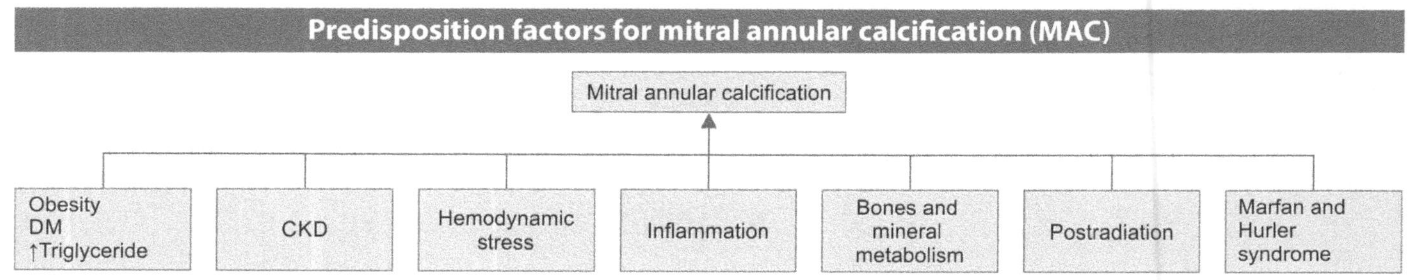

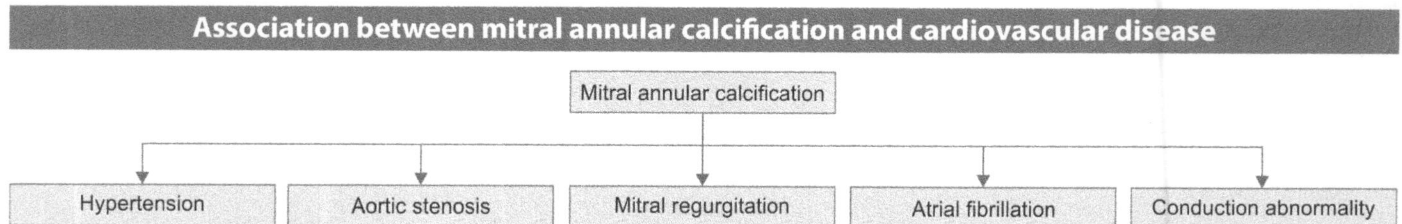

Valvular lesions due to of mitral annular calcification (MAC)[*]

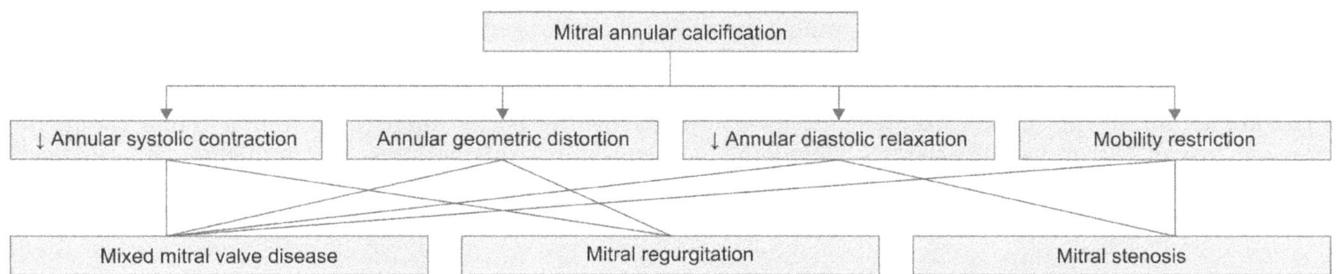

[*]In most of the cases, MAC in isolation is not responsible for valvular dysfunction. In Carpentier's series, in 93% cases, there were other pathologies for mitral valve dysfunction with MAC representing a bystander.[4]

Grading of mitral annular calcification (MAC)

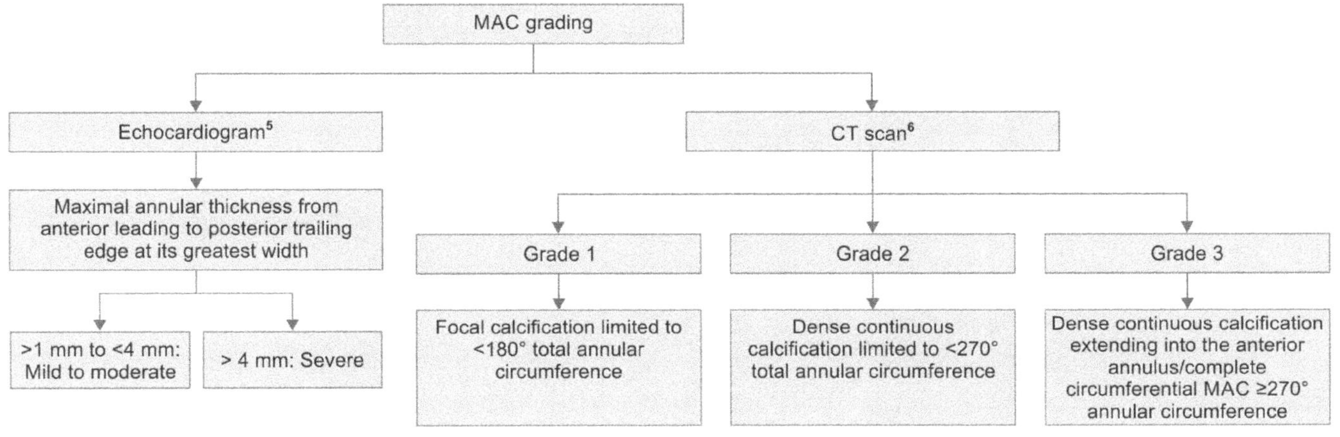

(CT: computed tomography; MAC: mitral annular calcification)

Intervention in mitral valve disease with mitral annular calcification (MAC)[7]

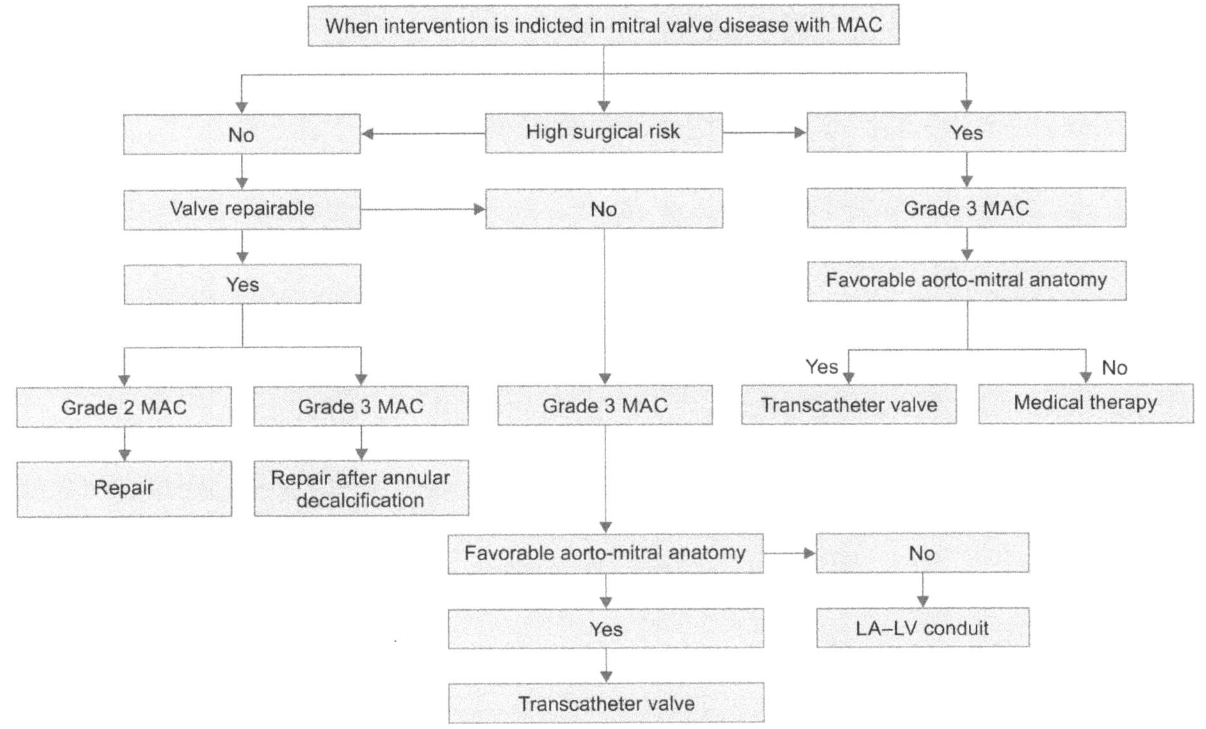

(LA: left atrial; LV: left ventricular; MAC: mitral annular calcification)

AORTIC VALVE SCLEROSIS

Aortic valve sclerosis (AVS) is an echocardiographic diagnosis, characterized by nonuniform thickening and calcification of the tricuspid aortic valve, clinically presented with a lower grade ejection systolic murmur at the aortic area. Prevalence of AVS is estimated up to 25–30% above the age of 65 years and up to 40% above the age of 75 years.[8] AVS is considered as a risk marker for all-cause and cardiovascular mortality, irrespective of age. There are common denominators in the pathophysiology of AVS and atherosclerosis, including lipid deposition, oxidative stress, inflammation, and calcification. The unique features of AVS are more intense calcium deposition and slow progression. AVS is an antecedent to clinically significant aortic stenosis. AVS progresses to significant aortic stenosis in 5.4% of patients over a period of 7 years.[9]

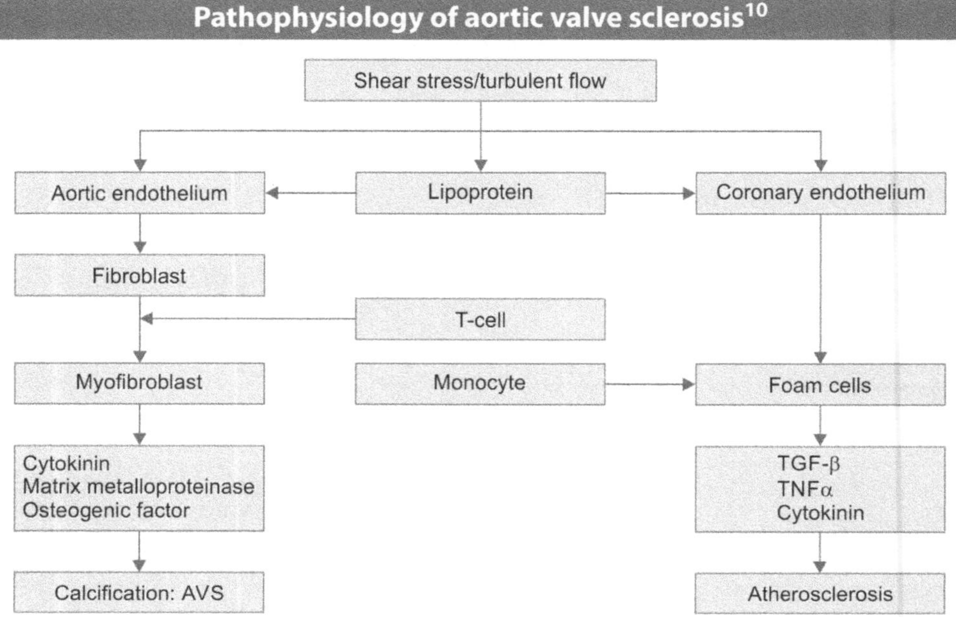

(TGF-β: transforming growth factor beta; TNFα: tumor necrosis factor alpha)

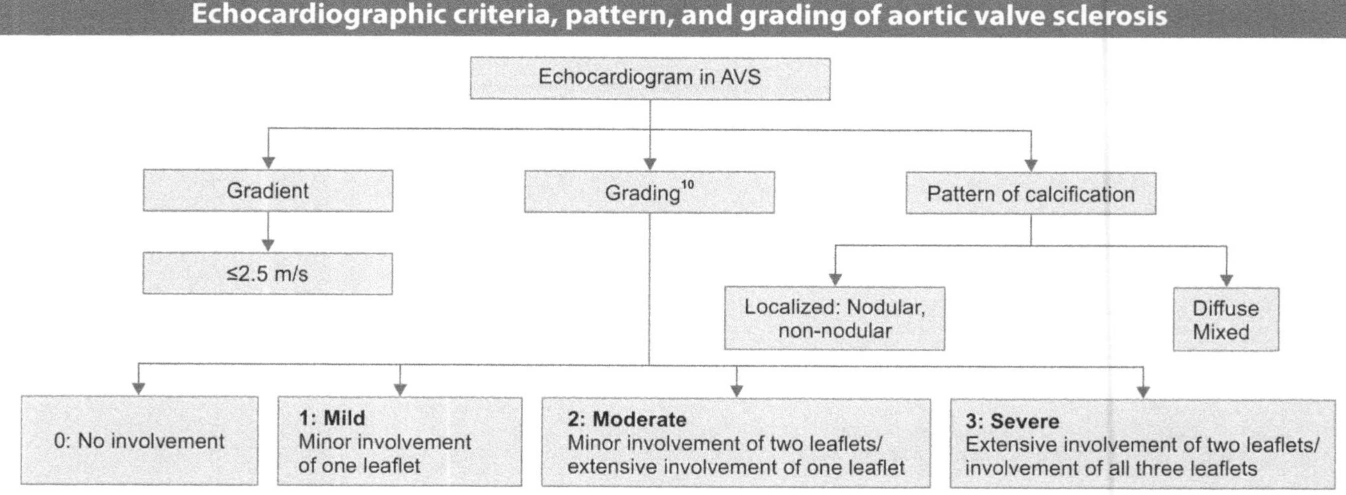

(AVS: aortic valve sclerosis)

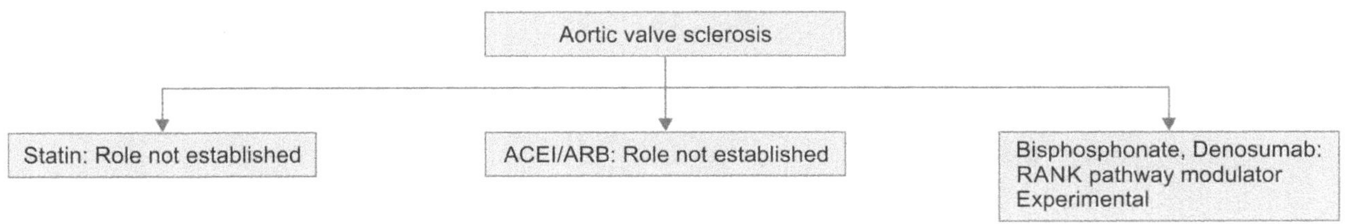

(ACEI: angiotensin-converting enzyme inhibitor; ARB: angiotensin receptor blocker; RANK: receptor activator of nuclear factor-κB)

SENILE CARDIAC AMYLOIDOSIS

Amyloidosis is a disorder characterized by a misfolded precursor protein that forms cross-β-sheet-rich amyloid fibrils extracellularly in several organs. The two most common types of amyloidosis are due to deposition of either transthyretin protein, known as transthyretin amyloid cardiomyopathy (ATTR-CM), or circulating immunoglobulin light chains, known as AL cardiomyopathy. In the nomenclature, A is used for amyloid, followed by the letter referring to the amyloid protein being deposited in the tissue. ATTR has two subtypes, according to transthyretin gene: wild-type with no mutation (ATTRwt) and hereditary with single-point mutation (ATTRm). ATTRwt is also known as senile systemic amyloidosis and is the most common type of cardiac amyloidosis. Up to 25% of persons over the age of 80 years have wild type of TTR fibril in myocardium, whereas 10% of elderly heart failure is due to ATTRwt. Median survival after the diagnosis of ATTRwt is between 43 and 67 months.[11]

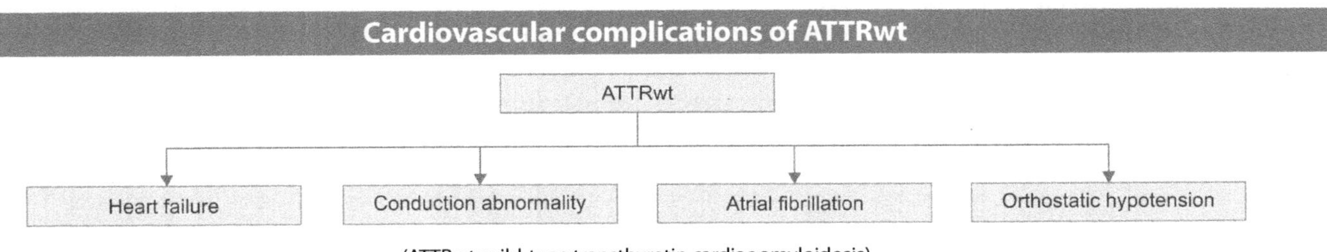

(ATTRwt: wild-type transthyretin cardiac amyloidosis)

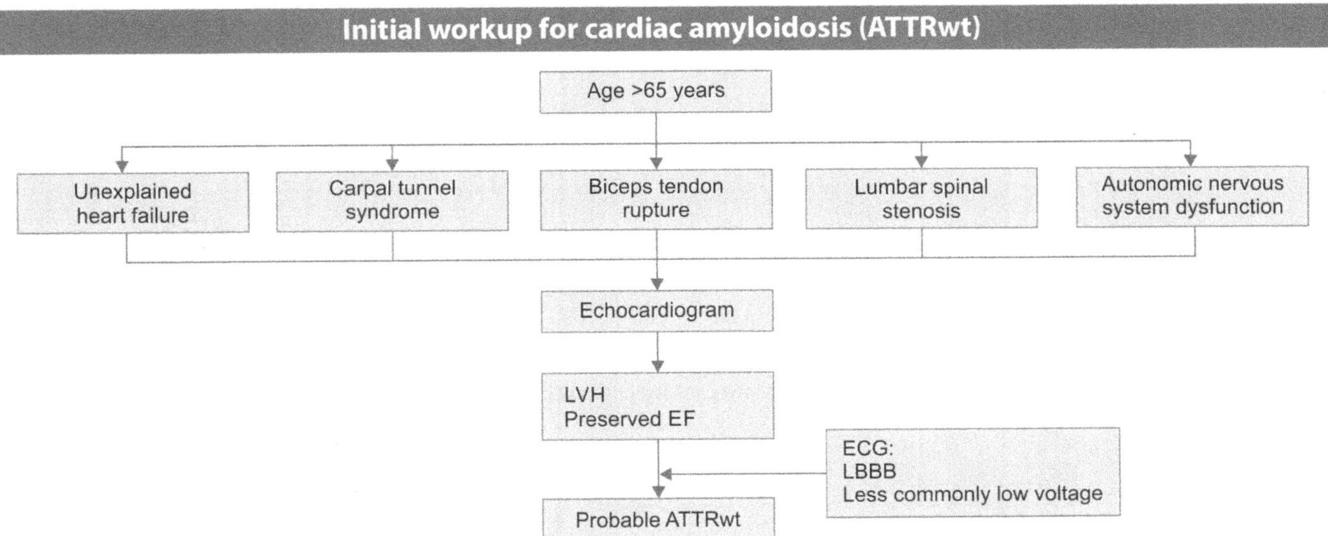

(ATTRwt: wild-type transthyretin cardiac amyloidosis; ECG: electrocardiogram; EF: ejection fraction; LBBB: left bundle branch block; LVH: left ventricular hypertrophy)

Imaging for cardiac amyloidosis (ATTRwt)

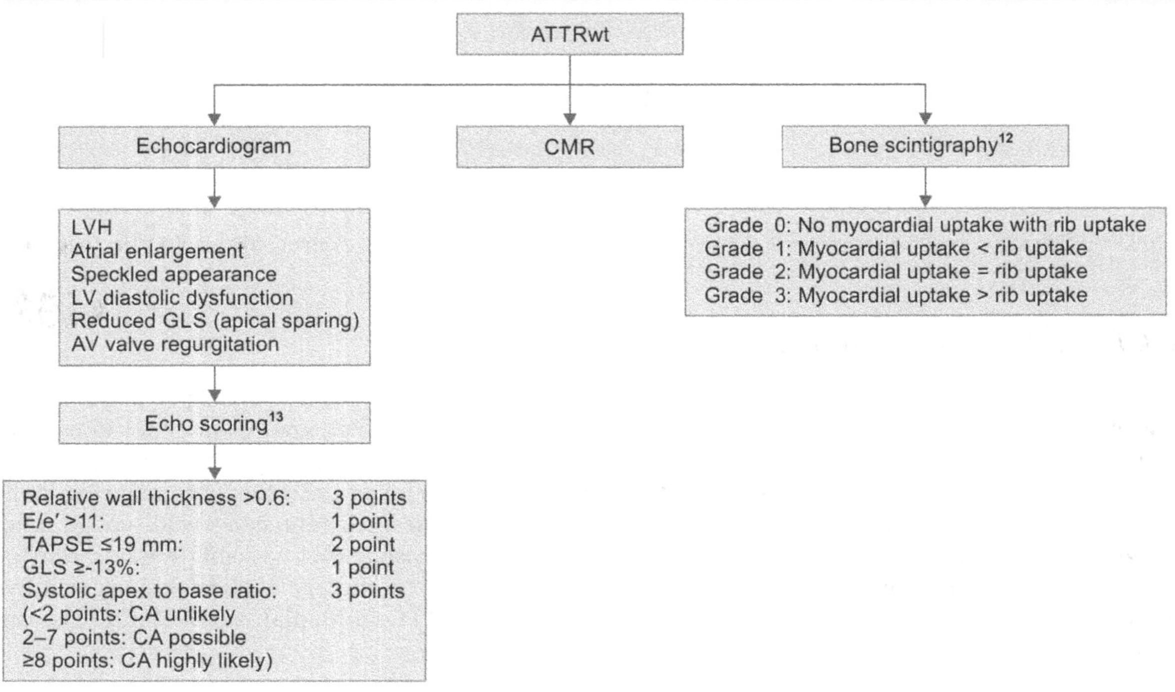

(ATTRwt: wild-type transthyretin cardiac amyloidosis; CA: cardiac amyloidosis; CMR: cardiac magnetic resonance; GLS: global longitudinal strain; TAPSE: tricuspid annular plane systolic excursion)

Confirmation of the diagnosis of cardiac amyloidosis

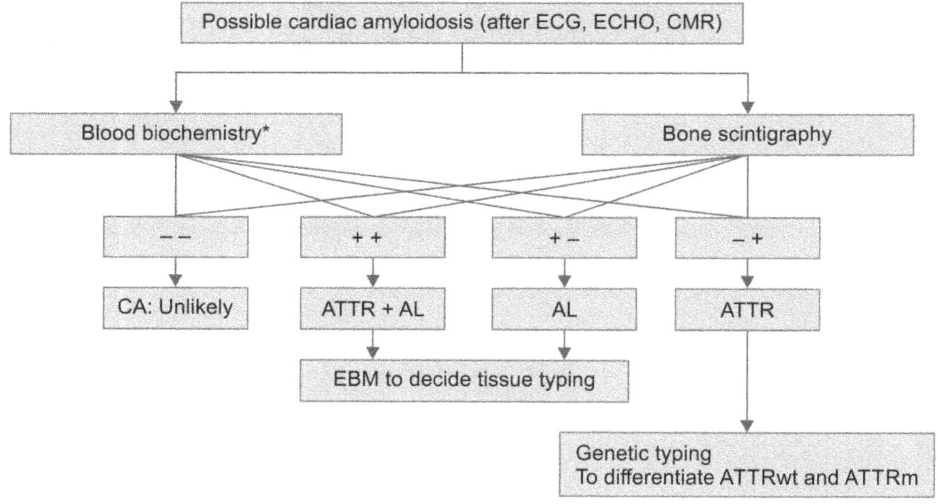

*Serum kappa/lambda free light chain ratio: Abnormal, if ratio is <0.26 or >1.65; serum or urine immunofixation electrophoresis: abnormal, if monoclonal protein is detected.
(ATTR: transthyretin amyloidosis; CA: cardiac amyloidosis; EBM: endomyocardial biopsy; ECG: electrocardiogram; ECHO: echocardiogram)

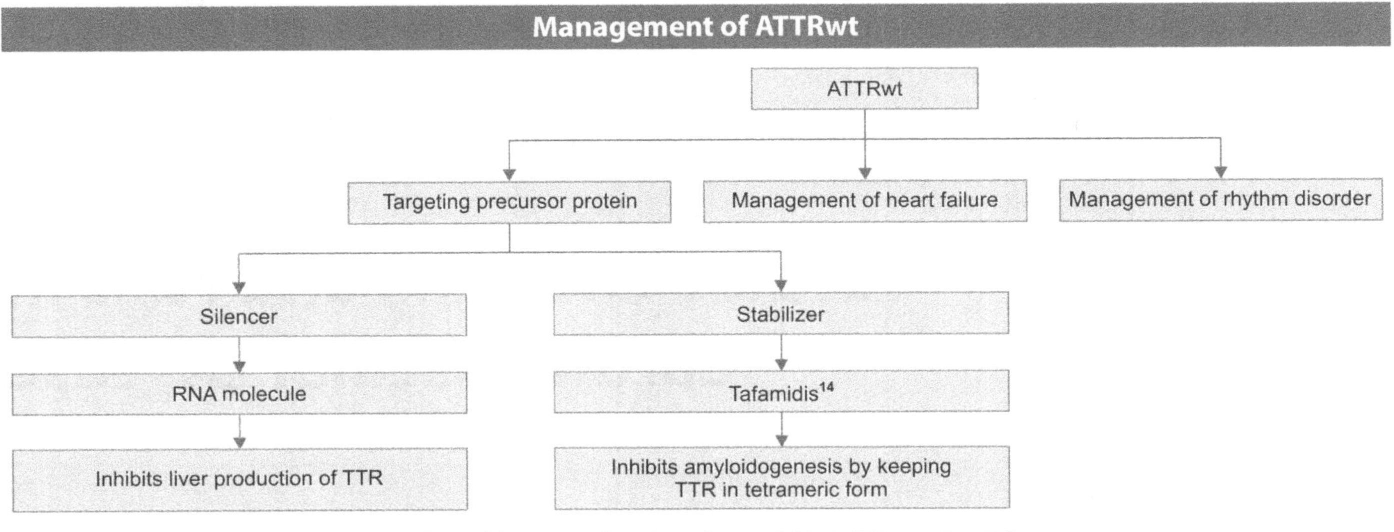

(ATTRwt: wild-type transthyretin cardiac amyloidosis; TTR: transthyretin)

REFERENCES

1. Gude NA, Broughton KM, Firouzi F, Sussman MA. Cardiac ageing: extrinsic and intrinsic factors in cellular renewal and senescence. Nat Rev Cardiol. 2018;15:523.
2. Linton PJ, Gurney M, Sengstock D, Mentzer RM Jr, Gottlieb RA. This old heart: cardiac aging and autophagy. J Mol Cell Cardiol. 2015;83:44-54.
3. Nestico PF, Depace NL, Morganroth J, Kotler MN, Ross J. Mitral annular calcification: clinical, pathophysiology, and echocardiographic review. Am Heart J. 1984;107:989-96.
4. Carpentier AF, Pellerin M, Fuzellier JF, Relland JY. Extensive calcification of the mitral valve anulus: pathology and surgical management. J Thorac Cardiovasc Surg. 1996;111:718-29; discussion 729-30.
5. Kohsaka S, Jin Z, Rundek T, Boden-Albala B, Homma S, Sacco RL, et al. Impact of mitral annular calcification o cardiovascular events in a multiethnic community: the Northern Manhattan study. JAACC cardiovascular. Imaging. 2008;1:617-23.
6. Field ME, Foley TA, Said SM, Pislaru SV, Rihal CS, et al. Severe Mitral Annular Calcification Multimodality Imaging for Therapeutic Strategies and Interventions. JAAC: Cardiovasc Imaging. 2016;9:1318-37.
7. Bedeir K, Kaneko T, Aranki S. Current and evolving strategies in the management of severe mitral annular calcification. J Thorac cardiovasc Surg. 2019;157:555-66.
8. Di Minno MND, Di Minno A, Ambrosino P, Songia P, Pepi M, Tremoli E, et al. Cardiovascular morbidity and mortality in patients with aortic valve sclerosis: a systematic review and meta-analysis. Int J Cardiol. 2018;260:138-44.
9. Cosmi JE, Kort S, Tunick PA, Rosenzweig BP, Freedberg RS, Katz ES, et al. The risk of the development of aortic stenosis in patients with "benign" aortic valve thickening. Arch Intern Med. 2002;162:2345-7.
10. Chandra HR, Goldstein JA, Choudhary N, O'Neill CS, George PB, Gangasani SR, et al. Adverse outcome in aortic sclerosis is associated with coronary artery disease and inflammation. J Am Coll Cardiol. 2004;43:169-75.
11. Witteles RM, Bokhari S, Damy T, Elliott PM, Falk RH, Fine NM, et al. Screening for transthyretin amyloid cardiomyopathy in everyday practice. JACC Heart Fail. 2019;7:709-16.
12. Gillmore JD, Maurer MS, Falk RH, Merlini G, Damy T, Dispenzieri A, et al. Nonbiopsydiagnosis of cardiac transthyretin amyloidosis. Circulation. 2016;133:2404-12.
13. Boldrini M, Cappelli F, Chacko L, Restrepo-Cordoba MA, Lopez-Sainz A, Giannoni A, et al. Multiparametric echocardiography scores for the diagnosis of cardiac amyloidosis. JACC: Cardiovascular Imaging. 2020;13:909-20.
14. Maurer MS, Schwartz JH, Gundapaneni B, Waddington-Cruz M, Kristen AV, Grogan M, et al. Tafamidis Treatment for Patients with Transthyretin Amyloid Cardiomyopathy. N Engl J Med. 2018;379:1007-16.

CHAPTER 68

Cardiac Cachexia and Falls in Cardiovascular Disease

CARDIAC CACHEXIA

Cardiac cachexia is a syndrome characterized by progressive loss of skeletal muscle and fat in patients with heart failure. It is often associated with increase in inflammation, insulin resistance, and anorexia. Cardiac cachexia is associated with increased mortality independent of functional status or ejection fraction. Cardiac cachexia is defined as unintentional weight loss >7.5% of dry body weight over at least 6-month period in the absence of any underlying cause.[1] Sarcopenia, frailty, and cardiac cachexia are three different forms of presentation of heart failure with a prevalence of 20%, 20–50%, and 15%, respectively.

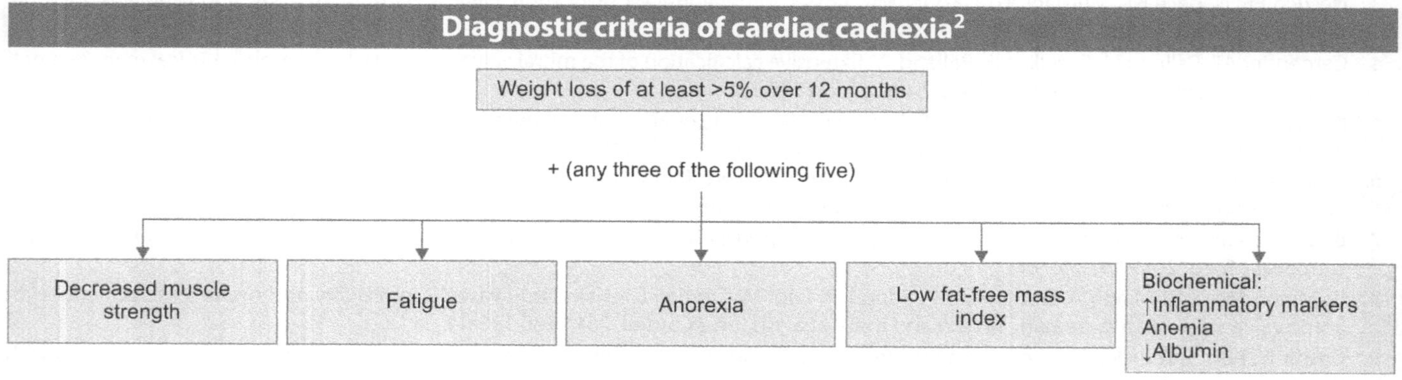

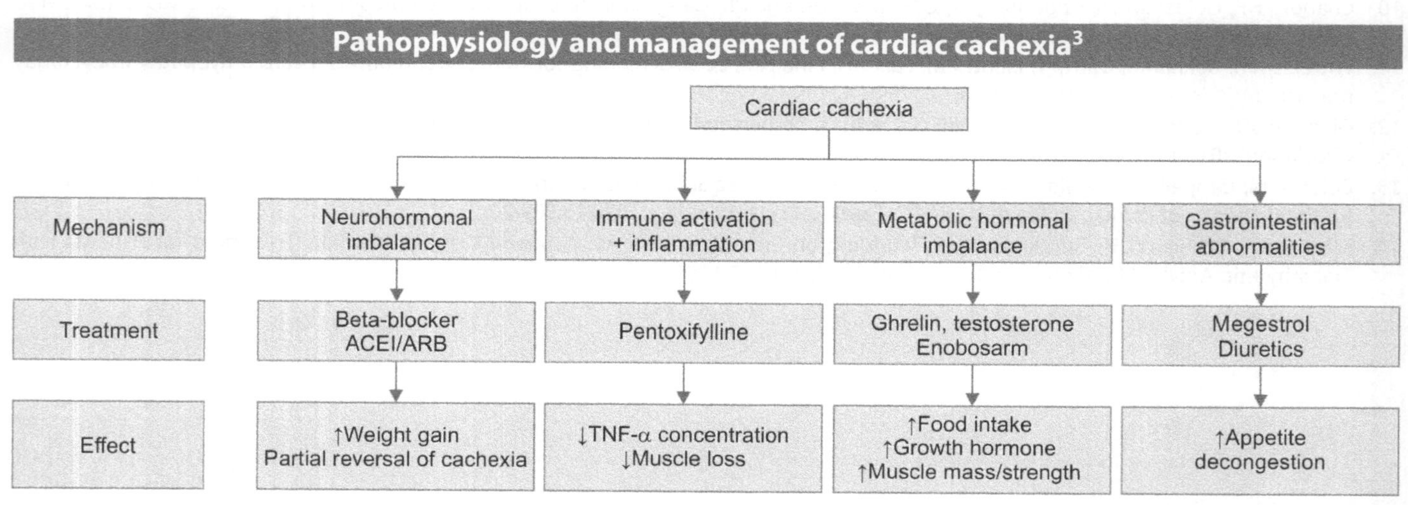

(ACEI: angiotensin-converting enzyme inhibitor; ARB: angiotensin receptor blocker; TNF-α: tumor necrosis factor-α)

FALLS AND CARDIOVASCULAR DISEASES

Falls are the world's second leading cause of accidental death. In a large series of falls,[4] 41% were accidental, 22% were due to medical causes, 19% were due to cognitive impairment, and 15% were unexplained. Falls are one of the common presentations of older persons, and 32% of all community-dwelling older persons fall every year. One-third of older persons fall every year and half of them are recurrent fallers, the criterion of which is falls two or more times per year. One of the most common presentations of sarcopenia and frailty is fall, which confers further limitation of physical activity of a person leading to enhancement of both sarcopenia and frailty.

Falls and syncope are both common in older patients and are often indistinguishable. Up to 30% of patients with loss of consciousness (LOC) have retrograde amnesia for LOC. Nearly 70% of patients with orthostatic hypotension presenting with falls deny LOC. As per guideline, unexplained fall should be treated as unexplained syncope.[5]

Treating cardiovascular disease alone does not prevent falls, the mechanism of which is multifactorial.

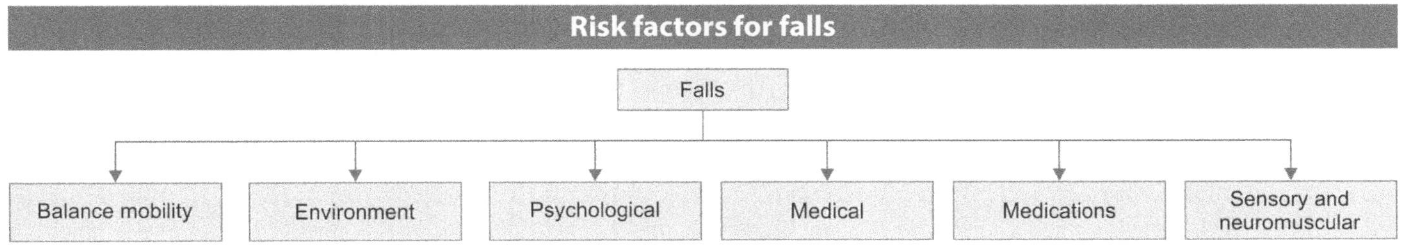

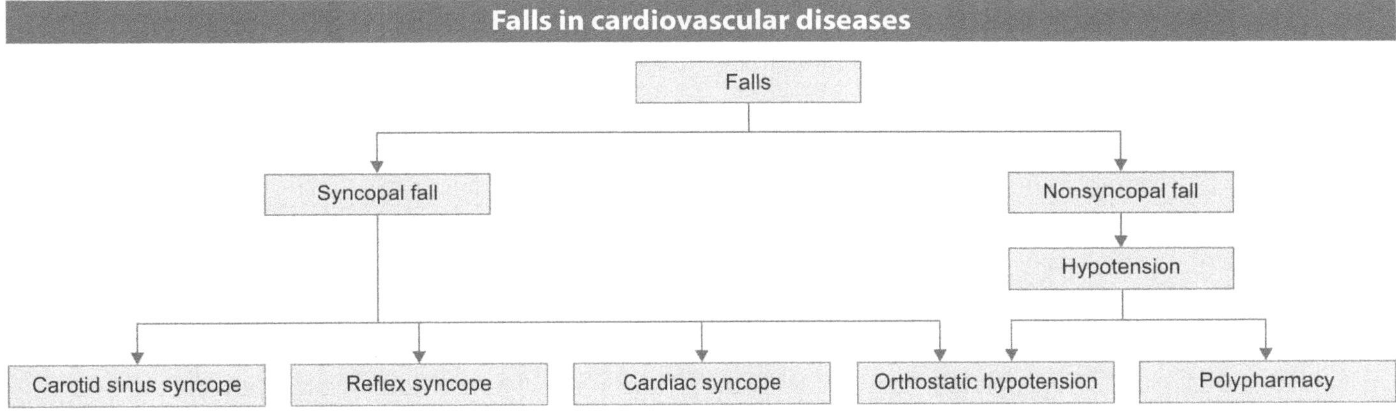

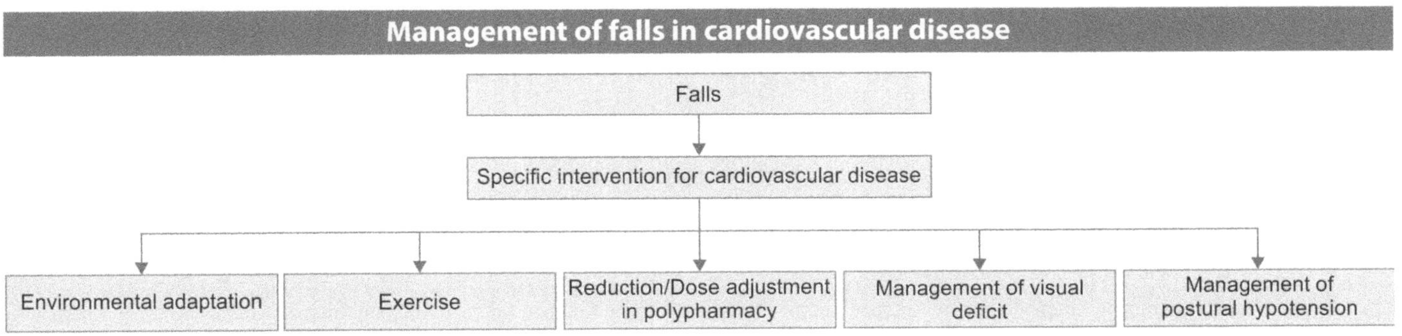

REFERENCES

1. Anker SD, Chua TP, Ponikowski P, Harrington D, Swan JW, Kox WJ, et al. Hormonal changes and catabolic/anabolic imbalance in chronic heart failure and their im- portance for cardiac cachexia. Circulation. 1997;96(2):526-34.
2. Evans WJ, Morley JE, Argilés J, Bales C, Baracos V, Guttridge D, et al. Cachexia: a new definition. Clin Nutr. 2008;27(6):793-9.
3. Rolfe M, Kamel A, Ahmed MM, Kramer J. Pharmacological management of cardiac cachexia: a review of potential therapy options. Heart Fail Rev. 2019;24(5):617-23.
4. Richardson DA, Bexton RS, Shaw FE, et al. Prevalence of cardioinhibitory carotid sinus hypersensitivity in patients 50 years or over presenting to the Accident and Emergency department with "unexplained" or "recurrent" falls. PACE. 1997;20:820-3.
5. Brignole M, Moya A, De Lange FJ, Deharo JC, Elliot PM, Fanciulli A, et al. 2018 ESC Guidelines for the di- agnosis and management of syncope. Eur Heart J. 2018;39:1883-948.

CHAPTER 69

Sarcopenia, Frailty, and Cardiovascular Disease

INTRODUCTION

Aging is a normal phenomenon and is accompanied by catabolism and degeneration of organs and their functions. The demographic shift with its enormous increase in the average age of population has led to evolution of a new branch of medicine, geriatric medicine, and one of its major subbranch of geriatric cardiology. Sarcopenia and frailty syndrome are the two most impressive expressions of aging. Sarcopenia can be described as a phenotype of physical frailty. It is twice as common as frailty, and it may lead to frailty. Over the age of 50 years, muscle mass starts declining by 1–2% per year, increasing 3% above the age of 60 years. The prevalence of sarcopenia above the age of 80 years is 11–50%.[1]

Frailty is three times more prevalent in older persons with heart disease as compared to those without heart disease. Frailty is 20% more common in older patients undergoing percutaneous coronary intervention (PCI) and is an independent predictor of mortality. Frailty is also a marker of morbidity and mortality in older patients who referred for coronary artery bypass graft (CABG) or transcatheter aortic valve replacement (TAVR).

Older patients with heart failure are sixfold more likely to be frail. At the same time, frail older persons have more chance of development of heart failure. Frailty confers more mortality and chance of hospitalization in older patients. Inflammation, metabolic, and autonomic abnormalities associated with heart failure lead to frailty.

SARCOPENIA

Sarcopenia, Greek meaning loss of flesh, has been defined as "a progressive and generalized skeletal muscle disorder that is associated with increased likelihood of adverse outcomes including falls, fracture, physical disability and mortality."[2] The importance of sarcopenia lies in the fact that it causes significant morbidity and mortality in middle-aged and older people.

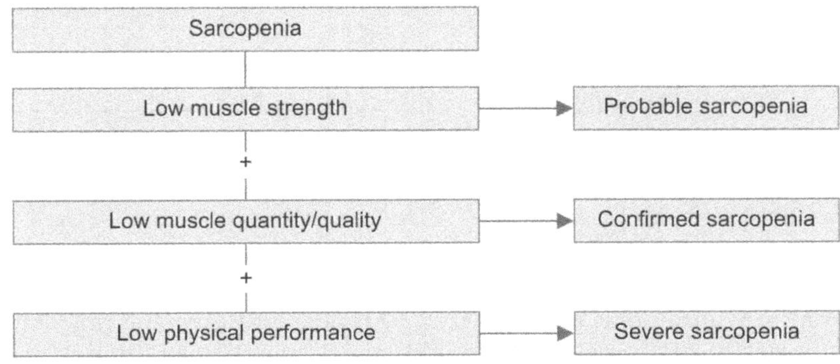

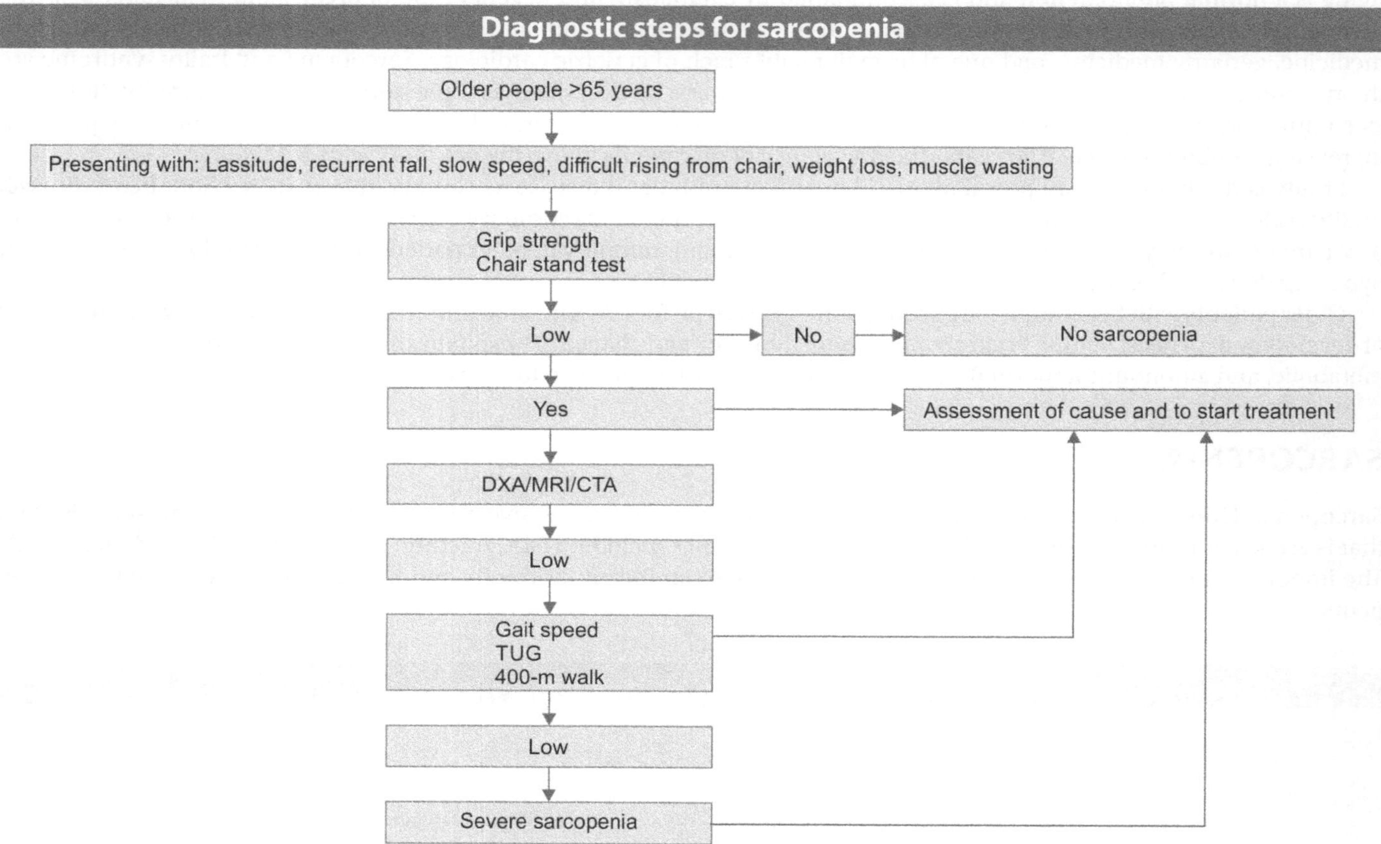

Note: Grip strength is measured by hand-held dynamometer; chair stand test measures the amount of time needed for a patient to rise 5 times from a seated position without using arm support; ASM mass is measured by dual-energy X-ray absorptiometry/MRI/CT scan; gait speed test is 4 m usual walking speed test; TUG patient is asked to rise from a chair, walk 3 m away, turn around, walk back, and sit again.

(ASM: appendicular skeletal muscle; TUG: timed-up and go test)

(CTA: computed tomography angiography; DXA: dual energy X-ray absorptiometry; MRI: magnetic resonance imaging; TUG: timed-up and go test)

FRAILTY SYNDROME

The frailty syndrome, a geriatric syndrome, is characterized by reduced reserve and reactivity to internal and external stressors physically, psychologically, and socially. The syndrome, a dynamic condition which may worsen or improve over time, is associated with increased morbidity, disability, and mortality.

Frailty screening questionnaires

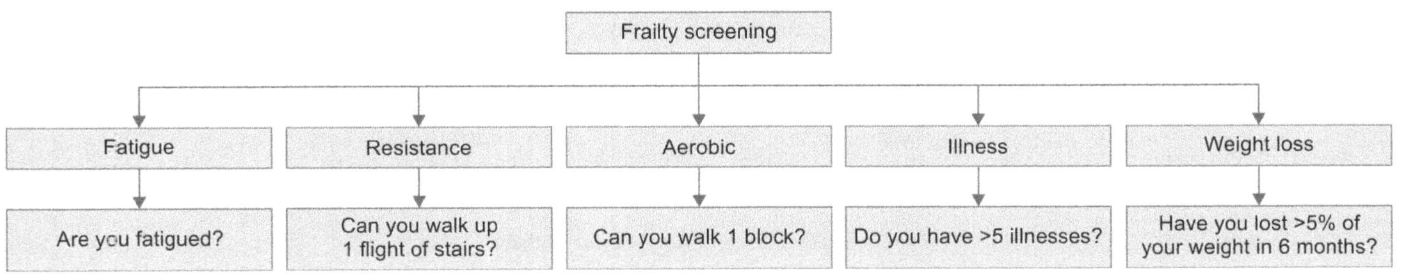

Note: 1 or 2: Prefrail; ≥3: frailty syndrome.

Frailty scoring parameters

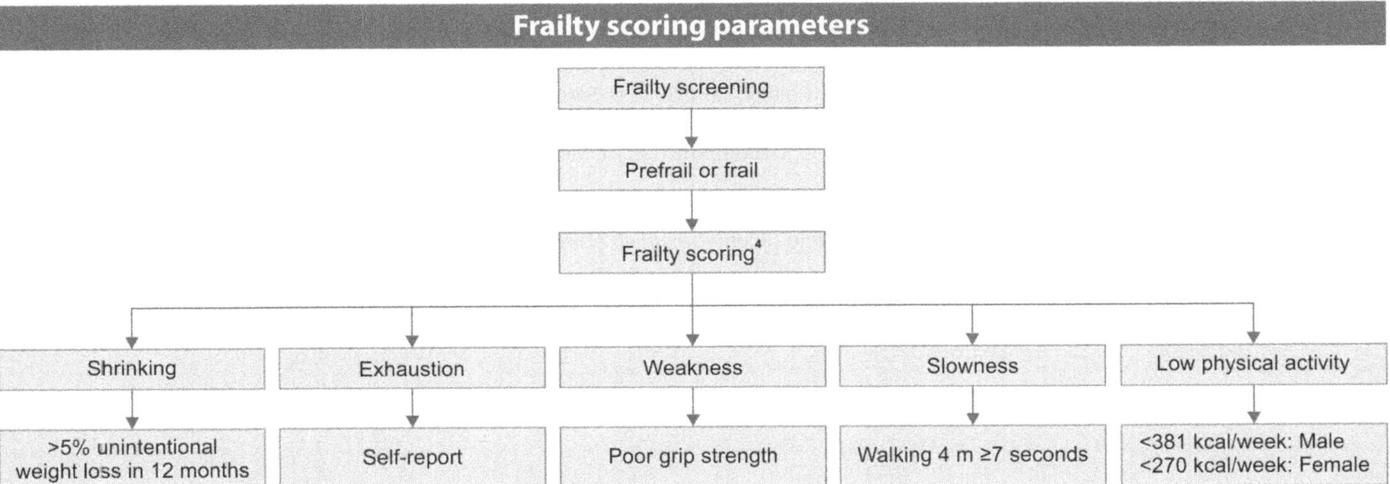

Note: 1 or 2: prefrail; ≥3: frailty syndrome

Pathophysiology of sarcopenia and frailty

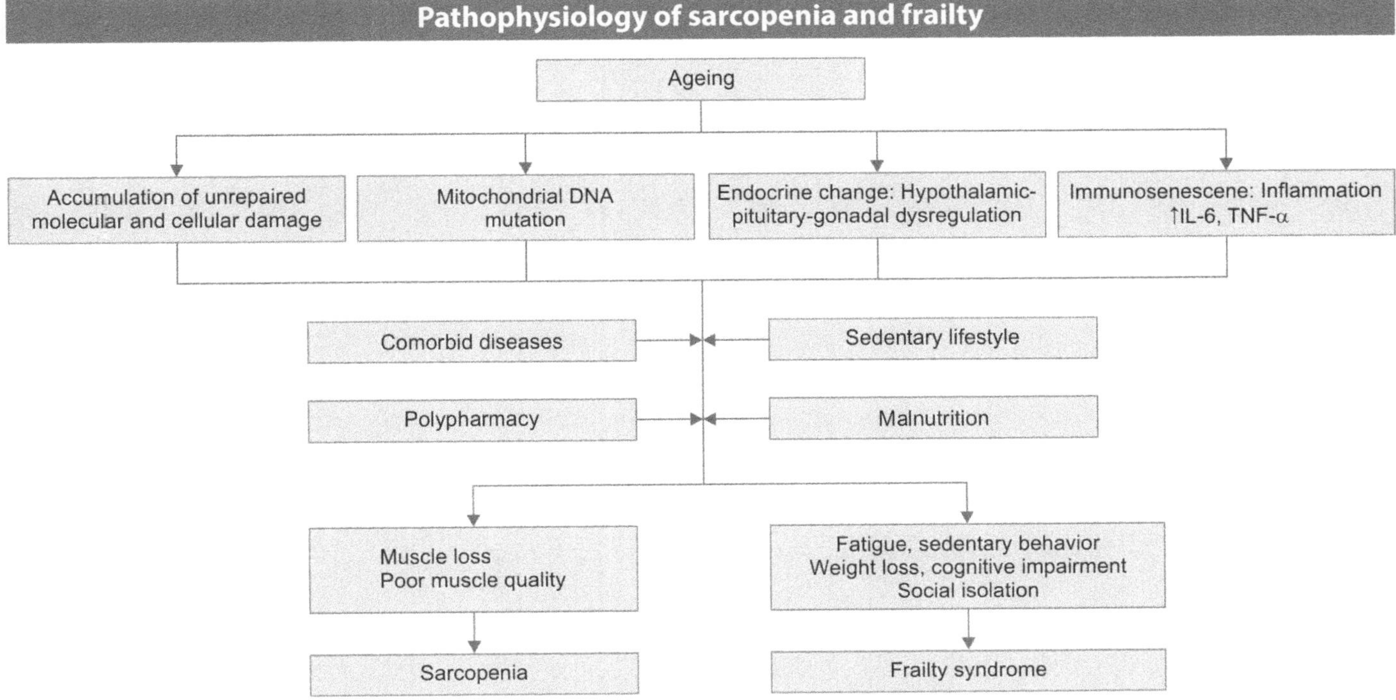

(DNA: deoxyribonucleic acid; TNF-α: tumour necrosis factor-alpha)

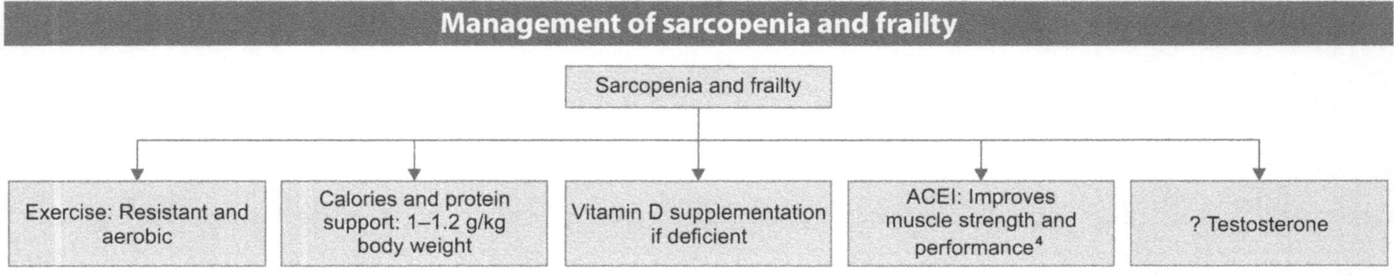

(ACEI: angiotensin-converting enzyme inhibitor)

REFERENCES

1. von Haehling S, Morley JE, Anker SD. An overview of sar- copenia: facts and numbers on prevalence and clinical impact. J Cachexia Sarcopenia Muscle. 2010;1:129-33.
2. Cruz-Jentoft AJ, Baeyens JP, Bauer JM, Boirie Y, Cederholm T, Landi F, et al. Sarcopenia: European consensus on dentition and diagnosis: report of the European working group on sarcopenia in older people. Age Ageing. 2010;39:412-23.
3. Cruz-Zentoft AJ, Bahat G, Bayur J, Boirie Y, Bruyère O, Cederholm T, et al. Sarcopenia: revised European consensus on definition and diagnosis. Age Ageing. 2019;48:16-31.
4. Onder G, Penninx BW, Balkrishnan R, Fried LP, Chaves PH, Williamson J, et al. Relation between use of angiotensin-converting enzyme inhibitors and muscle strength and physical function in older women: an observational study. Lancet. 2002;359:926-30.

Sport Cardiology

CHAPTER 70

Sport Cardiology and Athlete's Heart

INTRODUCTION

An athlete has been defined as "one who participates in an organized team or individual sport that requires competition against others as a central component, places a high premium on excellence and achievement, and requires some form of systematic (and usually intense) training."[1] Methodical systemic training leads to electrical, structural, and functional adaptation of the heart. This adapted heart is referred to as athlete's heart. In certain athlete's heart, this adaptation goes beyond normal variance, which is responsible for exercise-induced sudden cardiac death (SCD). Sporting discipline, sex, and race affect the grade of adaptation. Endurance training such as running or cycling causes a much more vigorous modulation than caused by static exercise such as strength exercise. Exercise has different effects on heart in male versus female and black versus white people.

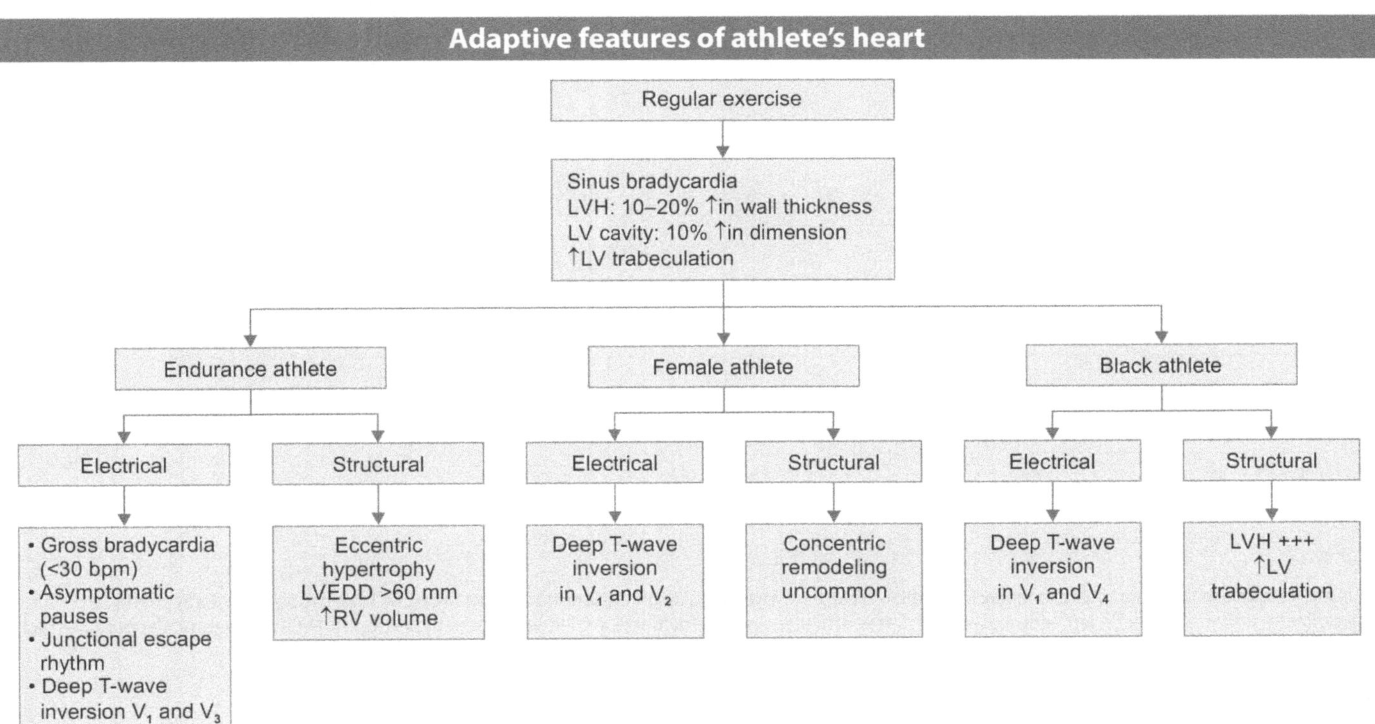

(LV: left ventricular; LVEDD: left ventricular end-diastolic dimension; LVH: left ventricular hypertrophy; RV: right ventricular)

Electrical remodeling in athlete's heart[2,3]

ECG changes

- Type 1 ECG (training related)
- Type 2 ECG (training unrelated)
  - Major
  - Minor

Type 1 ECG (training related):
Sinus bradycardia
Sinus arrhythmia
1st-degree AV block
Incomplete RBBB
Early repolarization
LVH/RVH
T-wave inversion
V_1 and V_4 associated with J-point elevation

Major:
T-wave inversion beyond V_4
ST depression
Pathological Q wave
Complete RBBB/LBBB
Pre-excitation
Long/short QT syndrome
Brugada syndrome-like ST elevation

Minor:
Left-axis deviation
Right axis deviation
Atrial enlargement

(AV: atrioventricular; ECG: electrocardiogram; LBBB: left bundle branch block; LVH: left ventricular hypertrophy; RBBB: right bundle branch block; RVH: right ventricular hypertrophy)

Structural remodeling in athlete's heart

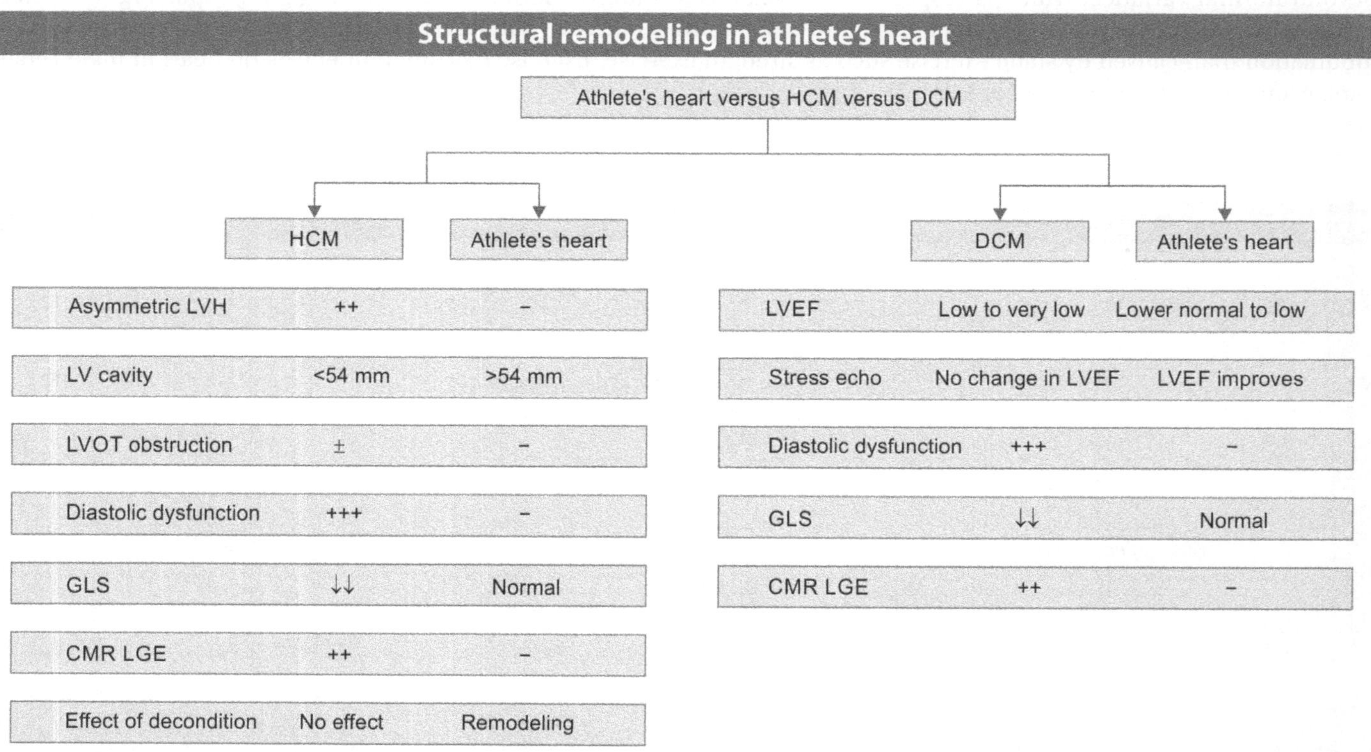

Athlete's heart versus HCM versus DCM

	HCM	Athlete's heart
Asymmetric LVH	++	–
LV cavity	<54 mm	>54 mm
LVOT obstruction	±	–
Diastolic dysfunction	+++	–
GLS	↓↓	Normal
CMR LGE	++	–
Effect of decondition	No effect	Remodeling

	DCM	Athlete's heart
LVEF	Low to very low	Lower normal to low
Stress echo	No change in LVEF	LVEF improves
Diastolic dysfunction	+++	–
GLS	↓↓	Normal
CMR LGE	++	–

(CMR: cardiovascular magnetic resonance; DCM: dilated cardiomyopathy; GLS: global longitudinal strain; HCM: hypertrophic cardiomyopathy; LGE: late gadolinium enhancement; LV: left ventricular; LVEF: left ventricular ejection fraction; LVH: left ventricular hypertrophy; LVOT: left ventricular outflow tract)

REFERENCES

1. Maron BJ, Douglas PS, Graham TP, Nishimura RA, Thompson PD. Task Force 1: Preparticipation screening and diagnosis of cardiovascular disease in athletes. J Am Coll Cardiol. 2005;45(8):1322-6.
2. Corrado D, Pelliccia A, Heidbuchel H, Sharma S, Link M, Basso C, et al. Recommendations for interpretation of 12-lead electrocardiogram in the athlete. Eur Heart J. 2010;31:243-59.
3. Corrado D, Calore C, Zorzi A, Migliore F. Improving the interpretation of the athlete's electrocardiogram. Eur Heart J. 2013;34:3600-9.

CHAPTER 71

Sudden Cardiac Death in Athlete

INTRODUCTION

Exercise is considered as good for overall health. Many of the epidemiological studies have shown the link between aerobic exercise and risk reduction for atherosclerotic heart disease. However, in a very small number of athletes, more specifically in younger athletes, exercise may cause sudden cardiac death (SCD) known as exercise paradox. The incidence of SCD in an athlete varies widely, ranging from 1 in 40,000 to 1 in 80,000.[1] The wide variability is due to different definitions of SCD: death during exertion or shortly (<1 hour) after exertion versus any sudden death in athlete during or outside exertion. A large autopsy database from the National College Athletic Association (NCCA) spanning from 2003 to 2013 showed that the most common cause of underlying disease was primary electrical disorders in 25% of cases, coronary artery anomalies in 11% of cases, and hypertrophic cardiomyopathy in 8% of cases.[2] The incidence of SCD is highest in male gender, black race, and basketball players.

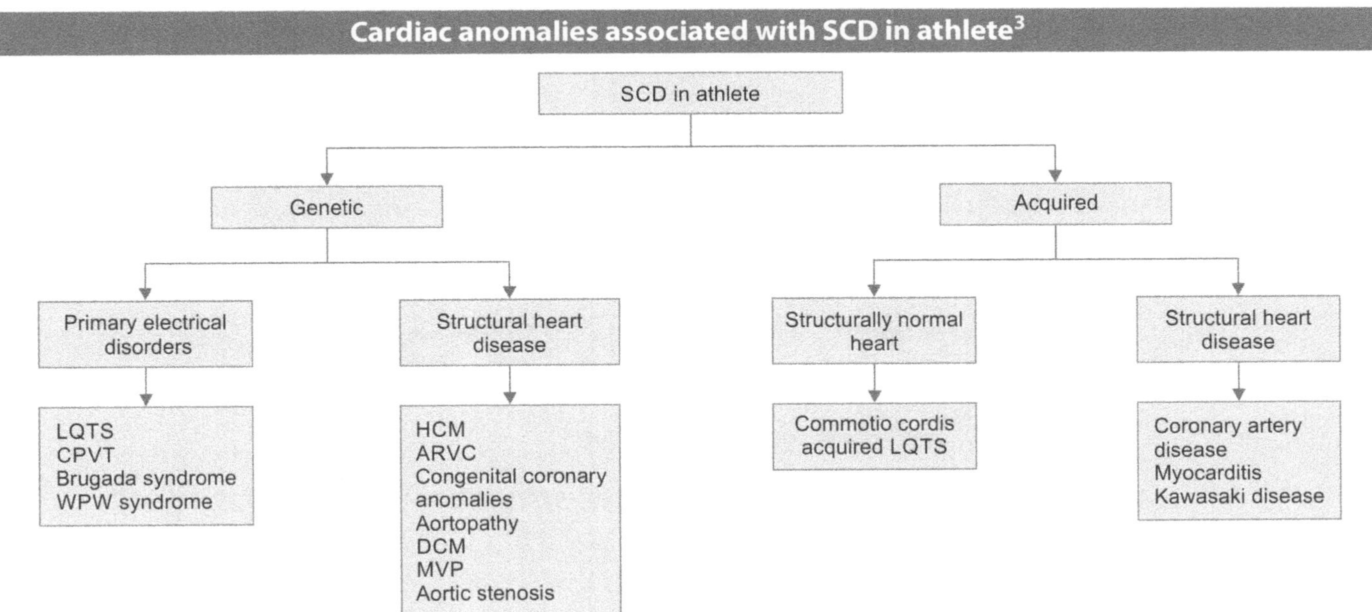

(ARVC: arrhythmogenic right ventricular cardiomyopathy; CPVT: catecholaminergic polymorphic ventricular tachycardia; DCM: dilated cardiomyopathy; HCM: hypertrophic cardiomyopathy; LQTS: long QT syndrome; MVP: mitral valve prolapse; SCD: sudden cardiac death; WPW: Wolff–Parkinson–White)

Mechanism of SCD on strenuous activity in athlete with underlying cardiac disease

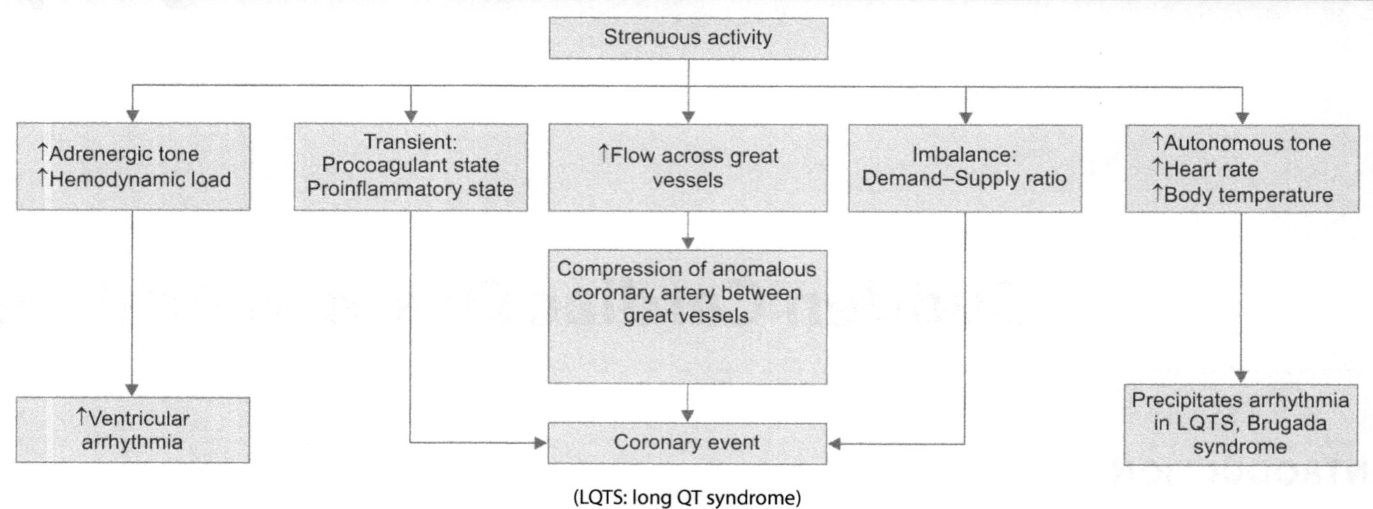

(LQTS: long QT syndrome)

Preparticipation screening for athletes[4]

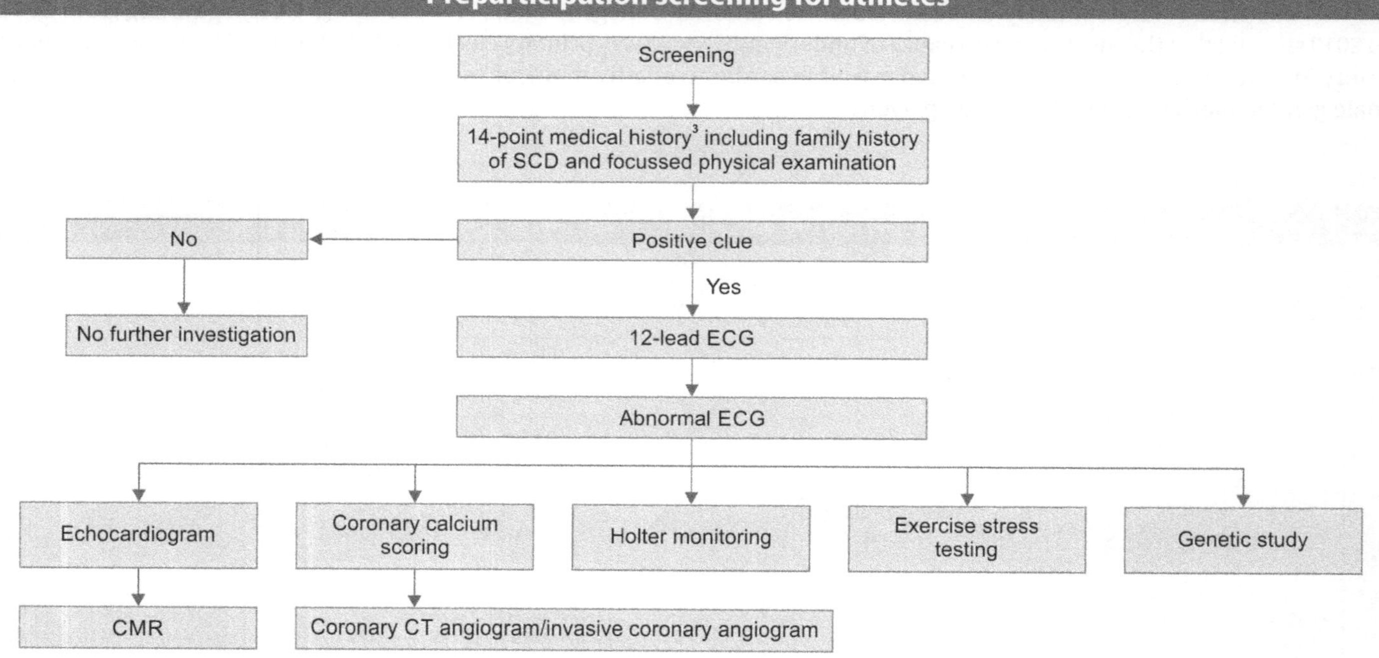

(CMR: cardiovascular magnetic resonance; ECG: electrocardiogram)

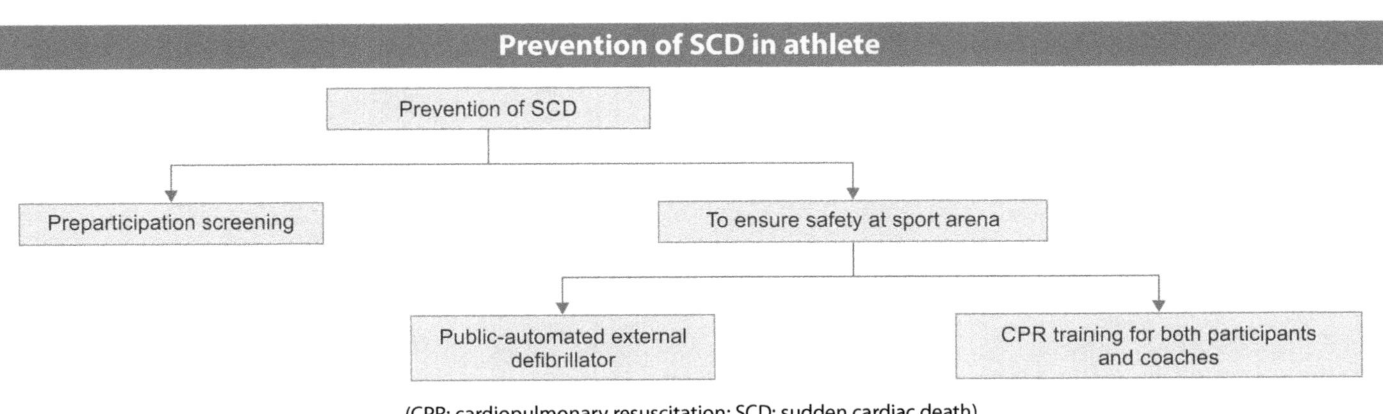

(AV: atrioventricular; ECG: electrocardiogram; LBBB: left bundle branch block; RBBB: right bundle branch block; RVH: right ventricular hypertrophy)

(CPR: cardiopulmonary resuscitation; SCD: sudden cardiac death)

REFERENCES

1. Harmon KG, Drezner JA, Wilson MG, Sharma S. Incidence of sudden cardiac death inathletes: a state-of-the-art review. Br J Sports Med. 2014;48(15):1185-92.

2. Harmon KG, Asif IM, Maleszewski JJ, Owens DS, Prutkin JM, Salerno JC, et al. Incidence, Cause, and Comparative Frequency of Sudden Cardiac Death in National Collegiate Athletic Association Athletes: A Decade in Review. Circulation. 2015;132(1):10-9.

3. Maron BJ, Thompson PD, Ackerman MJ, Balady G, Berger S, Cohen D, et al. American Heart Association Council on Nutrition, Physical Activity, and Metabolism. Recommendations and considerations related to preparticipation screening for cardiovascular abnormalities in competitive athletes: 2007 update: a scientific statement from the American Heart Association Council on Nutrition, Physical Activity, and Metabolism: endorsed by the American College of Cardiology Foundation. Circulation. 2007 Mar 27;115(12):1643-455.

4. Corrado D, Pelliccia A, Bjørnstad HH, Vanhees L, Biffi A, Borjesson M, et al. Study Group of Sport Cardiology of the Working Group of Cardiac Rehabilitation and Exercise Physiology and the Working Group of Myocardial and Pericardial Diseases of the European Society of Cardiology. Cardiovascular pre-participation screening of young competitive athletes for prevention of sudden death: proposal for a common European protocol. Consensus Statement of the Study Group of Sport Cardiology of the Working Group of Cardiac Rehabilitation and Exercise Physiology and the Working Group of Myocardial and Pericardial Diseases of the European Society of Cardiology. Eur Heart J. 2005;26(5):516-24.

Acute Vascular Syndrome

CHAPTER 72

Acute Pulmonary Embolism: General Approach

INTRODUCTION

Pulmonary embolism and deep vein thrombosis (DVT) are the two presentations of venous thromboembolism (VTE), which is the third most common cause of mortality among the three thrombotic conditions, after myocardial infarction and ischemic stroke. The incidence of VTE is overall 1–3 per 1,000 persons annually with a recurrence rate of 25% in 5 years and a 30-day case fatality rate of 5–10%.

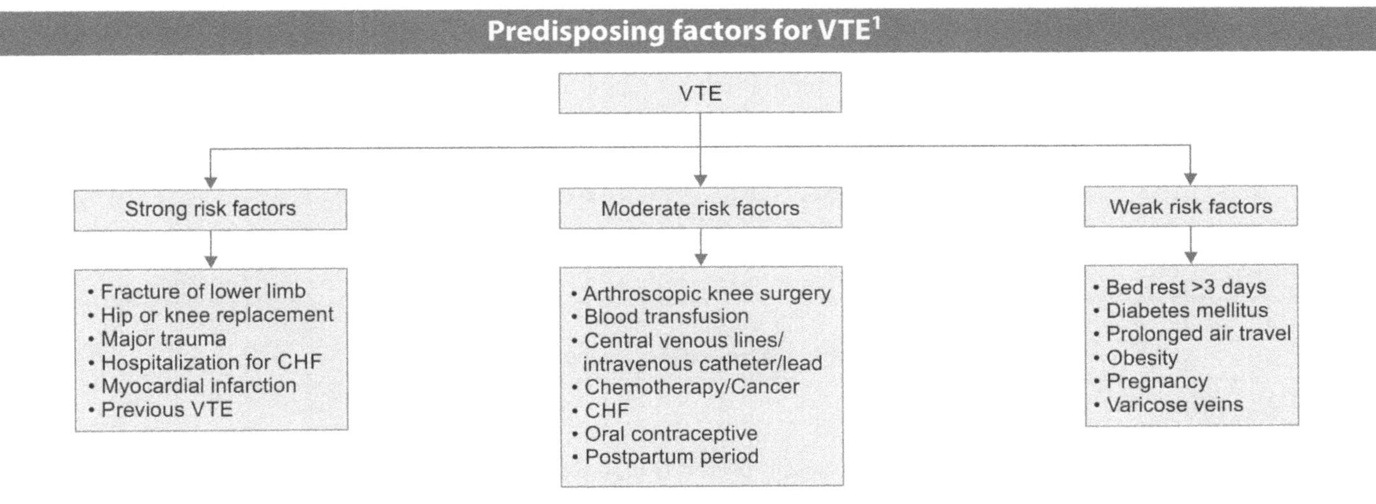

Wells clinical model to assess deep vein thrombosis (DVT)

DVT

1 point each:	1 point each:	1 point each:	−2 point:
Cancer Immobilization of lower limb Recently bedridden	Tenderness along deep veins Entire leg swollen Calf swelling >3 cm than other leg	Pitting edema Collateral nonvaricose superficial veins	Alternate diagnosis more probable

Note: Clinical probability: High: ≥3, moderate: 1–2 , low: ≤1.
(DVT: deep vein thrombosis)

Revised Geneva clinical model to assess acute pulmonary embolism[2]

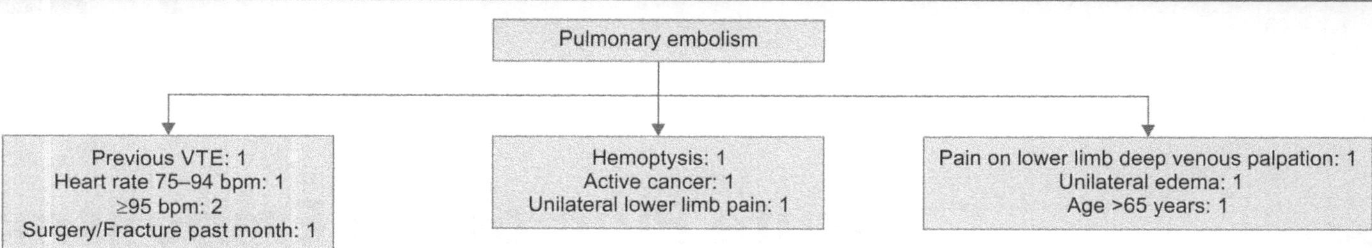

Note: Low probability: 0–1; intermediate probability: 2–4; high probability: ≥5.
(VTE: venous thromboembolism)

Diagnostic workup of acute pulmonary embolism[3]

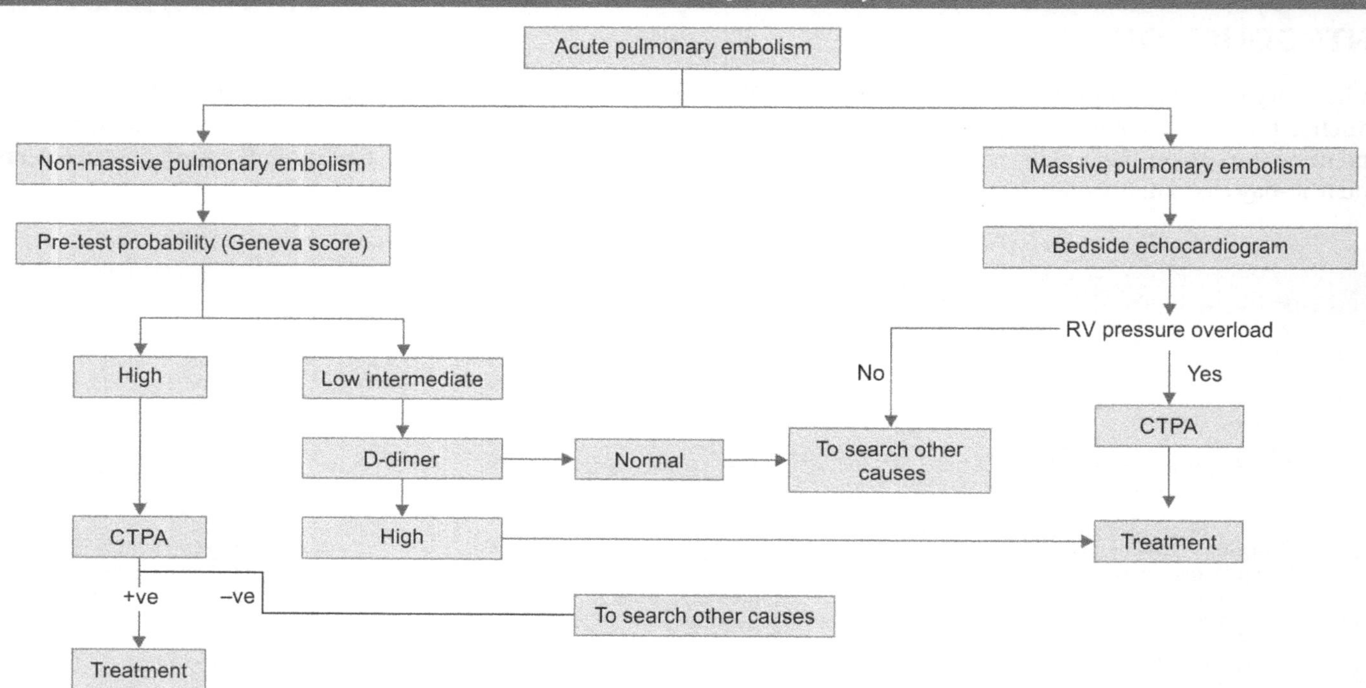

(CTPA: computed tomographic pulmonary angiography; RV: right ventricular)

Risk scoring of acute pulmonary embolism

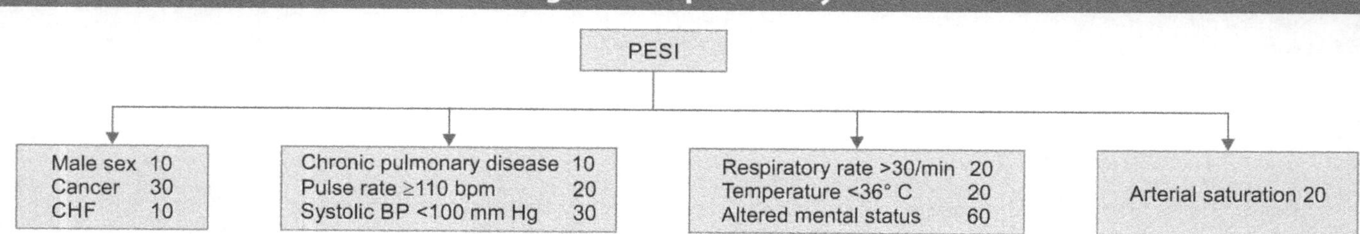

Note: Class I: <65; Class II: 66–85; Class III: 86–105; Class IV: 106–125; Class V: >125.
(BP: blood pressure; CHF: congestive heart failure; PESI: pulmonary embolism severity index)

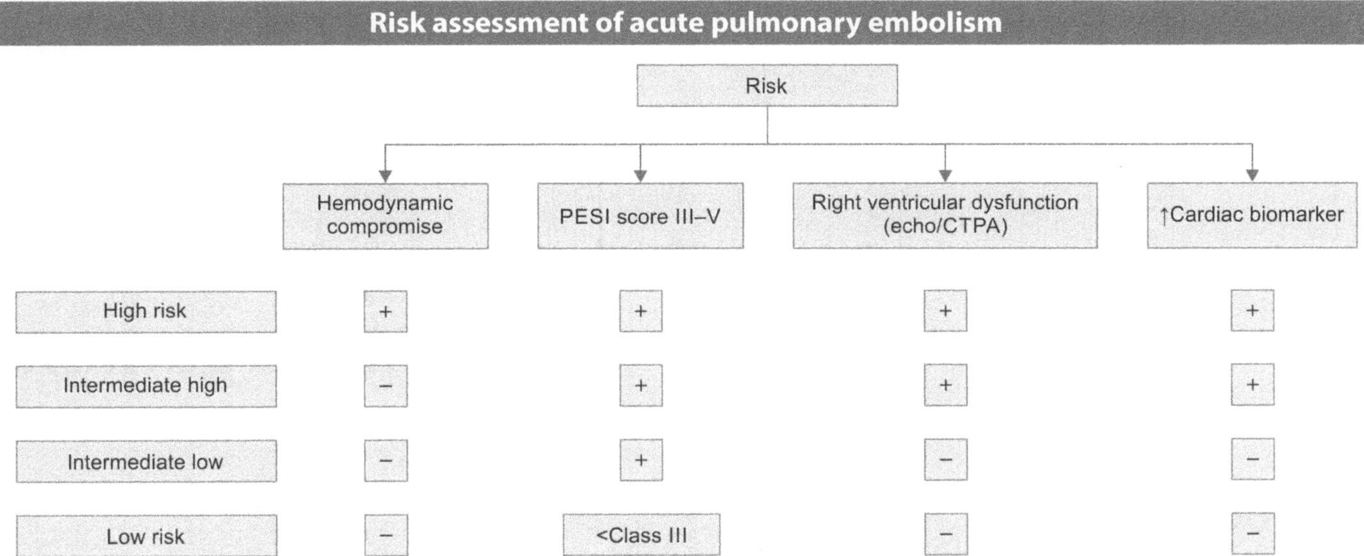

(CTPA: computed tomographic pulmonary angiography; PESI: pulmonary embolism severity index)

REFERENCES

1. Anderson FA Jr, Spencer FA. Risk factors for venous thromboembolism. Circulation. 2003;107:19-116.
2. Penaloza A, Verschuren F, Meyer G, Quentin-Georget S, Soulie C, Thys F, et al. Comparison of the unstructured clinician gestalt, the wells score, and the revised Geneva score to estimate pretest probability for suspected pulmonary embolism. Ann Emerg Med. 2013;62:117-24.
3. Konstantinides SV, Meyer G, Becattini C, Bueno H, Geersing GJ, Harjola VP, et al; ESC Scientific Document Group. 2019 ESC Guidelines for the diagnosis and management of acute pulmonary embolism developed in collaboration with the European Respiratory Society (ERS). Eur Heart J. 2020;41(4):543-603.

CHAPTER 73

Acute Pulmonary Embolism: Management

INTRODUCTION

Acute pulmonary embolism is the cause of death over 100,000 patients annually in USA and is the most preventable cause of death in hospitalised patients. Time-old anticoagulant therapy is the mainstay in its management. However, few complications like post-thrombotic syndrome, recurrent venous thromboembolism and chronic thromboembolic pulmonary hypertension are the sequelae even after successful anticoagulant therapy. Over two decades, endovascular intervention has been evolved as an important therapeutic armamentarium in the management of acute pulmonary embolism.

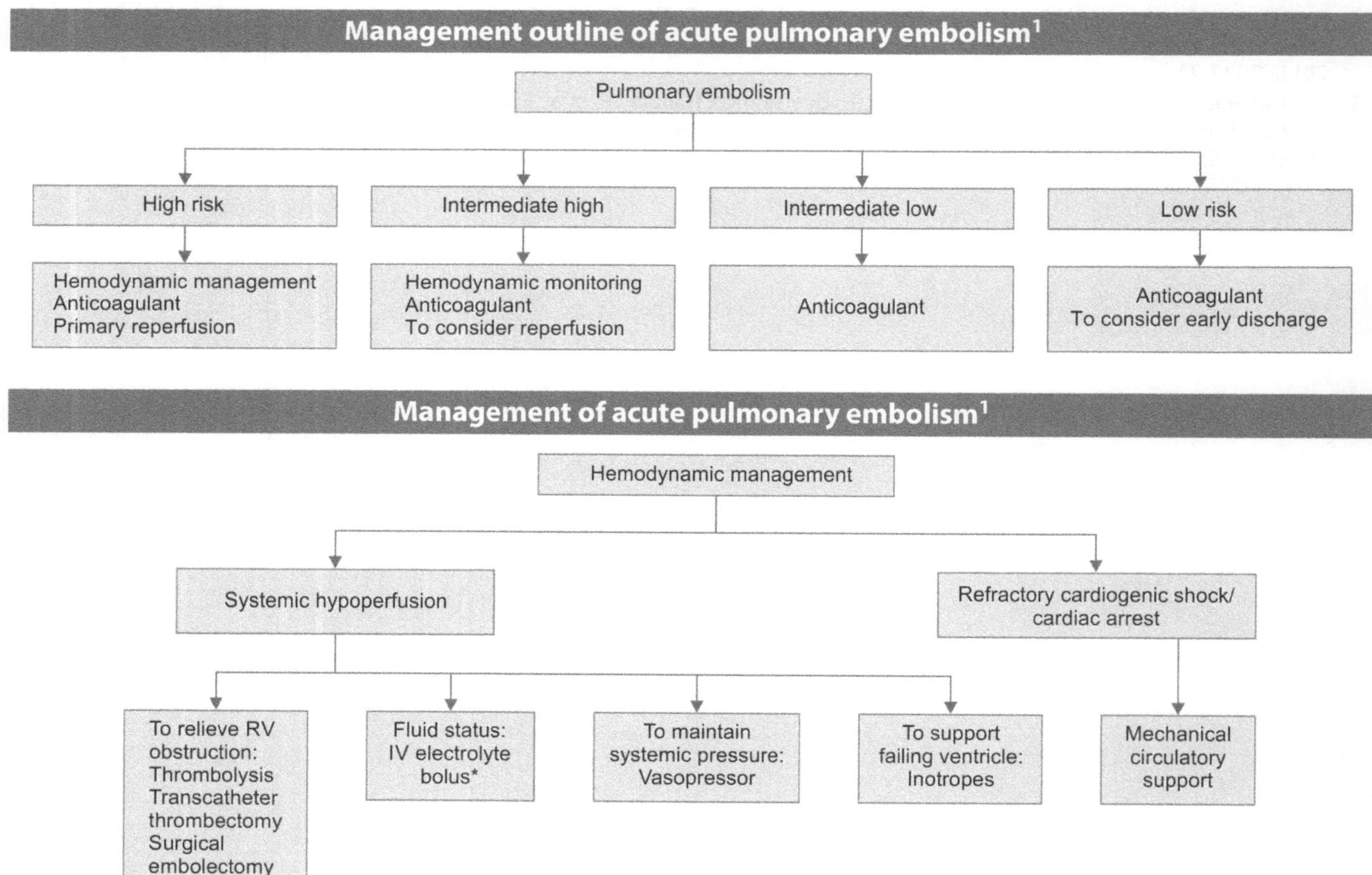

*Excess volume leading to right ventricular dilatation may be detrimental, because septal bulge may cause further low output state due to ventricular interdependence. Amount of fluid should be decided by the echocardiographic assessment of inferior vena cava diameter and collapsibility.

(IV: intravenous; RV: right ventricular)

Management of acute pulmonary embolism: Thrombolysis[1]

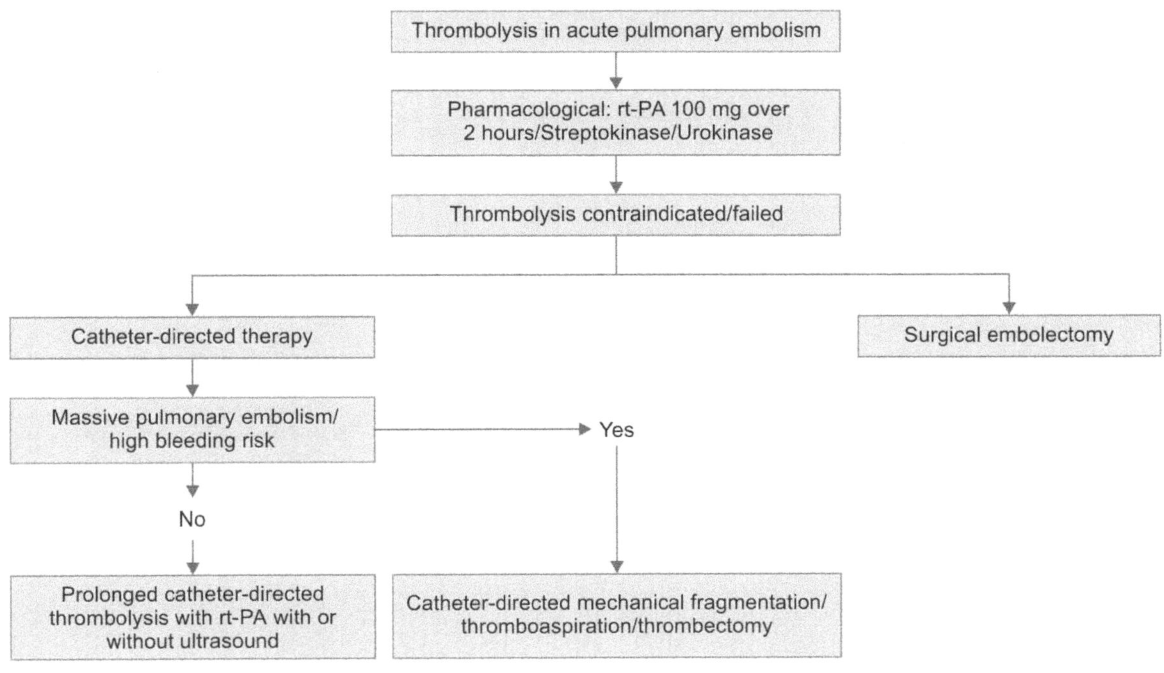

(rt-PA: recombinant tissue plasminogen activator)

Management of acute pulmonary embolism: Anticoagulation[1]

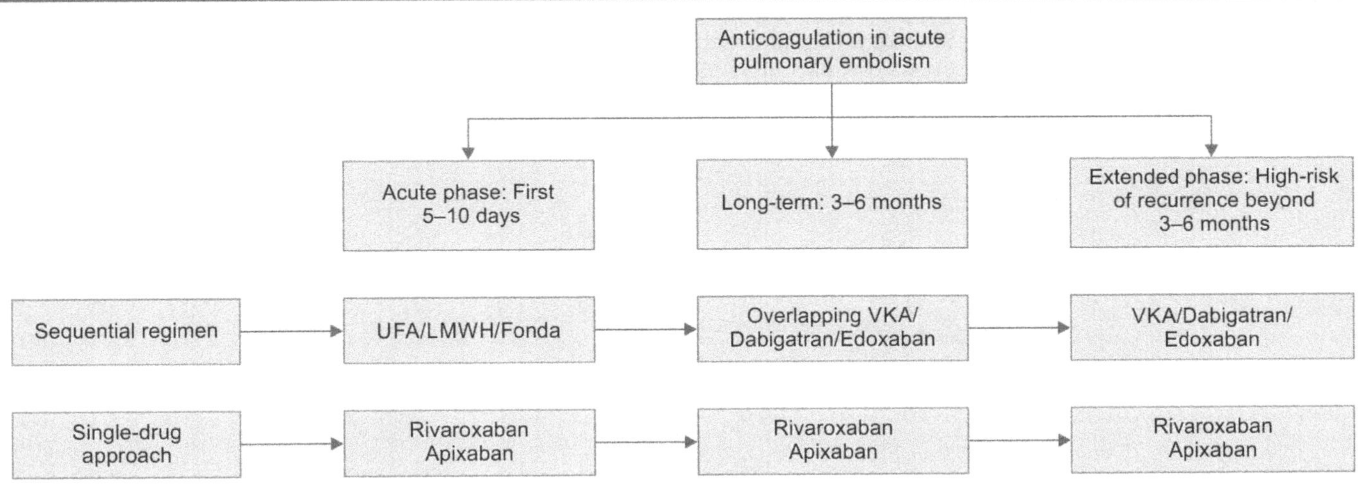

(Fonda: fondaparinux; LMWH: low molecular weight heparin; UFA: unfractionated heparin; VKA: vitamin K antagonist)

Duration of anticoagulants and risk of recurrence[2]

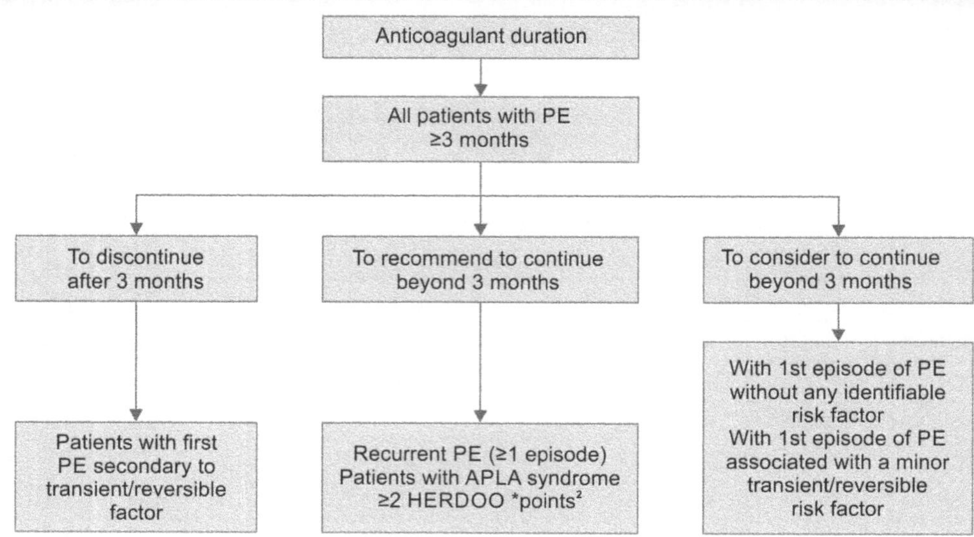

*HERDOO: 1 point: Hyperpigmentation, edema, or redness
1 point: D-dimer ≥250 µg/L
1 point: Obesity
1 point: Older age ≥65 years

(APLA: antiphospholipid antibody; PE: pulmonary embolism)

REFERENCES

1. Konstantinides SV, Meyer G, Becattini C, Bueno H, Geersing GJ, Harjola VP, et al. ESC Scientific Document Group. 2019 ESC Guidelines for the diagnosis and management of acute pulmonary embolism developed in collaboration with the European Respiratory Society (ERS). Eur Heart J. 2020;41(4):543-603.
2. Rodger MA, Le Gal G, Anderson DR, Schmidt J, Pernod G, Kahn SR, et al. Validating the HERDOO2 rule to guide treatment duration for woman with unprovoked venous thrombosis. BMJ 2017;365:j1065.

CHAPTER 74

Acute Aortic Syndrome: Approach

INTRODUCTION

Aorta, the "'greatest artery" of the body, carries nearly 200 million liters of blood to the body in average lifetime. Acute aortic syndrome (AAS) consists of an interrelated emergency condition involving the aorta with similar clinical patterns and challenges. The annual incidence of AAS is roughly 7.7 per 100,000 person-years.[1] The incidence in male is twice common than in female. The mean age of presentation is 66–72 years. AAS is an emergency, characterized by rapid evolvement toward major morbidity and mortality 1–2% per hour in untreated patients.

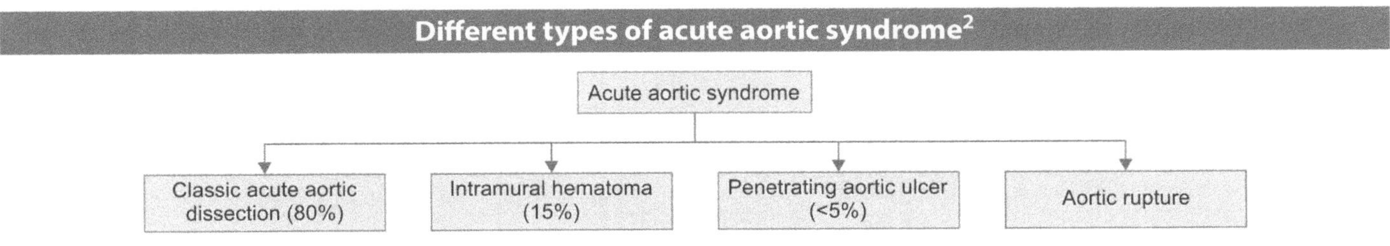

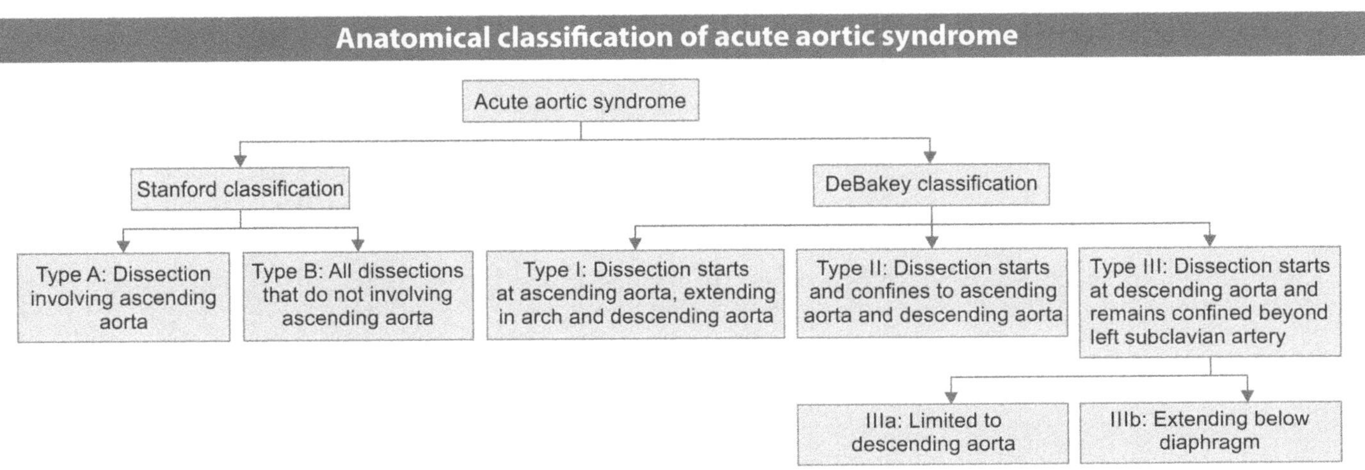

Pathophysiology of acute aortic syndrome

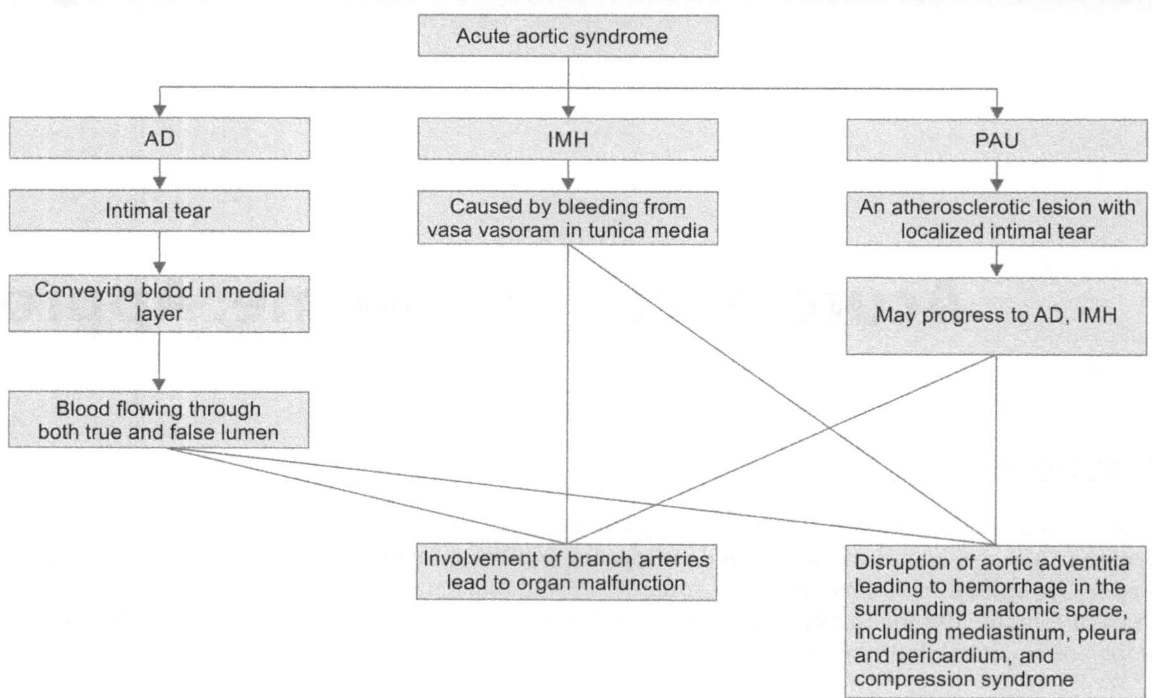

(AD: aortic dissection; IMH: intramural hematoma; PAU: penetrating aortic ulcer)

Precipitating factors in acute aortic syndrome[3]

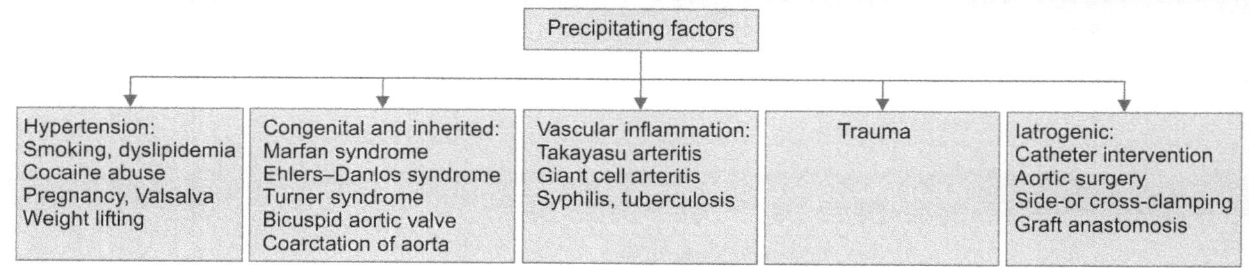

Clinical presentation of acute aortic syndrome[3]

Acute aortic syndrome

↓

Aortic dilatation, organ malperfusion
Aortic rupture with external hemorrhage
Inflammation/heart failure

↓

"Think-aorta" code: Truncal pain, syncope
Neurological deficit
Limb ischemia

Type A dissection	Type B dissection	IMH	Leaking thoracic aneurysm
Chest pain, syncope pulse difference, AR neurologic signs, tamponade	Chest/Back pain Distal pulse difference High BP, AKI Claudication	Chest/Back pain, high BP, tamponade	Diffuse chest/back pain, pallor, falling hemodynamic, exsanguination, sudden death

(AKI: acute kidney injury; AR: aortic regurgitation; BP: blood pressure; IMH: intramural hematoma)

REFERENCES

1. DeMartino RR, Sen I, Huang Y, Bower TC, Oderich GS, Pochettino A, et al. Population-based assessment of the incidence of aortic dissection, intramural hematoma, and penetrating ulcer, and its associatedmortality from 1995 to 2015. Circ Cardiovasc Qual Outcomes. 2018;11:1-12.
2. Erbel R, Aboyans V, Boileau C, Bossone E, Bartolomeo RD, Eggebrecht H, et al. 2014 ESC guidelines on the diagnosis and treatment of aortic diseases: Document covering acute and chronic aortic diseases of the thoracic and abdominal aorta of the adult. The Task Force for the Diagnosis and Treatment of Aortic Diseases of the European Society of Cardiology (ESC). Eur Heart J. 2014;35:2873-926.
3. Nienaber CA, Powell JT. Management of acute aortic syndromes. Eur Heart J. 2012;33(1):26-35.

CHAPTER 75

Acute Aortic Syndrome: Imaging and Management

INTRODUCTION

Diagnosis of acute aortic syndrome (AAS), a dramatic pathology is not very infrequently missed. The suspicion is very crucial. However, an expertise is most important. For this reason, aorta code, aorta center, and aorta team have been formulated.[1] Centralization of AAS care is necessary to achieve the best outcome. The concept is to ensure high-volume center with high-volume interventionist and surgeon. Surgical mortality for type A-AAS amounts to 10–35%. However, mortality only on medical management is nearing 50%.

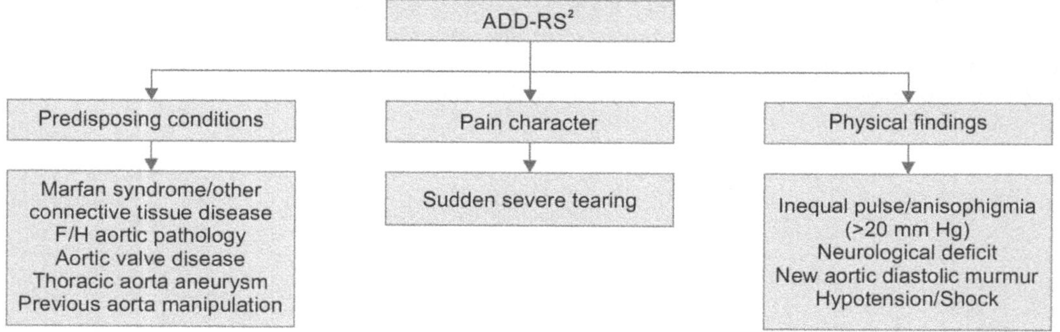

Notes: ADD-RS ranges from 0 to 3, depending on the number of categories where at least 1 risk factor is present. ADD-RS = 0 or low risk, ADD-RS = 1 or intermediate risk, ADD-RS = 2 or high-risk.

(ADD-RS: aortic dissection detection risk score: F/H: family history)

Diagnosis of acute aortic syndrome

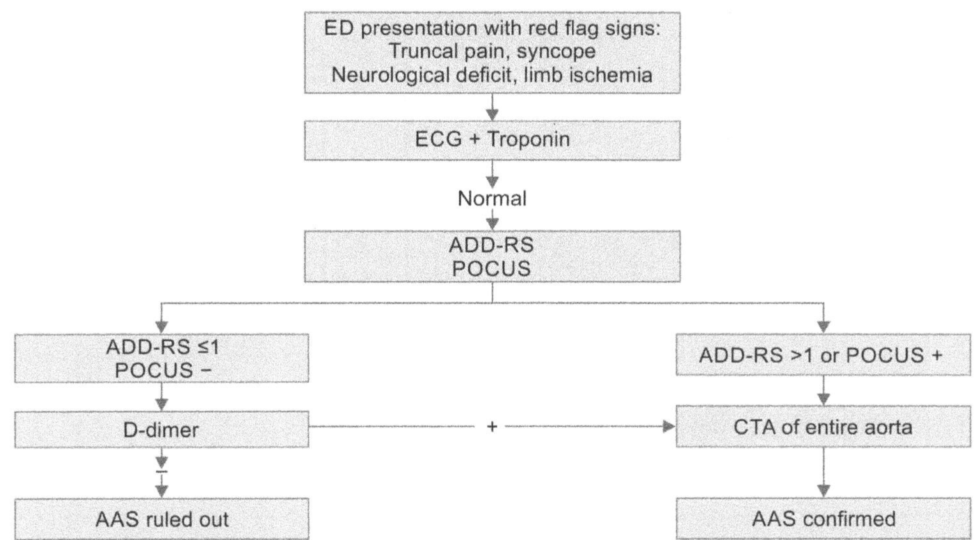

(AAS: acute aortic syndrome; ADD-RS: aortic dissection detection risk score; ECG: electrocardiogram; POCUS: point-of-care ultrasonography; CTA: computed tomography angiography)

Management of acute aortic syndrome: Medical management[3]

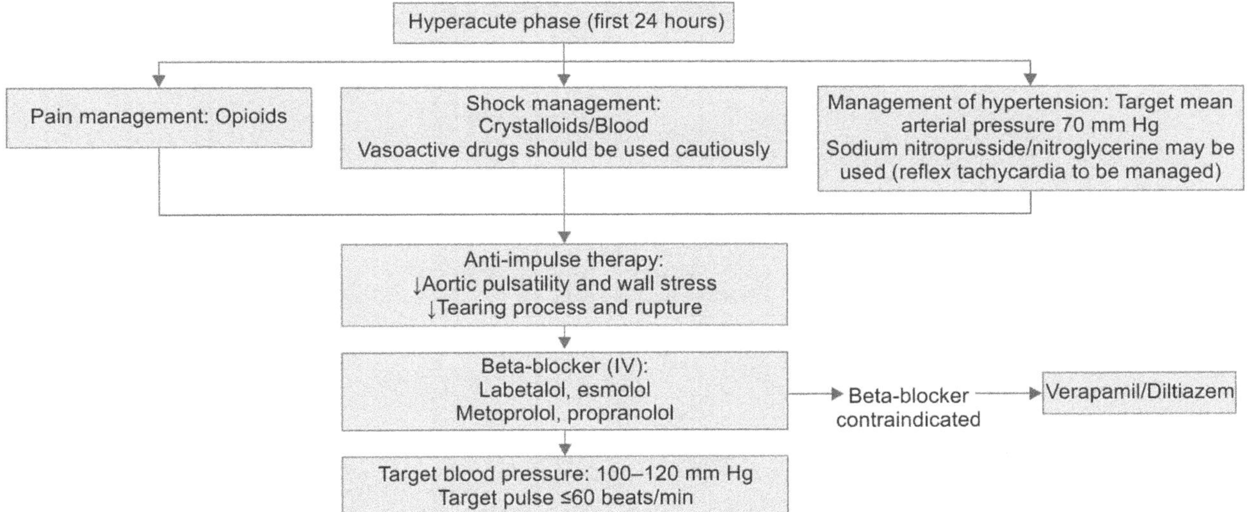

Surgical management of acute aortic syndrome

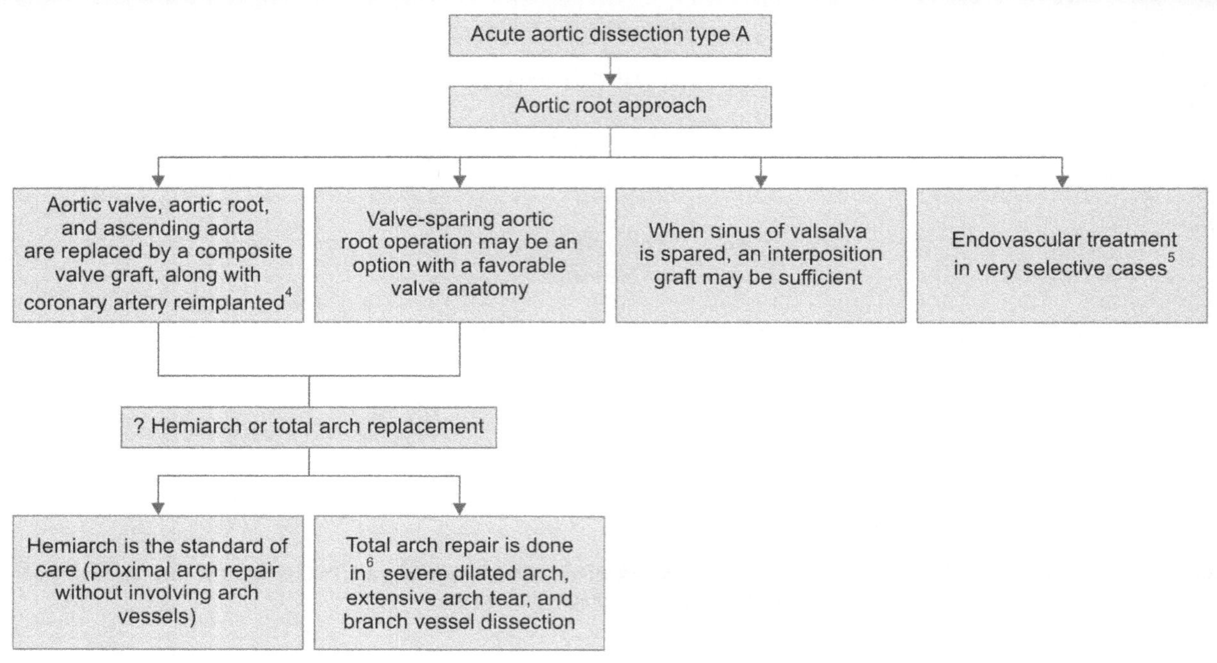

Management of type B aortic dissection[8]

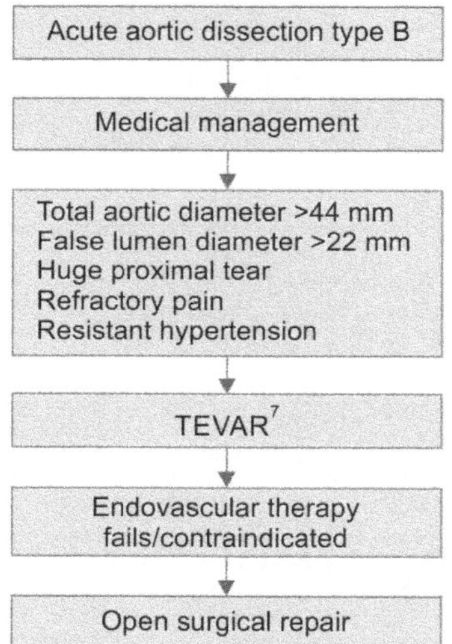

(TEVAR: thoracic endovascular aortic repair)

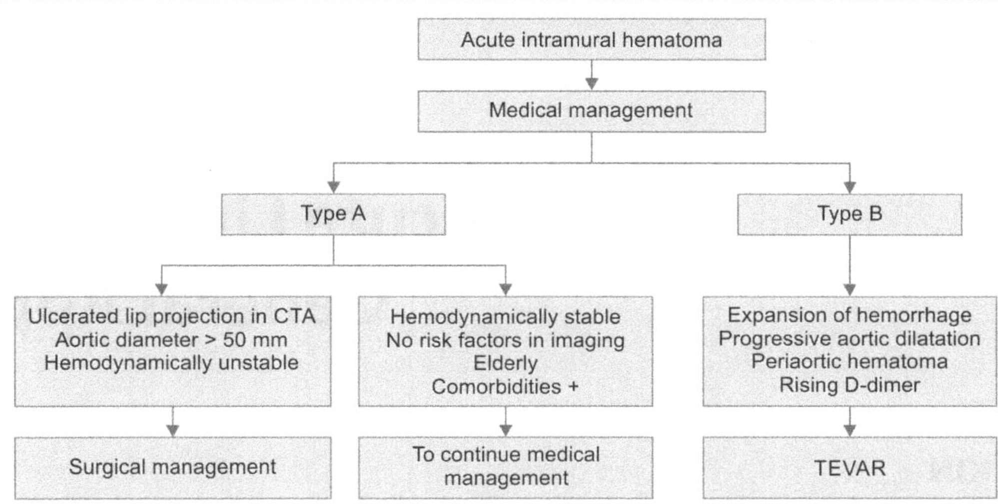

(CTA: computed tomography angiogram; TEVAR: thoracic endovascular aortic repair)

REFERENCES

1. Czearny M, Schmidli j, Adler S, van den Berg JC, Bertoglio L, Carrel T, et al. Current options and recommendations for the treatment of thoracic aortic pathologies involving the aortic arch: an expert consensus document of the Euro- pean Association for Cardio-Thoracic surgery (EACTS) and the European Society for Vascular Surgery (ESVS). Eur J Cardiothorac Surg. 2019;55:133-62.

2. Erbel R, Aboyans V, Boileau C, Bossone E, Bartolomeo RD, Eggebrecht H, et al. 2014 ESC guidelines on the diagnosis and treatment of aortic diseases: Document covering acute and chronic aortic diseases of the thoracic and abdominal aorta of the adult. The Task Force for the Diagnosis and Treatment of Aortic Diseases of the European Society of Cardiology (ESC). Eur Heart J. 2014;35:2873-926.

3. Morello F, Santoro M, Fargion AT, Grifoni S, Nazerian P. Diagnosis and management of acute aortic syndromes in the emergency department. Intern Emerg Med. 2021;16(1):171-81.

4. Khachatryan Z, Leontyev S, Magomedov K, Haunschild J, Holzhey DM, Misfeld M, et al. Management of aortic root in type Adissection: Bentall approach. J Card Surg. 2022;36:1779-85.

5. Swee W, Dake MD. Endovascular management of thoracic dissections. Circulation. 2009;117:1460-73.

6. Norton EL, Wu X, Kim KM, Fukuhara S, Patel HJ, Deeb GM, et al. Is hemiarch replacement adequate in acute type A aortic dissection repair in patients with arch branch vessel dissection withoutcerebral malperfusion? J Thorac Cardiovasc Surg. 2021;161:873-884.e2.

7. Ray HM, Durham CA, Ocazionez D, Charlton-Ouw KM, Estrera AL, Miller CC 3rd, et al. Predictors of intervention and mortality in patients with uncomplicated acute type B aortic dissection. J Vasc Surg. 2016;64:1560-8.

8. Vilacosta I, Roman AS, Bartolomeo RD, Eagle K, Estrera AL, Ferrera C, et al. Acute aortic syndrome revisited. J Am Coll Cardiol. 2021;78: 2106-25.

CHAPTER 76

Acute Limb Ischemia: General Approach

INTRODUCTION

Acute limb ischemia (ALI) is defined as sudden reduction in limb perfusion that threatens limb viability. Acuteness is defined as the clinical presentation within 2 weeks of symptoms. In contrast to critical limb ischemia or chronic limb-threatening ischemia in which there is collateral vessels to perfuse limbs, ALI threatens limb viability because ALI does not allow limb to develop collateral vessels due to a shorter period of the clinical tempo. The incidence of ALI is 1.5 cases out of 10,000 people per year.[1] ALI, a disease of elderly, is both limb-threatening and life-threatening. 30-day amputation and mortality are between 10 and 15%, respectively, despite early revascularization.[2] The embolic cause for ALI is falling, due to worldwide decrease in the incidence of rheumatic heart disease and improvement in the management of atrial fibrillation. As peripheral artery disease is common in 30% of people over the age of 70 years, acute on chronic limb ischemia is more common. Acute occlusion in a preconditioned limb, having chronic atherosclerotic obstruction with collaterals, may not produce overt ischemia or dramatic presentation.

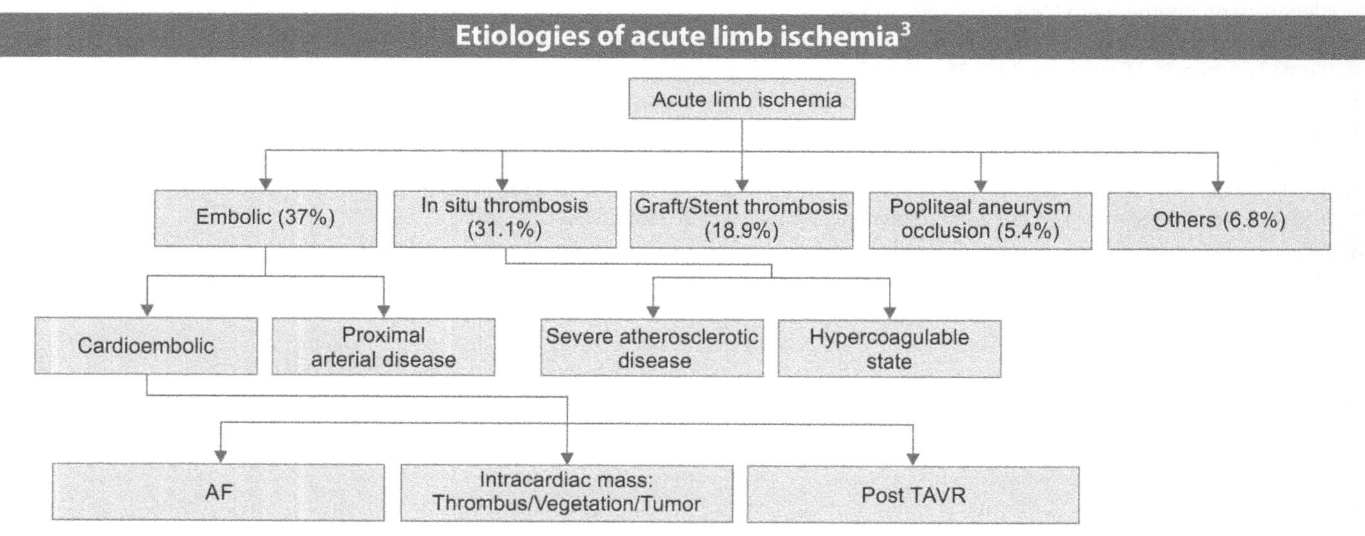

(AF: atrial fibrillation; TAVR: transcatheter aortic valve replacement)

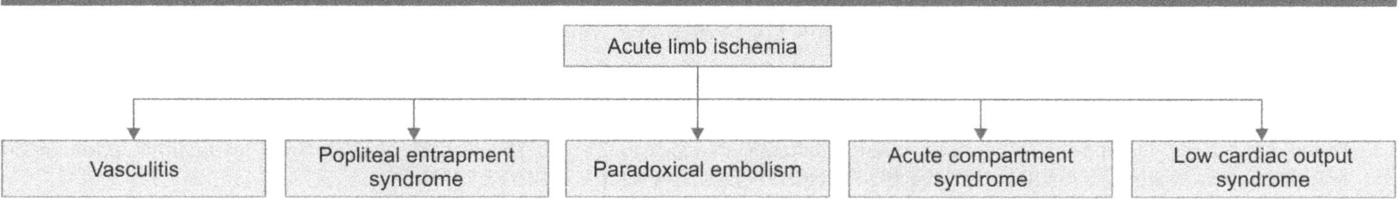

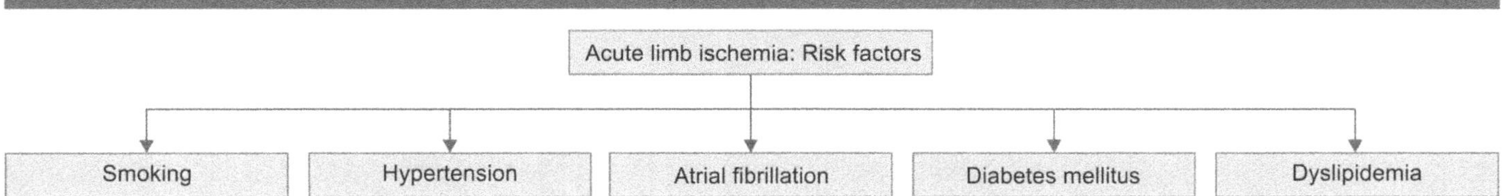

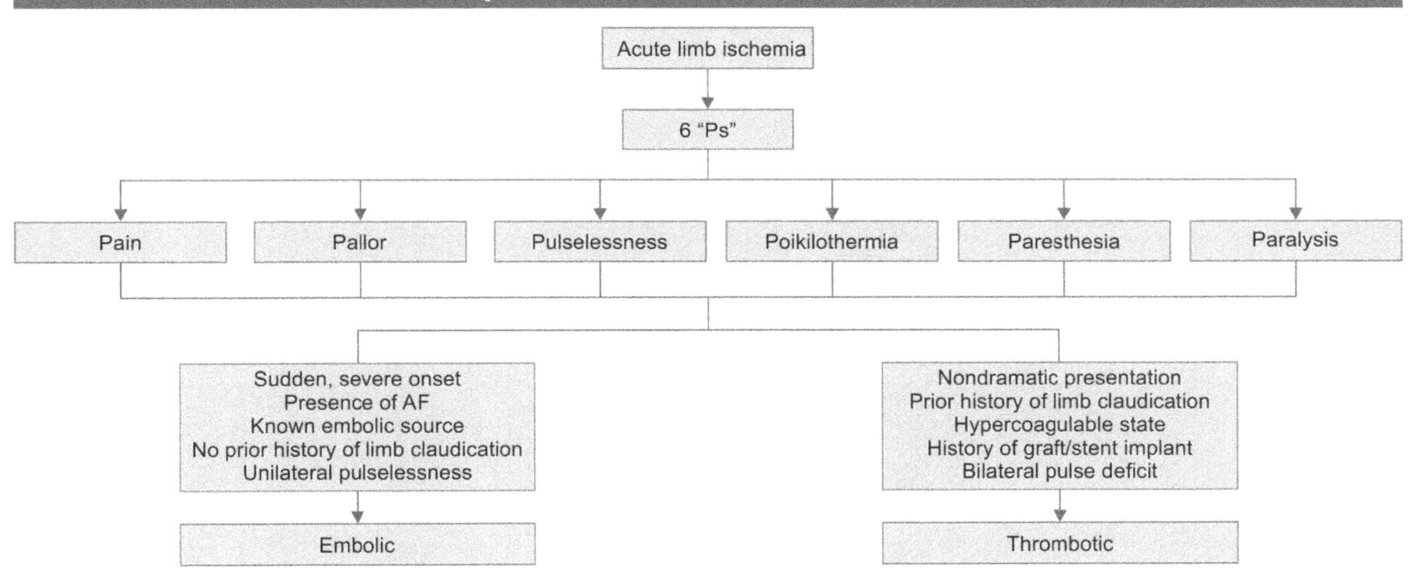

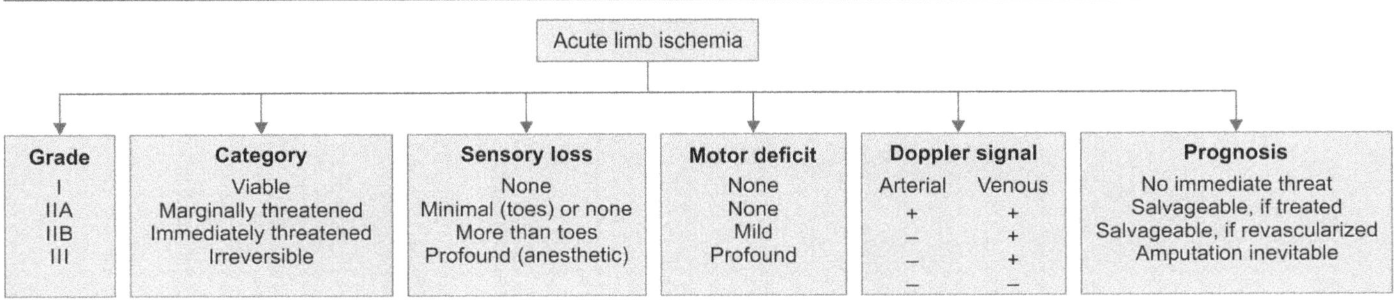

Grade	Category	Sensory loss	Motor deficit	Doppler signal		Prognosis
				Arterial	Venous	
I	Viable	None	None	+	+	No immediate threat
IIA	Marginally threatened	Minimal (toes) or none	None	−	+	Salvageable, if treated
IIB	Immediately threatened	More than toes	Mild	−	+	Salvageable, if revascularized
III	Irreversible	Profound (anesthetic)	Profound	−	−	Amputation inevitable

REFERENCES

1. Norgren L, Hiatt WR, Dormandy JA, Nehler MR, Harris KA, Fowkes FGR. Inter-society consensus for the management of peripheral arterial disease (TASC II). J Vasc Surg. 2007;45:S5-S67.
2. Earnshaw JJ, Whitman B, Foy C. National Audit of Thrombolysis for Acute Leg Ischemia (NATALI): Clinical factors associated with early outcome. J Vasc Surg. 2004;39:1018-25.
3. Duval S, Keo HH, Oldenberg NC, Baumgartner I, Jaff MR, Peacock JM, et al. The impact of prolonged lower limb ischemia on amputation, mortality and functional status: the FRENCH registry. Am Hear J. 2014;168:577-87.
4. Howard DP, Banerjee A, Fairhead JF, Hands L, Silver LE, Rothwell PM. Population-based study of incidence, risk factors, outcome, and prognosis of ischemic peripheralarterial events: implications for prevention. Circulation. 2015;132:1805-15.
5. Rutherford RB, Baker JD, Ernst C, Johnston KW, Porter JM, Ahn S, et al. Recommended standards for reports dealing with lower extremity ischemia: revised version. J Vasc Surg. 1997;26:517-38.

Acute Limb Ischemia: Imaging and Management

INTRODUCTION

In relation to cardiac muscle, the proverb is "muscle is time", which is also applicable to acute limb ischemia (ALI) and skeletal muscle, which can tolerate ischemia not more than 6 hours. Early revascularization depends on early diagnosis. This urgency of the diagnosis determines the mode of imaging in ALI. All imaging has been extensively used in chronic limb ischemia and many of the statistic in relation to ALI have been extrapolated.

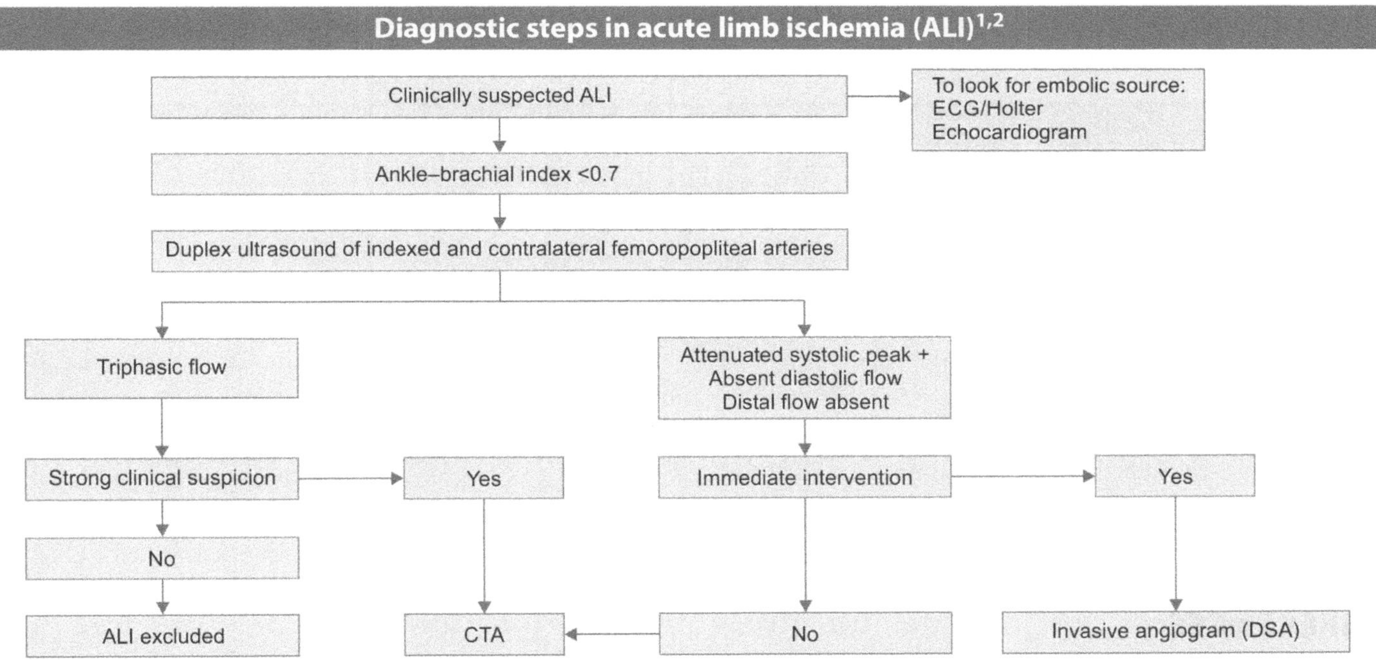

(ALI: acute limb ischemia; CTA: computed tomography angiography; DSA: digital subtraction angiography)

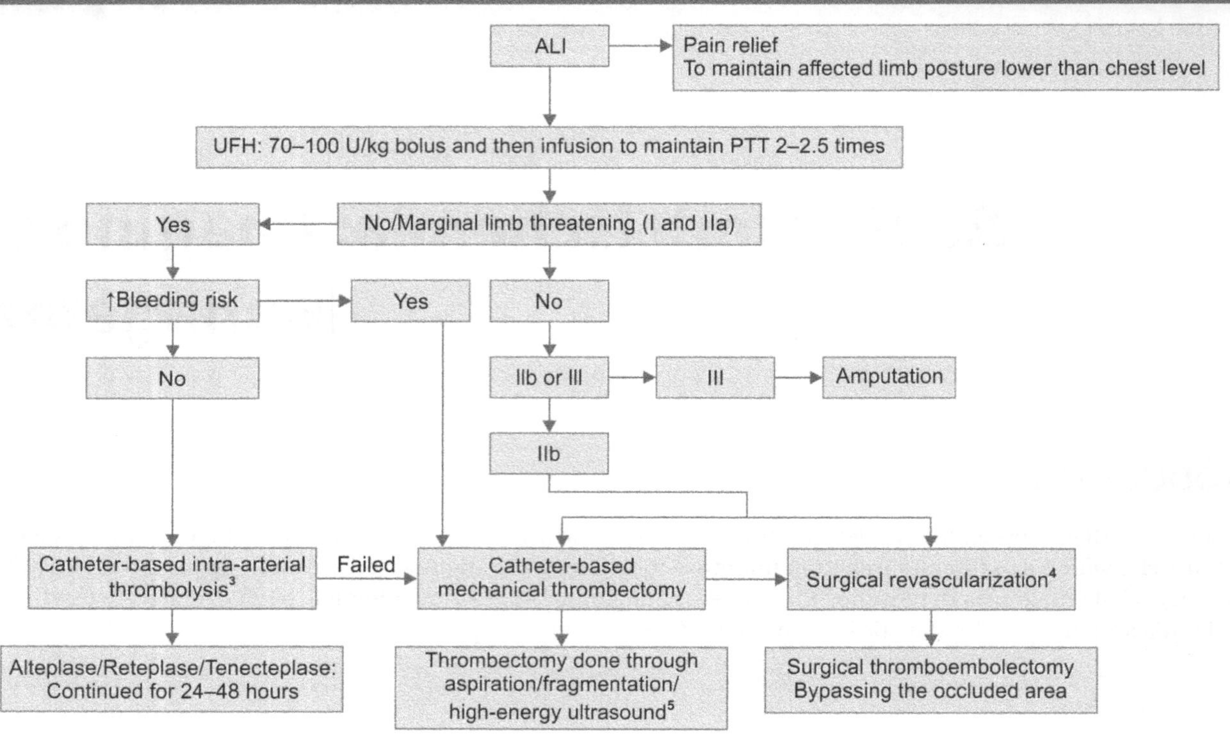

(ALI: acute limb ischemia; PTT: partial thromboplastin time; UFH: unfractionated heparin)

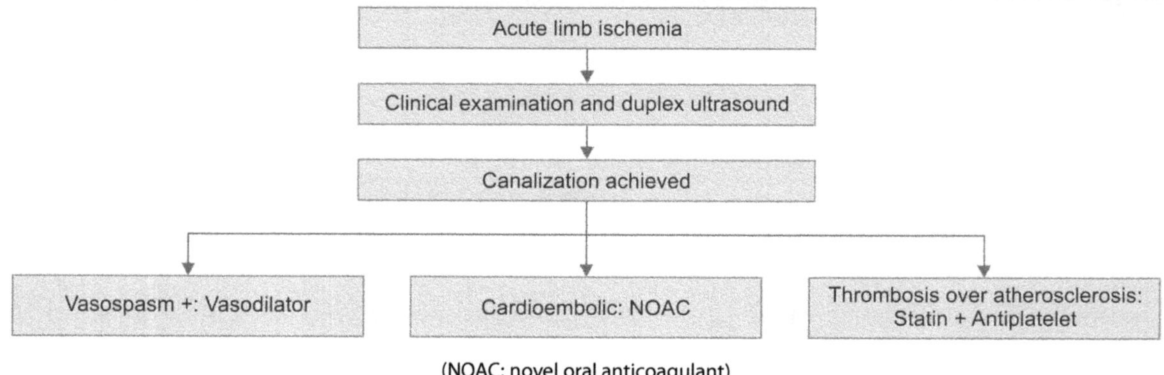

(NOAC: novel oral anticoagulant)

REFERENCES

1. Bandyk DF, Chauvapun JP. Duplex ultrasound surveillance can be worthwhile after arterial intervention. Perspect Vasc Surg Endovasc Ther. 2007;19:354-61.
2. Creager MA, Kaufman JA, Conte MS. Clinical practice. Acute Limb Ischemia. N Engl J Med. 2012;366:2198-206.
3. Ouriel K, Veith FJ, Sasahara AA. For the TOPAS Investigators. A comparison of recombinant urokinase with vascular surgery as initial treatment for acute arterial occlusion of the legs. N Engl J Med. 1998;16:1105-111.
4. Enezate TH, Omran J, Mahmud E, Patel M, Abu-Fadel MS, White C.J, et al. Endovascular versus surgical treatment for acute limb ischemia: A systematic review and meta-analysis of clinical trials. Cardiovasc Diagn. Ther. 2017;7:264-71.
5. Kronlage M, Printz I, Vogel B, Blessing E, Mueller OJ, Katus HA, et al. A comparative study on endovascular treatment of (sub) acute critical limb ischemia: Mechanical thrombectomy vs thrombolysis. Drug Des. Devel. Ther. 2017;11:1233-41.

www.ingramcontent.com/pod-product-compliance
Ingram Content Group UK Ltd.
Pitfield, Milton Keynes, MK11 3LW, UK
UKHW051542060425
457142UK00015B/677